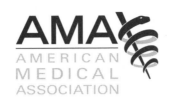

Introduction to CPT® Coding

Basic principles to learning, understanding, and applying the CPT® code set

Michelle Abraham, MHA, CCS-P

Danielle Pavloski, BS, RHIT, CCS-P

Arletrice Watkins, MHA, RHIA

Rejina L. Young

D1227656

ISBN: 978-1-60359-531-5
AC 24: 11-P-079:08/11

Acknowledgments

This book is dedicated to our late colleague and friend, Susan Tracy, MA, RHIT. Susan shared a special passion for coding education, which is reflected in many of the articles and chapters she wrote for CPT coding publications over the past years, and she was a dedicated professional to the health information management field. It is this dedication that has been the impetus for the publication of this book. We will miss Susan's contributions and miss working with her.

Table of Contents

Preface

Since 1966 the American Medical Association (AMA), through the CPT Editorial Panel, has maintained Current Procedural Terminology (CPT®) as a code set that clearly and comprehensively describes the clinically recognized and generally accepted services provided by health care professionals to individual patients and populations. The CPT code set is designed to communicate uniform information about medical services and procedures and to accurately describe medical, surgical, and diagnostic services among physicians, coders, patients, accreditation organizations, and payers for administrative, financial, and analytical purposes. Given the diverse uses and users of the CPT code set, the consistent and accurate application of the CPT codes and guidelines is important for everyone in the health care system.

Written by the AMA's CPT coding experts, *Introduction to CPT Coding: Basic Principles* addresses introductory coding skills by incorporating basic coding principles and coding scenarios with appropriate code assignments. The content of this book is designed to be used as a guide to learning and using the CPT code set and is not a substitute for the CPT codebook. Thus, it is recommended that this book be used in conjunction with the CPT codebook.

It is crucial to understand and correctly apply the CPT coding guidelines for each section and subsection of the CPT codebook. This book addresses the general guidelines for each section and subsection at the beginner's level and facilitates comprehension and application of the CPT coding guidelines.

Introduction to CPT Coding: Basic Principles is designed for use in community colleges, career colleges, and vocational school classrooms where future coders, medical students, medical assistants, medical insurance specialists, and other qualified health care providers are trained. It can also be used as an independent study tool for new medical office personnel, physicians, independent billing services personnel, and others in the health care field who want to learn additional coding skills.

Each chapter contains valuable features to provide further educational guidance on appropriate CPT coding, such as:

- Information about CPT coding format and conventions;
- Clarification of the CPT coding guidelines and their application with coding questions and operative procedures (topics covered include E/M, anesthesiology, surgery, radiology, pathology and laboratory, and medicine);
- Key Terms: fundamental terms are defined within the text for ease of use;
- Check Your Knowledges: feature questions and answers to check that students comprehend the preceding section of text;
- Coding Tips: provide even more help in assigning correct codes and extra information to help students differentiate and discern between similar or almost similar coding situations;
- Illustrations clarify anatomical structures relevant to the procedures and codes discussed;
- Exercises: exercises at the end of each chapter in several formats, such as true/false, multiple choice, and scenario reporting questions help students to test their understanding of the material covered in each chapter;
- Examples: real-life coding examples allow students to apply their newly acquired skills in every chapter.

Keep in mind that the information presented here is from the CPT coding perspective and conveys the CPT Editorial Panel's intent for various codes. Payment policies are set by third-party payers and not by CPT staff. Therefore, any specific payment-related questions or issues must be directed to the respective third-party payer.

Introduction to CPT® Coding

Chapter Objectives

- Understand section numbers and sequences
- Understand the format of the terminology in the CPT codebook
- Understand code symbols and guidelines
- Understand appendixes and index entries

Introduction

The Current Procedural Terminology (CPT) developed by the American Medical Association (AMA) is a set of codes, descriptions, and guidelines that describe procedures and services performed by physicians and other qualified health care providers. The use of CPT codes simplifies the reporting of services. In the beginning, learning the CPT coding system and guidelines can seem overwhelming. Therefore, it is important to have a solid foundation on which to build your CPT coding knowledge. Essential to learning to code correctly is a thorough understanding of both medical terminology and anatomy.

The intention of this introduction is to guide you through the very basics of CPT coding and jumpstart your knowledge base. To begin, become acquainted with the CPT codebook's layout, section numbers, and sequences. Next, look at the various code symbols that appear throughout the book. Learn how CPT codes and terminology are formatted. Taking the time to familiarize yourself with basic CPT coding concepts will help you develop that solid foundation you will need for assigning CPT codes as well as give you the tools to address the coding exercises in this book.

There are eight sections in the CPT codebook. The first six sections (see Table 1-1), which pertain to Category I CPT codes, include:

1. Evaluation and Management (E/M)
2. Anesthesiology
3. Surgery

TABLE 1-1 *Section Names and Code Sequences*

Section Name	Code Sequence
Evaluation and Management	99201-99499
Anesthesia	00100-01999
Surgery	10021-69990
Radiology	70010-79999
Pathology and Laboratory	80047-89398
Medicine	90281-99607

4. Radiology
5. Pathology and Laboratory
6. Medicine

The seventh and eighth sections pertain to the Category II, performance measurement CPT codes, and the Category III, new and emerging technology codes, respectively.

The majority of procedures and services listed in the CPT codebook are presented in numeric order, with the exception of the E/M section, which appears at the beginning of the book. (Because these codes are used by most physicians and other qualified health care providers in reporting a significant portion of their services, they were placed at the front of the book for easy reference.)

It is also important to note that some codes do not appear in numeric sequence in the listing of the CPT codes. These are the resequenced codes, and they are identified with the # symbol. Resequencing allows existing codes to be relocated to a location that is appropriate for the code's concept regardless of the numeric sequence. This reduces the need for deleting and renumbering codes. (Please refer to the discussion of resequenced CPT codes later in the chapter.)

Instructions for Reporting Medical Services and Procedures

When procedures and services by a physician are reported, the CPT code that most accurately identifies the service performed should be selected. Any service or procedure reported should be adequately documented in the medical record to support the specific code(s) reported. Do not select a CPT code that merely approximates the service provided. If a code for the exact procedure or service performed does not exist in the CPT code set, then report the service by using the appropriate "unlisted procedure or service" code. Some people maintain that they are discouraged from using unlisted procedure codes or not allowed to use them altogether. While the use of an unlisted procedure or service code will require a special report or documentation to describe the service, correct coding demands that a "square peg" not be fit into a "round hole."

Placement of a Code in the CPT Code Set

When procedures and services are evaluated for reimbursement or other purposes, it is important to consider each procedure and service on its own merits and not simply on the placement of the code in the CPT codebook. The listing of a procedure or service in a specific section of the CPT codebook does not restrict its use to a specific specialty group. Any procedure or service in any section of the book may be used to designate the services rendered by any qualified physician or other qualified health care professional.

Because the CPT code set is not a strict classification system, there may be some procedures that appear in sections other than in those in which you might expect to find them. From a historical perspective, CPT coding has always placed procedures in general sections according to where physicians will most conveniently find them.

EXAMPLE

The code for a diagnostic colonoscopy, although not involving an incision, is located in the Digestive System subsection. This was done because keeping the endoscopies involving a biopsy, tumor removal, or other operative intervention in proximity to the diagnostic procedure was considered important.

EXAMPLE

Cast applications are listed in the Musculoskeletal subsection in proximity to the fracture and dislocation treatments; however, a cast application is not a surgical procedure.

✓ Check Your Knowledge

1. How many sections are there in the CPT codebook?
2. What CPT code should be reported if no specific code exists in the CPT codebook?
3. Are the codes for procedures placed in sections according to a strict classification system?

Format of the Terminology

Without developing a basic understanding of the format of the code descriptions in CPT coding, appropriate use of the CPT codebook would be almost impossible. Understanding how to read the full description of a CPT code is a necessary and fundamental skill that you need in appropriate use of the CPT codebook.

Originally, each code was paired with a complete, stand-alone description of the medical procedure it referred to. However, to conserve space and avoid having to repeat information shared by several codes, some of the procedure descriptors in CPT coding are not printed in their entirety, but rather refer back to a code, called a ***parent code***, that contains a description of the portion of the procedure that is shared by the codes. When a code is indented in the codebook, you must refer back to the left-justified parent code that precedes that code to determine the full procedure descriptor of the indented code(s) that follows.

EXAMPLE

97010 Application of a modality to 1 or more areas; hot or cold packs

97012 traction, mechanical

97014 electrical stimulation (unattended)

97016 vasopneumatic devices

The shared part of the parent code **97010** (that part of the description to the left of the semicolon, "Application of a modality to 1 or more areas;") should be considered part of each of the following indented codes (**97012-97016**). Together, these codes (the parent code and the indented codes that follow it) are thought of as a series.

The full procedure descriptor represented by code **97012** actually reads:

97012 Application of a modality to 1 or more areas; traction, mechanical

---

Whether a code is indented or not has no bearing on whether those procedures would be performed together and also no bearing on whether or not they would be reported together. If two distinct procedures from the same series are performed, then both procedures can be reported. However, in such a case, the use of CPT modifiers becomes necessary. (See "Modifiers" later in this introduction for more information about using CPT modifiers.)

4. Which of the following codes is considered a parent code?

25100 Arthrotomy, wrist joint; with biopsy

25105   with synovectomy

5. Write down the full procedure code descriptor represented by code **25105**.

Code Symbols

Over the years, a number of code symbols have been incorporated into the CPT codebook to make it more user-friendly. It is important to know the various code symbols that appear throughout the CPT codebook.

- ● Whenever new procedure codes are added to the CPT code set, they are identified throughout the CPT codebook with the bullet symbol preceding the code number. Note that this symbol appears for only one year, the year the code is added.
- ▲ The triangle is used to designate codes with a substantially altered description. Once again, this symbol appears for only one year, the year the code is revised.
- ►◄ Sideways triangles are used throughout the CPT codebook to indicate new and revised text, such as new parenthetical notes and language added to guidelines. They do not apply to code descriptors (see ▲). These symbols appear for only one year, the year the new and revised text is added.
- ✚ Add-on codes (a special category of CPT codes) are identified with the plus symbol preceding the codes. This symbol was introduced in 1999. Add-on codes can also be identified by specific language in the code descriptor, such as "each additional" or "(List separately in addition to primary procedure)." A complete list of all add-on codes in the CPT code set can be found in Appendix D in the CPT codebook.
- ○ This symbol is used to indicate a reinstated or recycled code.
- ⊘ This symbol designates CPT codes that are exempt from the use of modifier 51, but have not been designated as CPT add-on procedures or services. As an added reference, Appendix E in the CPT codebook contains a complete list of the codes exempt from modifier 51 usage.

⊙ This symbol, introduced in 2005, is used to identify the CPT codes that include moderate (conscious) sedation. These codes are listed in Appendix G in the CPT codebook.

✗ This symbol, introduced in 2006, is used to identify codes for vaccines that are pending Food and Drug Administration (FDA) approval. They are listed in Appendix K of the CPT codebook.

\# This symbol, introduced in 2010, is used to denote a resequenced code. Resequenced codes, which are not placed numerically in the CPT codebook, are identified with this symbol. Resequencing is utilized to allow placement of related concepts in appropriate locations within the families of codes regardless of the availability of numbers for sequential numerical placement. These codes are listed in Appendix N of the CPT codebook.

EXAMPLE

11042 Debridement, subcutaneous tissue (includes epidermis and dermis, if performed); first 20 sq cm or less

\# + ● **11045** each additional 20 sq cm, or part thereof (list separately in addition to code for primary procedure)

References to AMA Resources

In addition to the symbols described above, the arrow (green and red in the CPT codebook) symbols ➔ ➔ appear throughout the CPT codebook to indicate that there are other AMA resources available regarding that particular code.

The ➔ indicates that the American Medical Association has published reference material in *CPT® Changes: An Insider's View* or the *CPT® Assistant* newsletter on that particular code. *CPT Changes* is published annually and includes educational instruction related to new, revised, and deleted codes. *CPT Assistant* is the AMA's monthly authoritative coding newsletter that contains educational instruction related to existing, revised, or new codes.

The ➔ refers to information regarding that code published in the quarterly newsletter *Clinical Examples in Radiology*. This publication is a collaboration of the American Medical Association and the American College of Radiology and features selected radiology procedure reports and information regarding coding in radiology.

EXAMPLE

72195 Magnetic resonance (eg, proton) imaging, pelvis; without contrast material(s)

➔ *CPT Assistant* Jul 01:7, Jun 06:17; *CPT Changes: An Insider's View* 2001

➔ *Clinical Examples in Radiology* Spring 06:8–9, Fall 06:7–8, Summer 07:4,5

An entry that reads *CPT Assistant* Jul 01:7 and appears after a specific code descriptor indicates that information regarding that code can be found in the July 2001 issue of *CPT Assistant* newsletter on page 7.

An entry that reads *Clinical Examples in Radiology* Spring 06:8–9 and appears after a specific code indicates that information regarding that code can be found in the Spring 2006 issue on pages 8 and 9.

Guidelines

Specific guidelines for reporting procedures and services can be found at the beginning of each of the six sections of the CPT codebook. These guidelines provide information that is necessary to appropriately interpret and report the procedures and services with the CPT codes found in that specific section. For example, the Medicine section guidelines contain specific instructions for handling unlisted services or procedures, special reports, and supplies and materials provided.

Guidelines also provide explanations pertaining to terms applicable in a particular section of the CPT codebook. For example, Radiology Guidelines provide a definition of the unique term, "radiological supervision and interpretation."

In addition to the guidelines that appear at the beginning of each section, several of the subheadings or subsections have special instructions that are unique to that section. These types of guidelines and instructional notes appear throughout the CPT codebook (eg, at the beginning of a category or subcategory of codes and in parenthetical notes either preceding or following a code). All of the guidelines and notes in the CPT codebook are there to assist users in appropriate interpretation and application of the codes throughout the book. These guidelines and notes are critical to using CPT codes correctly.

EXAMPLE

22864 Removal of total disc arthroplasty (artificial disc), anterior approach, single interspace; cervical

(Do not report 22864 in conjunction with 22861, 69990)

(For additional interspace removal of cervical total disc arthroplasty, use 0095T)

Modifiers

The CPT code set uses modifiers as an integral part of its structure. CPT modifiers are two-digit numeric indicators. Modifiers are appended to CPT codes to indicate that a performed service or procedure has been altered or modified by some specific circumstance, but not changed in its definition.

Modifiers may be used in many instances. Following are some examples:

- To report only the professional component of a procedure or service
- To report a service mandated by a third-party payer
- To indicate that a procedure was performed bilaterally
- To report multiple procedures performed at the same session by the same provider
- To report that a portion of a service or procedure is reduced or eliminated at the physician's discretion
- To report assistant surgeon services

Appending the appropriate modifier can be crucial for reimbursement when a CPT code is reported in a specific circumstance. Appendix A of the CPT codebook contains a complete listing of these modifiers and their definitions. For CPT 2004, hyphens were removed that previously appeared before the modifier numbers. The modifier is reported by a two-digit number placed after the five-digit CPT code, such as **27580 50**.

A detailed discussion and specific examples of the use of each of the modifiers can be found in Chapter 10.

Coding Tip

The code and modifier are reported as a one-line entry on the claim form.

Unlisted Procedure or Service

Because of advances in the field of medicine, there may be services or procedures performed by physicians or other health care professionals that have not yet been designated with a specific CPT code. To report unlisted procedures or services, a number of specific code numbers have been designated. Each of these unlisted procedure code numbers relates to a specific section of the CPT codebook and is referenced in the guidelines of that section. Unlisted codes provide the means of reporting and tracking services and procedures until a more specific code is established in the CPT code set.

It is very important that the CPT code accurately describe the service that was performed. For that reason, it is equally important that a code that is close to the procedure performed not be selected in lieu of an unlisted procedure.

As mentioned earlier, some people maintain that they are not allowed to use unlisted procedures or that the use of the codes is undesirable. Although the use of an unlisted procedure code will require a special report or documentation to describe the service, correct coding demands that a square peg not be fit into a round hole.

In some cases, alternative coding and procedural nomenclature that is contained in other code sets may allow for appropriate reporting of a more specific code. CPT references to use an unlisted procedure code do not preclude reporting an appropriate code that may be found in other code sets.

Appendixes

There are 14 appendixes located in the back of the CPT codebook:

- Appendix A contains a complete list of the CPT modifiers and their definitions.
- Appendix B contains a summary of additions, deletions, and revisions.
- Appendix C contains clinical examples for E/M codes.
- Appendix D contains a summary of CPT add-on codes. These codes are also identified throughout the text of the CPT codebook with the ✚ symbol placed before the code.
- Appendix E contains a summary of CPT codes that are exempt from the use of modifier 51. These codes, however, are not designated as CPT add-on codes. They are identified throughout the text of the CPT codebook with the ⊘ symbol placed before the code.
- Appendix F contains a summary of the CPT codes that are exempt from the use of modifier 63. (Modifier 63 is used to indicate a procedure performed on an infant less than 4 kg in size.)
- Appendix G contains a summary of the CPT codes that include conscious sedation.
- Appendix H is an alphabetical index of performance measures by clinical condition or topic.
- Appendix I contains a list of the genetic testing code modifiers.
- Appendix J contains a summary that assigns each sensory, motor, and mixed nerve with its appropriate nerve conduction study code.
- Appendix K contains a list of codes that are pending approval from the Food and Drug Administration (FDA).
- Appendix L contains the assignments of branches to first, second, and third order of vascular families.
- Appendix M includes a list of crosswalked deleted and renumbered codes and descriptors.
- Appendix N contains a list of resequenced CPT codes.

Following is additional information about each of the appendixes.

Appendix A: Modifiers

This appendix contains a complete list of the CPT modifiers and their definitions. Also, to provide a more complete reference for the hospital outpatient users of CPT coding, the Healthcare Common Procedure Coding System (HCPCS) Level II national modifiers that have been approved by the National Uniform Billing Committee for hospital outpatient reporting are included in this appendix. (Chapter 10 features a comprehensive discussion of modifiers.)

Appendix B: Summary of Additions, Deletions, and Revisions

This appendix summarizes the additions, deletions, and revisions applicable to the current edition of the CPT codebook.

Appendix C: Clinical Examples

This appendix contains the clinical examples of the CPT codes for E/M services. These clinical examples were developed in conjunction with the implementation of the new codes for E/M services, which were introduced in *CPT 1992*.

The explanatory paragraphs preceding the actual clinical examples provided contain very important information regarding the use of these clinical examples. The clinical examples, when used with the E/M code descriptors found in the full text of the CPT codebook, are intended to be used as a tool for reporting services provided to patients. Coders should take the time to read and understand the intent of these clinical examples, because the examples can lead to a deeper understanding of the services encompassed in the E/M codes.

Appendix D: Summary of CPT Add-on Codes

In this appendix, users will find a summary of the codes designated as CPT add-on codes for the current edition of the CPT codebook. These codes are also identified throughout the text of the CPT codebook with the ✚ symbol. (Refer to Chapter 4 for further discussion of add-on codes.)

Appendix E: Summary of CPT Codes Exempt From Modifier 51

The codes in the listing that appear in this appendix are exempt from the use of modifier 51 but have not been designated as CPT add-on codes. These codes are identified throughout the text of the CPT codebook with a ⊘ symbol placed before the code.

Appendix F: Summary of CPT Codes Exempt From Modifier 63

The codes in the listing that appear in this appendix are exempt from the use of modifier 63. These codes are identified throughout the text of the CPT codebook with the parenthetical instruction, "Do not report modifier 63 in conjunction with . . . ."

Appendix G: Summary of CPT Codes That Include Moderate (Conscious) Sedation

The procedure codes listed in this appendix include conscious sedation as an inherent part of providing the procedure. These codes are identified throughout the text of the CPT codebook with a ⊙ symbol placed before the code.

Appendix H: Alphabetical Clinical Topics Listing

This appendix provides an alphabetical index of performance measures categorized by clinical condition or topic. Prior to reporting a code, the user must review the complete description of the code in the Category II section of the CPT codebook and the complete description of its associated measure by accessing the measure developer's Web site provided in the footnoted reference of the table. This appendix is on the CPT Web site.

Appendix I: Genetic Testing Code Modifiers

The modifiers that appear in this appendix are intended for reporting with molecular laboratory procedures related to genetic testing. Genetic test modifiers should be used in conjunction with CPT and HCPCS codes to provide diagnostic granularity of service to enable providers to submit complete and precise genetic testing information without altering test descriptors.

Appendix J: Electrodiagnostic Medicine Listing of Sensory, Motor, and Mixed Nerves

This appendix contains a summary that assigns each sensory, motor, and mixed nerve with its appropriate nerve conduction study code in order to enhance accurate reporting of codes **95900**, **95903**, and **95904**. Each nerve constitutes one unit of service.

Appendix K: Product Pending FDA Approval

This appendix contains a list of vaccine product codes pending approval from the Food and Drug Administration (FDA). These codes are indicated with the ✔ symbol and will be tracked by the AMA to monitor FDA approval status.

Appendix L: Vascular Families

This appendix provides an assignment of first-, second-, and third-order branches in a vascular family. This table makes the assumption that the starting point is catheterization of the aorta. This categorization would not be accurate, for example, if a femoral or carotid artery were catheterized directly in an antegrade direction. Arteries highlighted in bold are those more commonly reported during arteriographic procedures.

Appendix M: Summary of Crosswalked Deleted CPT Codes

Appendix M is a summary of all deleted and renumbered codes as well as a list of *CPT Assistant* articles that refer to these codes.

Appendix N: Summary of Resequenced CPT Codes

Appendix N is a new feature that was introduced for the *CPT 2010 codebook*. It summarizes CPT codes that do not appear in numeric sequence within the section level. Rather than deleting and renumbering, resequencing allows codes to be located in proximity to related code concepts, regardless of the numeric sequence. The codes listed in this appendix are identified with a # symbol to help the user recognize them within a code family of related concepts. Numerically placed references (eg, **Code is out of numerical sequence. See . . .**) are used as navigational alerts to direct the user to the location of the out-of-sequence code.

✓ Check Your Knowledge

6. Which appendix contains a summary of codes that are pending approval from the FDA?

7. This appendix includes clinical examples for the E/M codes.

Alphabetical Index

The index is located after the appendixes in the CPT codebook. It is important to note that the alphabetical index is *not* a substitute for the main text of the CPT codebook. Even if only one code appears in the index, the user must refer to the main text of the CPT codebook to ensure that the code selection is accurate.

The index is organized by main terms. There are four primary classes of main index entries:

- **Procedure or service** (for example: Allergen Immunotherapy, Arthroscopy, Biopsy, Cardiac Catheterization, Debridement, Evaluation and Management, Laparoscopy, Osteopathic Manipulation, Physical Medicine/Therapy/Occupational Therapy, Vaccines)
- **Organ or other anatomic site** (for example: Abdomen, Bladder, Esophagus, Hip, Intestines, Malar Area, Olecranon Process, Prostate)
- **Condition** (for example: Abscess, Blepharoptosis, Dislocation, Esophageal Varices, Hemorrhage, Omphalocele, Varicose Vein)
- **Synonyms, eponyms, and abbreviations** (for example: Anderson Tibial Lengthening, CBC, Clagett Procedure, EKG).

A main term may be followed by a series of up to three indented terms that modify the main term. These modifying terms should be reviewed, as these subterms have an effect on appropriate code selection.

Cross-references provide additional instructions to the user. There are two types of cross-references in the index:

- *See.* This type of reference is used primarily for synonyms, eponyms, and abbreviations. As an added reference, a list of common abbreviations can be found on the back cover of the professional edition of the CPT codebook and inside the back cover of the standard edition.
- *See Also.* This reference directs the user to look under another main term if the procedure is not listed under the first main index entry.

Reviewing and understanding the basics of CPT coding is an important first step in this book. The next step in becoming a more effective coder is the application of these basics to each chapter of the CPT codebook.

Code Ranges

A code range is listed when more than one code applies to a given index entry. If several nonsequential codes apply, the codes are separated by a comma.

EXAMPLE

Esophagus

    Reconstruction   43300, 43310, 43313

✓ Check Your Knowledge Answers

1. There are eight sections in the CPT codebook.
2. Unlisted.
3. No, procedures in CPT are not placed in sections according to a strict classification system.
4. Code **25100**.
5. Arthrotomy, wrist joint; with synovectomy.
6. Appendix K.
7. Appendix C.

Chapter Exercises

Check your answers in Appendix B.

1. How many sections are in the CPT codebook?
2. Name each of the sections.
3. Where are the Appendixes located in the CPT codebook?
4. Explain the placement in the CPT code set.
5. What is an unlisted procedure code?
6. What is a modifier?
7. List common uses of modifiers.
8. What is the Format of Terminology?
9. Where is the Alphabetic Index in the CPT codebook?

Match the symbols below (a through j) with the proper description

10. New or revised text
11. Moderate sedation

12. Reinstated code
13. Resequenced code
14. Add-on code
15. Modifier 51 exempt
16. FDA approval pending
17. Revised code
18. *CPT Changes: An Insider's View*
19. New code

a. ⟋
b. ➲
c. ⊘
d. ✚
e. ▲
f. #
g. ●
h. ○
i. ▶◀
j. ⊙

Match the descriptions below (a through f) with the correct appendix

20. Appendix L
21. Appendix F
22. Appendix G
23. Appendix C
24. Appendix E
25. Appendix B

a. This appendix provides users with a table that shows the assignment of branches to first, second, and third order.
b. This appendix provides a listing of codes exempt from the use of the modifier that identifies procedures performed on infants.
c. This appendix provides examples related to the CPT codes for Evaluation and Management (E/M) services.
d. This appendix provides a listing of codes that have not been designated as CPT add-on codes and are exempt from the use of multiple procedures modifier.
e. This appendix provides a summary of codes identified with the ● symbol and ▲ symbol placed before the code number.
f. This appendix provides users with an indication that it would not be appropriate to separately report conscious sedation in addition to the procedure code.

Evaluation and Management Services

Chapter Objectives

This chapter will assist in accomplishing the following objectives:

- Understand the basic format of levels of Evaluation and Management (E/M) services
- Understand the key words, phrases, and definitions that pertain to E/M services
- Understand the Instructions for Selecting a Level of E/M

Understand the Guidelines for E/M categories

The Evaluation and Management (E/M) services codes were introduced into the Current Procedural Terminology (CPT®) nomenclature in 1992. These codes describe services provided by physicians and other qualified health care professionals to evaluate patients and manage their care. The E/M codes replaced "visit" codes that described services in general terms such as a brief, intermediate, or comprehensive visit, for example. The E/M codes are widely used by physicians of all specialties and describe a large portion of the medical care provided to patients of all ages. E/M services may also be reported by other qualified health care professionals who are authorized to perform such services within the scope of their practice. The following basic format of the levels of E/M services is the same for most categories:

A unique code number is listed. See Figure 2-1.

- Place and/or type of service (eg, office or inpatient setting)
- Content of service defined (eg, a problem-focused history, a problem-focused examination, straightforward medical decision making)

Counseling and/or coordination of care with other providers or agencies is/are included when an E/M service is reported, if appropriate.

- Nature of presenting problem associated with a given level
- Time typically required to provide the service (eg, 10 minutes)

FIGURE 2-1 *Diagram of an E/M Code*

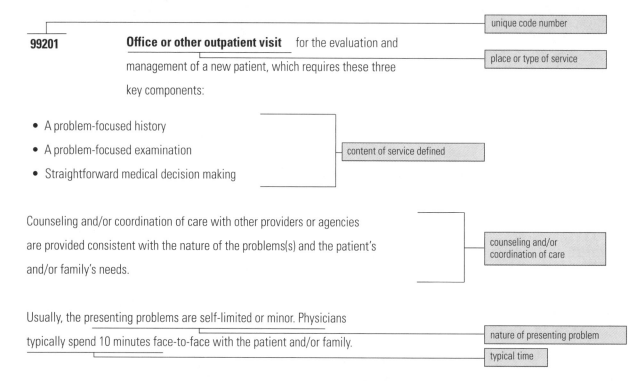

Categories and Subcategories of Service

To familiarize readers with the range and scope of E/M services, the following is an inclusive numeric listing of the categories and subcategories of E/M codes.

E/M codes are divided into the following categories and subcategories:

Office or Other Outpatient Services

Definitions of Commonly Used Terms

Words and phrases used throughout the E/M section are defined in the CPT code set to reduce the potential for differing interpretations and to increase consistency of reporting E/M services by physicians and other qualified health care professionals who are authorized to perform such services within the scope of their practice. It is very important to learn the definitions of these terms to appropriately report the codes within the E/M section.

New and Established Patients

Many of the E/M services CPT codes differentiate between new and established patients. A **new patient** is one who has not received any professional services from the physician or another physician of the same specialty who belongs to the same group practice within the past three years. An **established patient** is one who has received professional services from the physician or another physician of the same specialty who belongs to the same group practice within the past three years. Solely for the purpose of distinguishing between new and established patients, **professional services** are those face-to-face services rendered by a physician and reported by a specific CPT code(s). When a physician is on call for or covering for another physician, the patient's encounter is classified as it would have been by the physician who is not available. No distinction is made between new and established patients in the emergency department. E/M services in the Emergency Department Services category may be reported for any new or established patient who presents for treatment in the emergency department.

The definitions of new and established patient include professional services provided not only by a particular physician but also by other physicians of the same specialty belonging to the same group practice. This raises the question of subspecialty reporting within a given specialty (eg, electrophysiology specialists in a cardiology group, a hand surgeon in an orthopedic group). Although the CPT definitions do not explicitly address this question, it is possible for a patient receiving professional services from a subspecialist within the same group to be considered a new patient to another physician in the group. For example, if the subspecialists within the group practice have a separate tax identification number for their subspecialty different from the general group tax identification number, the patient receiving professional services from the subspecialist may be considered a new patient. See Figure 2-2.

Key Terms

New patient: one who has not received any professional services from the physician or another physician of the same specialty who belongs to the same group practice within the past three years.

Established patient: one who has received professional services from the physician or another physician of the same specialty who belongs to the same group practice within the past three years.

Professional services: face-to-face services rendered by a physician and reported by a specific CPT code.

FIGURE 2-2 *Decision Tree for New vs Established Patients*

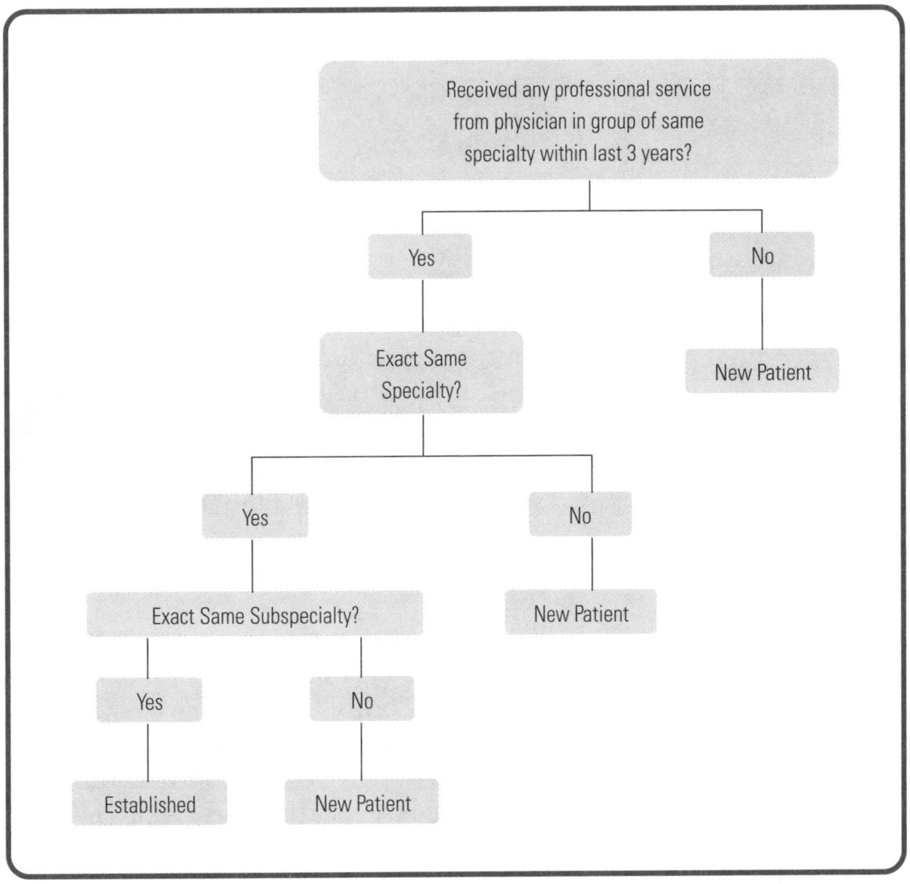

Coding Tip

Provided services such as telephone renewal of a prescription without a face-to face encounter are not considered when patients are identified as new or established.

Coding Tip

There are instances in which a physician is on call or covering for another physician. This patient encounter should be classified as it would have been by the physician who is not available.

✓ Check Your Knowledge

1. Define new and established patients.

2. Dr A leaves his group practice in Frankfort, Illinois, and joins a new group practice in Rockford, Illinois. When he provides professional services to his patients, whom he has seen within the past three years in the new Rockford practice, will he report these patients as new or established patients?

Concurrent Care and Transfer of Care

Concurrent care is the provision of similar services (eg, hospital visits) to the same patient by more than one physician on the same day. For CPT coding purposes, when concurrent care is provided, no special reporting is required. However, when concurrent care is provided, the *International Classification of Diseases, Ninth Revision, Clinical Modification* (ICD-9-CM) diagnosis code reported by each physician should reflect the need for the provision of similar services to the same patient by more than one physician on the same day. It is important to note that if the most specific ICD-9-CM diagnosis code is for the same condition, this does not preclude billing for concurrent care.

EXAMPLE

Dr A, an endocrinologist, provides a hospital visit to manage the patient's type 2 uncontrolled diabetes mellitus while Dr B, an infectious diseases specialist, provides a hospital visit to the same patient on the same day for management of the patient's pneumonia. Each physician reports the appropriate level of E/M service based on the content of the service provided (eg, extent of the history obtained, extent of the examination performed, and the complexity of the medical decision making). The ICD-9-CM diagnosis code reported by each physician should reflect his or her role in the management of the patient.

Transfer of care is the process whereby a physician who is providing management for some or all of a patient's problems relinquishes this responsbility to another physician who explicitly agrees to accept this responsibility and who, from the initial encounter, is not providing consultative services. The physician transferring care is then no longer providing care for these problems though he or she may continue providing care for other conditions when appropriate.

Key Terms

- Concurrent care
- Transfer of care

Coding Tip

Consultation codes should not be reported by the physician who has agreed to accept transfer of care before an initial evaluation but are appropriate to report if the decision to accept transfer of care cannot be made until after the initial consultation evaluation.

Key Terms

Concurrent care: provision of similar services (eg, hospital visits) to the same patient by more than one physician on the same day.

Transfer of care: process whereby a physician who is providing management for some or all of a patient's problems relinquishes this responsibility to another physician who explicitly agrees to accept this responsibility and who, from the initial encounter, is not providing consultative services.

Levels of E/M Services

Within each category or subcategory of E/M services, there are three to five levels of E/M services available for reporting purposes. Levels of E/M services are not interchangeable among the different categories or subcategories of service. The descriptors for the levels of E/M services recognize seven components, six of which are used in defining the levels of E/M services. These components are as follows:

- History
- Examination
- Medical decision making
- Counseling
- Coordination of care
- Nature of presenting problem
- Time

The first three of these components (history, examination, and medical decision making) are considered the **key components** in selecting a level of E/M service. As a general rule, these are the first components considered when the level of E/M service to report is determined. However, as with most rules, there are exceptions, eg, in the case of visits that consist primarily of counseling or coordination of care.

Key Term

- Key components

Key Term

Key components: history, examination, and medical decision making.

Selecting the Appropriate Level of E/M Services

E/M services are selected on the basis of either the key components or time. For the following categories and subcategories, all three of the key components (ie, history, examination, and medical decision making) must meet or exceed the stated requirements to qualify for a particular level of E/M service: office, new patient; hospital observation services; initial hospital care; office consultations, new or established patient;

inpatient consultations, new or established patient; emergency department services; initial nursing facility assessments; domiciliary care, new patient; and home services, new patient.

For the following categories and subcategories, two of the three key components (ie, history, examination, and medical decision making) must meet or exceed the stated requirements to qualify for a particular level of E/M services: office, established patient; subsequent hospital care; subsequent nursing facility care; domiciliary, rest home, or custodial care services, established patient; and home services, established patient.

When counseling and/or coordination of care dominate (more than 50%) the physician-patient and/or physician-family encounter (face-to-face time in the office or other outpatient setting or floor/unit time in the hospital or nursing facility), then time may be considered the key or controlling factor to qualify for selecting a particular level of E/M services. This includes time spent with parties who have assumed responsibility for the care of the patient or decision making, whether or not they are family members (eg, foster parents, persons acting in locum parentis, legal guardians). The extent of counseling and/or coordination of care must be documented in the medical record.

EXAMPLE

For several years, Dr C has been treating Mrs George for type 2 diabetes, hypertension, and obesity. Three days before this appointment, blood work was performed to determine the status of her diabetes. She presents to the physician's office, and the physician examines her for evidence of infection or circulatory problems. He then asks the patient about her compliance with the 1200-calorie diet she has been on for the past six months. After reviewing these findings, the physician indicates to the patient that she will have to begin using insulin, because her diabetes is not responding to the current treatment. Mrs George begins to sob uncontrollably. She tells Dr C that this means she is going to die because her grandmother got gangrene from this kind of diabetes and died from it. After calming her, Dr C explains that using insulin is not a death sentence. He discusses diet, insulin administration, and hypoglycemic reactions, as well as the symptoms of hyperglycemia. He refers Mrs George to an endocrinologist and provides instruction for proper foot and skin care and stresses the importance of seeing her ophthalmologist regularly. Mrs George is much calmer and feels that she will learn a lot from the booklets Dr C has given her.

The total time Dr C spent with Mrs George is 25 minutes, with 20 of those minutes spent providing counseling and/or coordination of care. Because more than 50% of the encounter was spent providing counseling and/or coordination of care, the total face-to-face time between Mrs George and Dr C may be considered the key factor in selecting the level of E/M service. Therefore, because Mrs George is an established patient and 25 total minutes were spent with the patient, it would be appropriate to report code **99214**.

Specific guidelines are also included in the categories and subcategories of the E/M services codes. It is important to also review these guidelines when selecting an appropriate E/M service code.

The following specific steps must be taken to select the appropriate level of E/M service:

1. Identify the category and subcategory of service.
2. Review the reporting instructions for the selected category or subcategory.
3. Review the E/M service code descriptors in the selected category or subcategory.
4. Determine the extent of history obtained.
5. Determine the extent of the examination performed.
6. Determine the complexity of medical decision making.
7. Select the appropriate level of E/M services.

Following is a comprehensive discussion of each of these steps.

Step 1: Identify the Category and Subcategory of Service

The first step in selecting a level of E/M service is to identify the appropriate category and subcategory of service provided. Refer to the table of Categories and Subcategories of E/M Services at the beginning of this chapter (eg, office or other outpatient services, new patient). A listing of the categories and subcategories of E/M services can also be found in the E/M guidelines of the CPT codebook.

Step 2: Review the Reporting Instructions for the Selected Category or Subcategory

Once the appropriate category and subcategory of service have been identified, it is important to review the reporting instructions for the selected category and/or subcategory. Most of the categories and many of the subcategories of E/M services have special guidelines or instructions unique to that category or subcategory. It is important for users to read and be guided by these special instructions.

Step 3: Review the E/M Service Code Descriptors in the Selected Category or Subcategory

Remember, the descriptors for the levels of E/M services recognize seven components (history, examination, medical decision making, counseling, coordination of care, nature of presenting problem, and time). The first six are used in defining the levels of E/M services. Take a minute to review the E/M code descriptors in the category or subcategory selected.

Step 4: Determine the Extent of History Obtained

To select the appropriate level of E/M service, it is necessary to determine the extent of the key components performed (ie, extent of history obtained, extent of the examination performed, and the complexity of medical decision making). Start by determining the extent of history obtained.

The medical history provides essential information for diagnosis and management and varies based on the clinical judgment of the physician and each individual patient and problem(s).

The following are included in obtaining the history:

- Chief complaint (CC)
- History of present illness (HPI)
- Review of systems (ROS)
- Past, family, and/or social history (PFSH)

When some patient groups are considered (eg, newborn infants), not all components are available or appropriate to consider.

The CC is a concise statement describing the symptom, problem, condition, diagnosis, or other factor that is the reason for the encounter, usually stated in the patient's (or the patient's parent's) words.

The HPI is a chronological description of the development of the patient's present illness from the first sign and/or symptom to the present.

Patients usually express their problems as symptoms (eg, pain or discomfort) or signs (eg, a noticeable physical abnormality such as a lump, cut, bruise, or murmur), with the exception of a newborn, whose presenting complaint may be related to his or her mother's (eg, maternal fever during labor). The further elaboration of any symptom requires attention to some or all of the dimensions of the HPI. Signs are better described by physical findings. Problems can also be described as the status of one or more chronic condition.

The CPT guidelines recognize seven dimensions of the HPI, including a description of the following:

- Location
- Quality
- Severity
- Timing
- Context
- Modifying factors
- Associated signs and symptoms

When an HPI is obtained, elaborating on the patient's CC(s) and other symptoms is most often accomplished by asking questions that focus on the seven dimensions. Following are examples of questions that the clinician may ask to elicit specific information regarding the dimensions of the HPI.

Location. What is the location of the pain or discomfort? Ask the patient to point to the specific symptomatic area. Is the pain diffuse or localized? Unilateral or bilateral? Does it radiate, or is it referred to other location(s)?

Quality. Include a description of the quality of the symptom. For example, is the pain described as sharp, dull, throbbing, stabbing, constant or intermittent, acute or chronic, or stable, improving, or worsening?

Severity. The patient may be asked to describe the severity of the pain by using a crude self-assessment scale to measure subjective levels (ie, on a scale of 1 to 10, with 1 being no pain and 10 the worst pain experienced). Or the patient may be asked to compare the pain quantitatively with a previously experienced pain (eg, kidney stone or labor pains).

Timing. Timing involves establishing the onset of the pain and a rough chronology of the development of the pain. To accomplish this, the physician may ask if there is a repetitive pattern for the pain or if the pain primarily occurs in the evening or during daylight hours or if it is continuous.

Context. Where is the patient, and what is he or she doing when the pain begins? Is the patient at rest or involved in an activity? Is the pain aggravated or relieved or does it recur with a specific activity? Has situational stress or some other factor preceded or accompanied the pain?

Modifying factors. What has the patient attempted to do to obtain relief or make himself or herself better? What makes the pain worse? For example, does the local application of heat or cold relieve or exacerbate the pain? Does eating relieve or exacerbate abdominal discomfort? Does coughing irritate the pain? Have over-the-counter or prescribed medications been attempted—with what results?

Associated signs and symptoms. A clinician's impressions formulated during the interview may lead to questioning about additional sensations or feelings. Examples might include diaphoresis (marked sweating) associated with indigestion or chest pain; tremulousness, weakness, and hunger pains in patients with diabetes; or blurring of vision accompanying a headache.

The following scenario is provided to further explain the elements of the HPI.

EXAMPLE

A 27-year-old man presents for evaluation of episodic cough and shortness of breath of two years' duration. He notes the latter to be exacerbated with exposure to smoke or dust. He has been employed at a feed mill for four years, which is dusty and exacerbates the symptoms. He has used no respiratory protection. He notes shortness of breath primarily with activity (eg, running up stairs) but otherwise feels he is able to keep pace with others his age and size without difficulty. He has noted some mild wheezing and has tried albuterol, which does not achieve prompt symptomatic relief. He is a lifelong nonsmoker with no history of asthma or other pulmonary disorder.

When the status of a chronic condition is being described, many of the same elements may apply as well as issues such as frequency of medication use, compliance, and associated measurements the patient reports (eg, home blood pressure, glucose). It is also common, especially in geriatric patients, to ascertain functional status related to activities of daily living (ADLs) (eg, ability to feed and clothe one's self, walk, shop, prepare food). For the child with chronic disease, the effects on the child's growth and development are also commonly evaluated.

The ROS is an inventory of body systems obtained through a series of questions asked by the physician seeking to identify signs and/or symptoms that the patient may be experiencing or has experienced. This helps define the problem, clarify the differential diagnosis, identify testing needed, or serve as baseline data on other systems that might be affected by any possible management (treatment) options. An ROS may be highly dependent on the age of the patient and irrelevant for newborns and young infants.

The following elements of a system review have been identified in the CPT code set:

- Constitutional symptoms (fever, weight loss, etc)
- Eyes
- Ears, nose, mouth, throat
- Cardiovascular
- Respiratory
- Gastrointestinal
- Genitourinary
- Musculoskeletal
- Integumentary (skin and/or breast)
- Neurologic
- Psychiatric
- Endocrine
- Hematologic/lymphatic
- Allergic/immunologic

The past, family, and/or social history (PFSH) includes a review of past medical experiences of the patient and the patient's family.

Past history is a review of the patient's past experiences with illnesses, injuries, and treatments that may include significant information about the following:

- Prior major illnesses and injuries
- Prior operations
- Prior hospitalizations
- Current medications
- Allergies (eg, drug, food)
- Age-appropriate immunization status
- Age-appropriate feeding/dietary status
- Birth history (eg, birth weight, Apgar score)
- Growth and developmental history

Family history is a review of medical events in the patient's family, including significant information about the following:

- The health status or cause of death of parents, siblings, and children
- Specific diseases related to problems identified in the CC or HPI and/ or ROS
- Diseases of family members that may be hereditary or place the patient at risk

Social history is an age-appropriate review of past and current activities that includes significant information about the following:

- Marital status and/or living arrangements
- Current/previous employment

- Use of drugs, alcohol, and tobacco
- Level of education
- School progress or failure
- Sexual history
- Domestic violence
- Other relevant social factors

The levels of E/M services recognize four types of history. The types of history and their respective definitions are provided in Table 2-1.

Step 5: Determine the Extent of the Examination Performed

The next key component to consider is the extent of the examination performed. It depends on the clinical judgment of the physician and the nature of the patient's presenting problems.

The levels of E/M services recognize four types of examination. The types of examination and their respective definitions are provided in Table 2-2.

TABLE 2-1 *E/M Patient Histories*

Type of History	Definition
Problem-focused	CC; brief HPI
Expanded problem-focused	CC; brief HPI; problem-pertinent ROS
Detailed	CC; extended HPI; problem-pertinent ROS including review of a limited number of additional systems; pertinent PFSH (directly related to the patient's problems)
Comprehensive	CC; extended HPI; ROS directly related to problem(s) identified in HPI plus review of all additional body systems; complete PFSH

TABLE 2-2 *E/M Patient Examinations*

Type of Examination	Definition
Problem-focused	A limited examination of the affected body area or organ system
Expanded problem-focused	A limited examination of the affected body area or organ system and other symptomatic or related organ system(s)
Detailed	An extended examination of the affected body area(s) and other symptomatic or related organ system(s)
Comprehensive	A general multisystem examination or a complete examination of a single organ system

For the purposes of the CPT definitions provided in Table 2-2, the following body areas are recognized:

- Head, including the face
- Neck
- Chest, including breasts and axillae
- Abdomen
- Genitalia, groin, buttocks
- Back
- Each extremity

For the purposes of the CPT definitions provided in Table 2-2, the following organ systems are recognized:

- Eyes
- Ears, nose, mouth, and throat
- Cardiovascular
- Respiratory
- Gastrointestinal
- Genitourinary
- Musculoskeletal
- Skin
- Neurologic
- Psychiatric
- Hematologic/lymphatic/immunologic

Step 6: Determine the Complexity of Medical Decision Making
The final key component is the complexity of medical decision making. Medical decision making refers to the complexity of establishing a diagnosis and/or selecting a management option as measured by the three following elements:

- The number of possible diagnoses and/or the number of management options that must be considered
- The amount and/or complexity of medical records, diagnostic tests, and/or other information that must be obtained, reviewed, and analyzed
- The risk of significant complications, morbidity, and/or mortality as well as comorbidities associated with the patient's presenting problem(s), the diagnostic procedure(s), and/or the possible management options

Comorbidities or underlying diseases in and of themselves are not considered in selecting the level of E/M services unless their presence significantly increases the complexity of the medical decision making.

Four types of medical decision making are recognized in the CPT code set. Table 2-3 lists them and the elements required to qualify for each type.

To qualify for a given type of medical decision making, two of the three elements in Table 2-3 must be met or exceeded.

A limited number of diagnoses or management options, a moderate amount and/or complexity of data to be reviewed, and a low risk of complications and/or morbidity or mortality constitute low-complexity medical decision making.

TABLE 2-3 *Definitions of Types of Medical Decision Making*

Type of Medical Decision Making	Number of Diagnoses or Management Options	Amount and/ or Complexity of Data to Be Reviewed	Risk of Complications and/or Morbidity or Mortality
Straightforward	Minimal	Minimal or none	Minimal
Low complexity	Limited	Limited	Low
Moderate complexity	Multiple	Moderate	Moderate
High complexity	Extensive	Extensive	High

Step 7: Select the Appropriate Level of E/M Services

Now that the appropriate category and subcategory of services have been identified, the guidelines for that specific category and/or subcategory have been reviewed, and the key components have been determined, it is time to select the appropriate level of E/M service. This selection is based on the key components performed by the physician and the number of key components required for the particular category or subcategory identified.

Some of the categories and subcategories of E/M services require all of the key components to meet or exceed requirements stated in the code descriptor to qualify for a level of E/M service. Other categories and subcategories of E/M services require only two of the three key components to meet or exceed the stated requirements to qualify for a particular level of service.

Table 2-4 indicates the categories and subcategories of service requiring all of the key components (ie, history, examination, and medical decision making) to meet or exceed the requirements stated in the code descriptor to qualify for a particular level of service.

Finally, before selecting the level of E/M service, the content of the E/M service provided must be given careful consideration. This is true whether the E/M service involves a new or an established patient visit. If counseling and/or coordination of care do not constitute more than 50% of the encounter, the level of service is selected on the basis of the key components that have been met.

A Review of the Categories and Subcategories of E/M Services

Within the E/M section of the CPT codebook there are several categories and subcategories of services. See Table 2-4. Generally, the categories of service vary depending on the site of service (eg, office or other outpatient, hospital inpatient services, emergency department services). Every category of E/M service has guidelines and instructional notes at the beginning of the category. Many of the subcategories

TABLE 2-4 *Categories and Subcategories of Service*

Category	Subcategory	CPT Codes
Office or Other Outpatient Services		
	New Patient	99201-99205
Hospital Observation Services		99218-99220
Hospital Inpatient Services		
	Initial Hospital Care	99221-99223
Observation or Inpatient Care Services (Including Admission and Discharge Services)		99234-99236
Consultations		
	Office or Other Outpatient Consultations	99241-99245
	Initial Inpatient Consultations	99251-99255
Emergency Department Services		99281-99285
Nursing Facility Services		
	Initial Nursing Facility Care	99304-99306
	Other Nursing Facility Services	99318
Domiciliary, Rest Home (eg, Boarding Home), or Custodial Care Services		
	New Patient	99234-99238
Home Services		
	New Patient	99341-99345

have guidelines and instructional notes in addition to those that appear at the beginning of the category. Refer to the CPT codebook for the complete guidelines pertaining to each category and subcategory of service.

Office or Other Outpatient Services

The Office or Other Outpatient Services codes (**99201-99215**) are used to report E/M services provided in the physician's office or other outpatient/ambulatory settings, including E/M services provided in an urgent care setting. Office and Other Outpatient Services include the subcategories of new and established patient visits. When new patient visits are reported, all three key components must meet or exceed the stated requirements to qualify for a particular level of E/M service. When established patient visits are reported, two of the three key components must meet or exceed the stated requirements to qualify for a particular level of E/M service.

If a patient is admitted to the hospital in the course of the office encounter, all E/M services provided by the physician in conjunction with the admission are considered part of the initial hospital care when performed on the same date as the admission. A separate code for the office visit is not reported. The initial hospital care level of service reported by the admitting physician should include the services related to the admission provided in the physician's office as well as the E/M services the physician provided on that same date in the inpatient setting.

EXAMPLE

A patient presents to Dr D's office with complaints of fever, chills, malaise, and a cough. The physician obtains the history from the patient, performs an examination, and orders a chest X ray. The patient is admitted to the hospital by Dr D on that same day for intravenous antibiotic therapy for treatment of pneumonia. After completion of his office hours that day, Dr D provides an E/M service to the patient in the hospital.

In the example, Dr D will not separately report the office visit and the initial hospital care. Rather, the initial hospital care level of service reported should include all the services related to the admission he provided in the office as well as in the inpatient setting.

Hospital Observation Services

Hospital Observation Services codes (**99217-99226**) are used to report E/M services provided to patients designated or admitted as "observation status" in a hospital. These patients are to be observed to determine whether they should be admitted to the hospital, transferred to another facility, or sent home. Because not all hospitals have a specific area designated for observation patients, the patient does not have to be located in an observation area designated by the hospital. Instead, the patient can be designated or admitted as observation status in the medical record. Codes in this category are not used to report hospital observation services involving admission and discharge services provided on the same date. Hospital Observation or Inpatient Services involving admission and discharge services provided on the same date are reported with codes **99234-99236**.

Codes **99218-99220** are used to report the initial observation care and are reported for new or established patient visits. When these codes are reported, it is necessary for all three of the key components to meet or exceed the requirements stated in the code descriptor to qualify for a particular level of service. Codes **99224-99226** are used to report the subsequent observation care and are reported for new or established patient visits. When these codes are reported, it is necessary to meet at least two of the three key components stated in the code descriptor to qualify for a particular level of service.

Code **99217** is used to report observation care discharge-day management. This code is used by the physician to report final examination of the patient, discussion of the observation stay, instructions for continuing care, and preparation of discharge records. This code is reported only if the discharge from observation status is on a date other than the initial date of observation status. In the event that an observation stay exceeds two days, the appropriate initial observation care code is reported for the initial day, code **99217** is reported for the observation care discharge day. If the physician provides an E/M service on a given date in another site (eg, physician's office, hospital emergency department, nursing facility) and subsequently initiates observation status in a hospital for that patient on the same date, the physician reports only an initial observation care code for all E/M services provided on that date. The level of initial observation care reported by the physician should include the services provided in the other site of service as well as those provided in the observation setting. If a patient is designated as observation status on a given date and is subsequently admitted to the hospital on that date by the same physician, only an initial hospital care code is reported for both of these E/M services provided on that date. The initial hospital care level of service reported should include all E/M services provided on that date.

The hospital observation codes are not intended to be used to report physician services related to postoperative recovery of a patient. No E/M code is reported for E/M services provided by the physician who performs a surgery and then routinely evaluates the patient in an observation area postoperatively. The global surgical package generally includes those evaluations immediately after surgery.

Hospital Inpatient Services

The Hospital Inpatient Services codes (**99221-99239**) are used to report E/M services provided to hospital inpatients. Services include the following three subcategories of codes: Initial Hospital Care, Subsequent Hospital Care, and Hospital Discharge Services. Patients in a partial hospital setting are also included in this range of codes. A partial hospital setting is used for crisis stabilization, intensive short-term daily treatment, or intermediate-term treatment of psychiatric disorders.

Initial Hospital Care

Initial Hospital Care codes (**99221-99223**) are used to report new or established patient E/M services. These codes are intended to be reported for the first hospital inpatient encounter by the admitting physician. This date may not be the same as the date the patient was admitted to the hospital.

EXAMPLE

The physician provided an E/M service to the patient in the office on Wednesday and subsequently admitted the patient to the hospital on that same day. However, the physician did not have an inpatient encounter with that patient until Thursday morning. In this scenario, the appropriate code for office or other outpatient level of E/M service is reported for the E/M services provided on Wednesday. The date of service and appropriate code for the initial hospital care would be Thursday's date—the date the admitting physician had the first hospital inpatient encounter with the patient.

The initial hospital care level of service reported by the admitting physician should include all E/M services provided to that patient in conjunction with that admission on the same date. For example, if the physician provides an E/M service to the patient in the office (or other site of service) on Wednesday, admits the patient to the hospital, and subsequently has an inpatient encounter with that patient all on the same date (Wednesday), then the initial hospital care level of service reported should include all E/M services provided on that date. A separate code would not be reported for the E/M services provided in the office (or other site of service) on that date.

The initial hospital care level of service codes include all E/M services provided to that patient in conjunction with that admission on the same date. A separate code would not be reported for the E/M services provided in the office (or other site of service) on that same date.

Subsequent Hospital Care

Subsequent Hospital Care codes (**99231-99233**) are reported to identify services provided by the admitting physician on dates subsequent to the provision of initial hospital care. When subsequent hospital care is reported, at least two of the three key components must meet or exceed the stated requirements to qualify for a particular level of E/M service.

Hospital Discharge Services

The Hospital Discharge Services codes (**99238** and **99239**) are reported for the total time spent by the attending physician for hospital discharge of the patient provided the date of discharge is different from the date of admission. These codes include final examination of the patient; discussion of the hospital stay; instructions for continuing care to all relevant caregivers; and preparation of discharge records, prescriptions, and referral forms. The Hospital Discharge Services codes may be used to report discharge services provided to patients who die during the hospital stay.

Consultations

A *consultation* is defined as a type of service provided by a physician whose opinion or advice regarding evaluation and/or management of a specific problem is requested by another physician or other appropriate source. Types of consultations include the following:

- Office or Other Outpatient Consultations
- Inpatient Consultations

A consultation must include the following elements:

- A written or verbal request for a consultation made by a physician or other appropriate source must be documented in the patient's medical record.
- The consultant must document his or her opinion and any services ordered or performed.
- The consultant may initiate diagnostic and/or therapeutic services at the same or a subsequent visit.
- The consultant must communicate in a written report the opinion and any services ordered or performed to the requesting physician or other appropriate source.

Office or Other Outpatient Consultations

The Office or Other Outpatient Consultations codes (**99241-99245**) are used to report consultations provided in the office or other outpatient setting, including the physician's office; a hospital observation service; home services; domiciliary, rest home, or custodial care; emergency department; or other ambulatory facility. There is no differentiation between new and established patient visits. When the codes in this subcategory of service are reported, all three key components must meet or exceed the stated requirements to qualify for a particular level of service.

A consultation that is initiated by a patient and/or family and not requested by a physician or other appropriate source (eg, physician assistant, nurse practitioner, doctor of chiropractic, physical therapist, occupational therapist, speech-language pathologist, psychologist, social worker, lawyer, or insurance company) is not reported using the consultation codes but may be reported using the office visit, home service, or domiciliary/rest home care codes.

Follow-up visits provided in the consultant's office or other outpatient facility that are initiated by the consulting physician or patient are reported by using the appropriate codes for established patients: office visits (**99211-99215**); domiciliary, rest home (**99334-99337**); or home (**99347-99350**). If an additional request for an opinion or advice regarding the same or a new problem is received from another physician or other appropriate source and documented in the medical record, the office consultation codes may be used again.

Inpatient Consultations

The Inpatient Consultations codes (**99251-99255**) are used to report consultations provided to hospital inpatients or residents of nursing facilities or patients in a partial hospital setting. Within this series of codes there is no differentiation between new and established patient visits. When the codes in this subcategory are reported, all three key components must meet or exceed the requirements of the code descriptor to qualify for a particular level of service. Only one consultation should be reported by a consultant per admission. Subsequent services during the same admission are reported using Subsequent Hospital Care codes (**99231-99233**) or Subsequent Nursing Facility Care codes (**99307-99310**), including services to complete the initial consultation, monitor progress, revise recommendations, or address a new problem.

EXAMPLE

The physician provided a consultation for a patient in the hospital on Wednesday. However, the consulting physician performed a follow-up consultation on Thursday afternoon. In this scenario, the appropriate Subsequent Hospital Care codes (**99231-99233**) should be reported as only one consultation and should be reported by a consultant per admission.

Consultation vs Referral

From a CPT coding perspective, the terms *consultation* and *referral* are not used interchangeably. When a physician refers a patient to another physician, it is not automatically a consultation. A consultation would be appropriate if the E/M service provided meets the previous criteria for reporting a consultation. If a physician sends a patient to another physician for specialized care that is not in his or her domain and the physician to whom the patient is referred does not communicate his or her opinion or advice to the requesting physician, then this is not a consultation.

Emergency Department Services

An *emergency department* (ED) is defined as an organized hospital-based facility for the provision of unscheduled episodic services to patients who present for immediate medical attention. E/M services provided in the emergency department, regardless of whether the patient is new or established, are reported with the codes in this series (**99281-99285**). When the codes in this category of service are reported, all three key components must be met. These codes are not limited to use by emergency department physicians. Time is not a descriptive component for emergency department levels of service because services are typically provided on a variable-intensity basis, often involving multiple encounters over an extended period. The descriptor of code **99285** is differentiated in that it indicates that three key components are required "within the constraints imposed by the urgency of the patient's clinical condition and/or mental status." This allows code **99285** to be reported even if the patient's condition precludes the completion of the comprehensive history and/or the comprehensive examination. Code **99285** can also be reported when the patient's condition normally requires this level of service but the physician is unable to complete a comprehensive-level history or examination.

Critical Care Services

The Critical Care Services codes (**99291** and **✚99292**) are time-based codes for reporting the total duration of time on a given date spent by a physician providing critical care services to a critically ill or critically injured patient, even if the time spent by the physician on that date is not continuous. Critical care is defined as the direct delivery of medical care for a critically ill or critically injured patient by a physician or physicians. A critical illness or injury acutely impairs one or more vital organ systems such that there is a high probability of imminent or life-threatening deterioration in the patient's condition. For a given period of time, the physician must devote full attention to the patient, providing critical care services, and cannot provide services to any other patient during the same period. The time that can be reported as critical care is the time spent engaged in work directly related to the individual patient's care, whether that time was spent at the immediate bedside or elsewhere on the floor or unit. Time spent with the individual patient should be recorded in the patient's record. Although critical care is usually given in a critical care area such as the coronary care unit, intensive care unit (ICU), respiratory care unit, or emergency care facility, it is not required that the patient be physically located in such an area to receive critical care services.

Code **99291** is reported once per date for the first 30 to 74 minutes of critical care, even if the time spent by the physician is not continuous on that date. Critical care of less than 30 minutes in total duration on a given date should be reported with the appropriate E/M code. Code **✚99292** is used to report additional blocks of time of up to 30 minutes each beyond the first 74 minutes. When critical care services are provided in the outpatient setting, code **99291** or **✚99292** is reported regardless of the age of the patient.

Services included in the critical care codes when performed during the critical period by the physician(s) providing critical care are as follows:

- Interpretation of cardiac output measurements (**93561, 93562**)
- Chest X rays (**71010, 71015, 71020**)
- Pulse oximetry (**94760, 94761, 94762**)
- Blood gases and information data stored in computers (eg, ECGs, blood pressures, hematologic data, **99090**)
- Gastric intubation (**43752, 43753**)
- Temporary transcutaneous pacing (**92953**)
- Ventilator management (**94002-94004, 94660, 94662**)
- Vascular access procedures (**36000, 36410, 36415, 36591, 36600**)

Any services performed that are not in the preceding list should be reported separately.

Nursing Facility Services

The Nursing Facility Services codes (**99304-99318**) are reported for services provided to patients in nursing facilities (formerly called skilled nursing facilities, intermediate care facilities, or long-term care facilities).

There are four subcategories of Nursing Facility Services codes: Initial Nursing Facility Care, Subsequent Nursing Facility Care, Nursing Facility Discharge Services, and Other Nursing Facility Services. Nursing facilities have the responsibility to conduct comprehensive assessments of each resident's functional capacity by means of a resident assessment instrument (RAI). An RAI is a form composed of a uniform minimum data set and resident assessment protocols.

Initial Nursing Facility Care

The Initial Nursing Facility Care codes (**99304-99306**) are reported for the physician's involvement in providing admission or readmission services to nursing facility patients. There are three codes in this subcategory, one for each level of care that is provided dependent upon the patient's condition (eg, low, moderate, or high severity) and services provided (eg, whether the history taken and examination done were detailed or comprehensive, and what level of medical decision was performed) by the physician.

Subsequent Nursing Facility Care

Subsequent Nursing Facility Care codes (**99307-99310**) are reported for the services provided to a patient subsequent to the physician's initial and/or previous assessment. There are four levels of subsequent nursing facility care services involving straightforward to high-complexity medical decision making and requiring at least two of the three key components (history, examination, medical decision making) ranging in intensity from problem-focused to comprehensive.

Nursing Facility Discharge Services

The Nursing Facility Discharge Services codes (**99315** and **99316**) are time based and are intended to be reported for the total duration of time spent by the physician for the final nursing facility discharge of the patient, even if the time spent providing the service is not continuous. Only one code is reported: code **99315** if the total time is 30 minutes or less or code **99316** if the total time is more than 30 minutes. Like the Hospital Discharge Services codes, the Nursing Facility Discharge Services codes may be used to report discharge services provided to patients who die during the nursing facility stay.

Chapter 2

The attending physician would perform the final examination of the patient (pronouncing the patient dead), discuss the nursing facility stay with family members or others, and prepare discharge records.

Other Nursing Facility Services

The Other Nursing Facility Services code (**99318**) is used to report the annual assessment required by the nursing facility for its residents. This service requires a detailed interval history, a comprehensive examination, and medical decision making that is of low to moderate complexity.

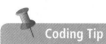

Coding Tip

Code **99318** should not be used in conjunction with any of the other nursing facility service codes and should occur as a separate service entailing only the annual nursing facility assessment dictated by the facility.

Domiciliary, Rest Home (eg, Boarding Home), or Custodial Care Services

The Domiciliary, Rest Home (eg, Boarding Home), or Custodial Care Services codes (**99324-99337**) are used to report E/M services in a facility that provides room, board, and other personal assistance services, generally on a long-term basis. There are separate codes for reporting new (**99324-99328**) and established (**99334-99337**) patient visits. When new patient visits are reported, all three key components must meet or exceed the requirements of the code descriptor to qualify for a particular level of service. When established patient visits are reported, two of the three key components must meet or exceed the requirements of the code descriptor to qualify for a particular level of service.

Domiciliary, Rest Home (eg, Assisted Living Facility), or Home Care Plan Oversight Services

The Domiciliary, Rest Home (eg, Assisted Living Facility), or Home Care Plan Oversight Services codes (**99339** and **99340**) are intended to be reported for care plan oversight services of patients in the home, domiciliary, or rest home (eg, assisted living facility) under the individual supervision of a physician.

Home Services

The Home Services codes (**99341-99350**) are used to report provision of E/M services in the patient's private residence by the physician. There are separate subcategories of codes for new patient and established patient visits. For nonphysician health care professionals providing services in the home setting, codes **99500-99602** in the Home Health Procedures/ Services subsection of the Medicine section should be reported.

Prolonged Services

The Prolonged Services codes (**99354-99360**) are used to report the provision of prolonged services by a physician that are beyond the usual services provided in either an inpatient or outpatient setting. There are three separate subcategories of codes used to distinguish prolonged services involving direct (face-to-face) patient contact (**99354-99357**), prolonged physician services without direct (face-to-face) patient contact (**99358** and **99359**), and physician standby services (**99360**).

Prolonged Physician Services With Direct (Face-to-Face) Patient Contact

The Prolonged Physician Services With Direct (Face-to-Face) Patient Contact codes (**99354-99357**) are used when a physician provides prolonged service involving direct (face-to-face) patient contact that is beyond the usual service (ie, beyond the typical time) in either the inpatient or outpatient setting. The term *face-to-face* refers only to patient face-to-face contact. These are time-based codes and are reported for the total duration of face-to-face time spent by a physician providing prolonged services on a given date. It is not necessary for the time spent by the physician providing the prolonged service to be continuous. These codes are all add-on codes and are reported separately, in addition to the appropriate code for the E/M service provided.

Codes **✚99354** and **✚99355** are reported for the office or other outpatient setting. Codes **99356** and **99357** are reported for the inpatient setting.

Codes **✚99354** and **✚99356** are used to report the first hour of prolonged service. These codes may also be used to report a total duration of prolonged service of 30 to 60 minutes on a given date. Prolonged service of less than 30 minutes in total duration on a given date is not reported separately. Less than 30 minutes of prolonged service is included in the E/M code reported for that date. Codes **✚99355** and **✚99357** are used to report each additional 30 minutes beyond the first hour of prolonged services. These codes may also be used to report the final 15 to 30 minutes of prolonged service on a given date.

Prolonged service of less than 15 minutes beyond the first hour or less than 15 minutes beyond the final 30 minutes is not separately reported.

Prolonged Physician Services Without Direct (Face-to-Face) Patient Contact

The Prolonged Physician Services Without Direct (Face-to-Face) Patient Contact codes (**99358** and **99359**) are used to report prolonged services without direct (face-to-face) patient contact in either the inpatient or outpatient setting. The total duration of time spent providing these services on a given date is reported, even if the time spent by the physician on that date is not continuous. Prolonged services of less than 30 minutes in total duration on a given date are not reported. These codes are considered add-on codes and are reported separately, in addition to the code(s) for other physician services and/or inpatient or outpatient E/M service. Code **99358** is intended to be reported separately in addition to code(s) for other physician service(s) and/or an inpatient or outpatient E/M service. Code **99358** must first be reported to report code **+99359**.

Code **99358** is used to report the first hour of prolonged service on a given date, regardless of the place of service. This code may also be used to report a total duration of prolonged service of 30 to 60 minutes on a given date. It should be reported only once per patient per date, even if the time spent by the physician is not continuous on that date.

Code **+99359** is used to report each additional 30 minutes beyond the first hour of prolonged physician services, again regardless of the place of service. It may also be used to report the final 15 to 30 minutes of prolonged service on a given date. Prolonged service of less than 15 minutes beyond the first hour or less than 15 minutes beyond the final 30 minutes is not reported separately.

Physician Standby Services

The Physician Standby Services code (**99360**) is used to report physician standby services requiring prolonged physician attendance without direct (face-to-face) patient contact. Physician standby services are provided at the request of another physician. This code is used to report a total duration of 30 minutes of physician standby service on a given date. Standby services of less than 30 minutes on a given date are not reported separately. If an additional full 30 minutes of a standby service are provided, it is appropriate to report code **99360** for each full 30 minutes of standby service.

To report code **99360**, the physician must be available to provide care to the patient but may not actually provide any care. The physician providing the standby services cannot provide care or services to other patients during the period of standby.

This code is not reported by the standby physician if the period of standby ends with his or her performance of a procedure subject to a surgical package. It is also not appropriate to report this code for time spent proctoring another physician.

Case Management Services

Physician case management is a process in which a physician is responsible for directly caring for a patient, coordinating and controlling access to health care services needed by the patient, and initiating and/or supervising other health care services needed by the patient. The Case Management Services codes include the following subcategories: Anticoagulant Management and Medical Team Conferences.

Anticoagulant Management

The Anticoagulant Management codes (**99363-99364**) are intended to describe the outpatient management of warfarin therapy, including ordering, reviewing, and interpreting of international normalized ratio (INR) testing; communicating with patient; and adjusting dosage as appropriate. When reporting these services, the work of anticoagulant management may not be used as a basis for reporting an E/M service or Care Plan Oversight time during the reporting period.

Any period less than 60 continuous outpatient days is not reported. If less than the specified minimum number of services per period are performed, do not report the anticoagulant management services (**99363** and **99364**).

Medical Team Conferences

Medical Team Conferences codes (**99366-99368**) are intended to describe participation by a minimum of three qualified health care professionals from different specialties or disciplines. These are time-based codes, and they differentiate between direct (face-to-face) contact with the patient (**99366**) and without direct (face-to-face) contact with the patient (**99367-99368**).

Care Plan Oversight Services

Care Plan Oversight Services codes (**99374-99380**) are reported for physician supervision of patients under the care of a home health agency, hospice, or nursing facility.

All the codes are time based and used to report the complexity and approximate physician time of the care plan oversight services provided within a 30-day period (within a calendar month).

Preventive Medicine Services

The Preventive Medicine Services codes (**99381-99429**) include initial preventive medicine E/M services for new patient visits and periodic preventive medicine reevaluation and management services for established patient visits. The codes for initial and periodic preventive medicine E/M services are categorized by patient age. There are also codes for preventive medicine counseling for individuals and groups.

The preventive medicine E/M codes for new and established patients include a comprehensive history and a comprehensive examination. The comprehensive nature of the Preventive Medicine Services codes reflects an age- and gender-appropriate history/examination and is not synonymous with the comprehensive examination required in E/M codes **99201-99350**.

The comprehensive history obtained as part of the preventive medicine E/M service is not problem oriented and does not involve a chief complaint or present illness. It does, however, include a comprehensive system review and comprehensive or interval past, family, and social history, as well as a comprehensive assessment/history of pertinent risk factors. The comprehensive examination performed as part of the preventive medicine E/M service is multisystem, but the extent of the examination is based on the age of the patient and the risk factors identified.

If an abnormality is encountered or a preexisting problem is addressed in the process of performing the preventive medicine E/M service and the problem is significant enough to require additional work for the physician to perform the key components of a problem-oriented E/M service, then the appropriate Office or Other Outpatient Service code (**99201-99215**) should be reported in addition to the appropriate code for the preventive E/M service. **Modifier 25** should be appended to the office/outpatient code reported. Appending **modifier 25** indicates that a significant, separately identifiable E/M service (above and beyond the preventive medicine E/M service) was provided by the same physician on the same day as the preventive medicine service. If in the process of performing the preventive medicine E/M service a physician encounters an insignificant or trivial problem or abnormality that does not require additional work and the performance of the key components of a problem-oriented service, then it would not be appropriate to report the problem-oriented service in addition to the preventive services.

The codes for new and established patient preventive medicine E/M services include counseling, anticipatory guidance, and risk factor reduction interventions that are provided at the time of the initial or periodic preventive medicine service. Counseling and/or risk factor reduction interventions provided at a separate encounter for the purpose of promoting health and preventing illness or injury are reported with codes **99401-99412**. Immunizations and ancillary studies involving laboratory, radiology, other procedures, or screening tests identified with a specific CPT code are reported separately.

Non-Face-to-Face Physician Services (99441-99444)

The non-face-to-face E/M services provided by a physician include telephone services and online medical evaluation services, and are explained in more detail below.

Telephone Services

There are three codes within the Non-Face-to-Face Physician Services subcategory (**99441-99443**) for reporting telephone calls by a physician. These are non-face-to-face E/M services provided by a physician to a patient using the telephone. Each code includes examples of the type of service that may be provided when the code is reported. These are time-based codes and are reported based upon the total time the physician spent on the telephone with the patient. It would not be appropriate to report these codes in the event the telephone service provided ends with a decision to see the patient within 24 hours or on the next available urgent visit appointment. This encounter would be considered part of the pre-service work of the subsequent E/M service, procedure, and visit. If the telephone call refers to an E/M service performed and reported by the physician within the previous seven days (either physician requested or unsolicited patient follow-up) or within the postoperative period of the previously completed procedure, then the service(s) are considered part of that previous E/M service or procedure.

Codes **99441-99443** should not be reported for telephone services provided by a qualified nonphysician health care professional. These types of services should be reported with codes **98966-98968** in the Non-Face-to-Face Nonphysician Services subsection in the Medicine section.

On-Line Medical Evaluation

Code **99444** is reported for a non-face-to-face physician E/M service to a patient utilizing Internet resources in response to a patient's on-line inquiry. This involves the physician's personal timely response to the patient's inquiry and permanent storage (electronic or hard copy) of the encounter. The service is reported only one time for the same episode of care during a seven-day period. It would not be appropriate to report this service if the on-line medical evaluation refers to an E/M service previously performed and reported by the physician within the previous seven days. The reporting of code **99444** encompasses the sum of communication (eg, related telephone calls, prescription provision, laboratory orders) pertaining to the on-line patient encounter.

It would not be appropriate to report code **99444** for an on-line medical evaluation service provided by a qualified nonphysician health care professional. This type of service should be reported with code **98969** in the Non-Face-to-Face Nonphysician Services subsection in the Medicine section.

Newborn Care Services

Newborn Care Services codes (**99460-99463**) are used to report E/M services provided to newborns (birth through the first 28 days) in several different settings. Use of the normal newborn codes is limited to the initial care of the newborn in the first days after birth prior to home discharge. E/M services provided to newborns who are other than normal are reported with the Hospital Inpatient Services (**99221-99233**) or with the neonatal intensive and critical care services (**99466-99469, 99477-99480**).

The E/M services for the newborn include maternal and/or fetal and newborn history, newborn physical examination(s), ordering of diagnostic tests and treatments, meetings with the family, and documentation in the medical record. Procedures (eg, **54150**) are not included with the normal newborn codes and should be reported separately, when performed. Code **99460** is used to report the initial evaluation and management of a normal newborn infant in the hospital or birthing center care setting. Code **99461** is reported for the initial evaluation and management of a normal newborn in settings other than the hospital or birthing room center.

Both codes **99460** and **99461** are reported only once per day of service. If the initial E/M services are provided to a normal newborn who is admitted and discharged on the same date of service in a hospital or birthing care center, then code **99463** would be reported.

Hospital discharge services provided to a normal newborn on a date subsequent to the admission date are reported with the Hospital Discharge Services codes (**99238-99239**), as appropriate. When normal newborns are seen in follow-up after the date of discharge in the office or other outpatient setting, then this service should be reported with codes **99201-99215**, **99381**, **99391**, as appropriate.

Inpatient Neonatal Intensive Care Services and Pediatric and Neonatal Critical Care Services

This subsection of the E/M section of the CPT codebook includes codes for reporting transport for pediatric critical care patients, critical care for neonatal and pediatric patients in the inpatient setting, and codes for reporting initial and continuing intensive care services.

Pediatric Critical Care Patient Transport

The Critical Care Patient Transport codes **99466-99467** are time-based codes reported for pediatric patients (24 months of age or less) who are critically ill or critically injured who receive face-to-face critical care services delivered by a physician during interfacility transport.

Only the time the physician spends in direct face-to-face contact with the patient during the transport should be reported. Face-to-face care begins when the physician assumes primary responsibility of the pediatric patient at the referring hospital or facility, and ends when the receiving hospital or facility accepts responsibility for the pediatric patient's care. Procedure(s) or service(s) performed by other members of the transporting team may not be reported by the supervising physician.

Code **99466** is reported for the first 30 to 74 minutes of direct face-to-face time with the transport pediatric patient. Code **+99467** is reported for each additional 30 minutes. Both codes should be reported only once on a given date. It is important to note that face-to-face pediatric patient transport services of less than 30 minutes should not be reported with codes **99466-99467**. These types of services should be reported with the appropriate E/M code.

Inclusive Services

The following services are included in the Inpatient Neonatal and Pediatric Critical Care codes (**99468-99476**), and the Initial and Continuing Intensive Care Services codes (**99477-99480**) and may not be reported separately:

Invasive or noninvasive electronic monitoring of vital signs, vascular access procedures (**36000, 36140, 36620, 36510, 36555, 36400, 36405, 36406, 36420, 36600, 36660**), airway and ventilation management (**31500, 94002-94004, 94375, 94610, 94660**), monitoring or interpretation of blood gases or oxygen saturation (**94760-94762**), transfusion of blood components (**36430, 36440**), oral or nasogastric tube placement (**43752**), suprapubic bladder aspiration (**51100**), bladder catheterization (**51701, 51702**), and lumbar puncture (**62270**).

Any services performed that are not in the preceding list should be reported separately.

Inpatient Neonatal and Pediatric Critical Care

The Inpatient Neonatal Critical Care codes (**99468-99469**) are reported for services provided by a physician directing the inpatient care of a critically ill neonate 28 days of age or less. Code **99468** is reported for the initial E/M service, whereas code **99469** is reported for the subsequent E/M service. These codes may be reported only once per day, per patient by a single physician.

The Pediatric Critical Care codes (**99471-99476**) are reported for services provided by a physician directing the inpatient care of a critically ill infant or young child from 29 days of postnatal age through 5 years of age. Codes **99471** and **99475** are reported for the initial E/M service provided to a pediatric critical care patient in the inpatient setting. Codes **99472** and **99476** are reported for subsequent E/M services provided to a pediatric critical care patient in the inpatient setting. Critical care services provided to a pediatric patient 6 years of age or older are reported with the critical care codes **99291, 99292**.

Critical care services provided to either a neonate or pediatric patient in an outpatient setting are also reported with the critical care codes **99291, 99292**. Critical care services provided by a second physician when one is reporting the per diem critical care code are reported with **99291, 99292**.

In the instance when critical care services are provided to neonates or pediatric patients less than 5 years of age at two separate institutions by a physician from a different group on the same date of service, the receiving institution should report the appropriate global admission code (**99468-99476**) whereas the physician from the referring institution should report their critical care services with the critical care codes **99291, 99292**.

Initial and Continuing Intensive Care Services

The Initial and Continuing Intensive Care Services codes (**99477-99480**) are noncritical care codes for low birth weight infants who require intensive observation, frequent interventions, or other intensive management services. Examples of such care include continuous cardiac and/or respiratory monitoring, continuous and/or frequent vital signs, temperature maintenance, enteral and/or parenteral nutritional adjustments, and laboratory and oxygen monitoring.

Code **99477** is reported for the initial E/M service of the neonate who is not critically ill but requires intensive observation, frequent interventions, and other intensive care services in the hospital setting. This code should be reported once per date of service per patient by a single physician.

The subsequent E/M services provided by a physician directing the continuing intensive care of an infant who does not meet the definition of critically ill are reported with codes **99478-99480**. These codes are reported based upon the present body weight of the infant and should be reported only once per date of service per patient by a single physician.

The subsequent care of a sick neonate who is less than 28 days of age but more than 5000 grams who does not require intensive or critical care services should be reported with the Subsequent Hospital Care codes **99231-99233**.

✓ Check Your Knowledge Answers

1. A new patient is a patient who has not received any professional services from the physician or another physician of the same specialty who belongs to the same group practice within the past three years. An established patient is one who has received professional services from the physician or another physician of the same specialty who belongs to the same group practice within the past three years.

2. Established patient visit. Since Dr A has provided professional services to that patient within the past three years, the patient would be considered an established patient to Dr A.

Chapter Exercises

Check your answers in Appendix B.

1. A patient is referred by his physician to see an orthopedic surgeon for a consultative service. During the first visit with the orthopedic surgeon, the physician initiates diagnostic or therapeutic

service upon completion of the visit, opinion, or advice rendered back.

   a. Is this encounter considered a consultation?

   b. This encounter should be reported with a code from the Office or Other Outpatient Services code series (**99201-99205**), because it was the first time the patient saw the orthopedic surgeon.

   c. The encounter should be reported with code **99499**, Unlisted Evaluation and Management Service.

   d. The encounter service may be coded as a consultation with a code from the series **99241-99245**.

2. If a patient is admitted to the hospital on October 23 and discharged on October 26, what is the appropriate E/M code to report for the October 26 discharge date?

3. **Preventive Medicine:** An 18-month-old boy was brought to his regular physician's office for his 18-month checkup. According to his mother, he was doing fine. He was eating table food and sleeping through the night. Progress note indicates the following:

   Subjective: Patient is here for his 18-month checkup. His mother reports no problems and no recent illnesses. He is eating table food, sleeping through the night, and going to a play group twice a week. He is walking and running without difficulty and does not tire easily. He plays appropriately with others his age.

   Objective: Weight, 22 lb; length, 31 in; temperature, 98.6°F

   HEENTN: Nl, ears Nl, pharynx Nl

   Lungs: Clear

   Heart: Heart tones normal, no extra sounds, no thrill

   Abdomen: No masses; no organomegaly; no tenderness

   Genitourinary: Both testicles descended

   Extremities: Normal, legs straight

   Central nervous system: Normal for age

   Skin: No lesions

   Denver Developmental Screening Test: Passes all

   Assessment: Normal 18-month check

   Plan: DTaP-4. Anticipatory guidance and accident prevention discussed with mother.

   How is this procedure reported?

4. **Preventive Medicine:** A 22-year-old male established patient came to the physician's office seeking information about HIV. He did not want an examination but said he wanted to learn all he could from "an expert" rather than from his friends. The physician's progress note stated the following:

   Patient came in asking to learn about HIV. He said he is not sure if what he hears on the street is true and has come here to learn the facts. He said he is not sexually active but that he may become sexually active in the near future. He said that he is heterosexual. HIV was discussed with the patient in terms of what it is, how it affects the immune system, how it is spread, how to decrease the chance of becoming infected, and safer sex. Total length of time spent counseling the patient was 30 minutes.

How is this procedure reported?

5. **Emergency Department (ED):** A 20-year-old male was dropped off in front of the hospital ED with a knife hilt sticking out of his midleft anterior chest. The patient was not fully conscious. No one accompanied him. The patient was transported into the ED and the attending emergency department physician began the evaluation. Physical examination was less than comprehensive, but it was noted that whenever there was a peripheral pulse, the knife handle quivered. The attending ED physician initiated trauma team mobilization and ordered necessary diagnostics and fluid/blood replacement products. A partial history was obtained and documented by the attending ED physician. Care of the patient proceeded under the attending ED physician's management. Twenty minutes after the patient was brought into the ED, the on-call trauma surgeon arrived in the emergency department, and the attending ED physician transferred care of the patient to the surgeon. The patient's need for a high-level E/M service and inability to provide a comprehensive history, as well as the unsuitability of an initial comprehensive examination, was evident in the medical record.

How is this procedure reported?

6. **Emergency Department (ED)—Critical Care:** A 61-year-old patient walked into the ED complaining of "pressure on my chest." The attending ED physician evaluated the patient, including a full interpretation of a 12-lead electrocardiogram (ECG). Among the findings of the ECG interpretation were signs of acute cardiac damage but no arrhythmia. The attending ED physician provided appropriate initial management and contacted the attending admitting physician, who happened to be in the hospital. Arrangements were made to admit the patient to the cardiac care unit. When the attending admitting physician came to the ED, the attending ED physician transferred care of the patient to her. Unfortunately, there were no beds immediately available in the cardiac care unit so the patient had to be held in the ED. After evaluating the patient, the admitting physician left the ED.

Three hours later, the patient was still in the ED and, during a period of 80 minutes, experienced acute difficulty breathing, increased chest pain, arrhythmias (as noted on a cardiac monitor), and a cardiopulmonary arrest. During this 80-minute period, the attending ED physician provided critical care services for the patient, provided a full interpretation of a new 12-lead ECG at the beginning of the 80 minutes, performed endotracheal intubation, directed hospital personnel's efforts to restore the patient's breathing and circulation for 20 minutes, and interpreted one lead of a third ECG printout. The resuscitation attempt was unsuccessful. The physician noted a total critical care service provision time of 44 minutes, exclusive of other separately reportable services.

What code(s) should the emergency department physician report?

7. **Prolonged Services:** A 55-year-old male was referred to a neurologist because of leg weakness and sensory loss that had begun after surgery two years earlier. On the basis of his evaluation, the neurologist suspected a thoracic myelopathy. He was most concerned about a spinal cord infarct or space-occupying lesion in the thoracic cord. The patient arrived at the appointment without medical records from the surgery and the many physicians he had seen in the intervening two years. The neurologist suggested that the patient make another appointment, requesting that he bring copies of the medical records and imaging studies. The patient returned in one month toting two inches of paper records and a large number of X-ray jackets containing plain X rays, magnetic resonance imaging scans, computed tomography scans, and a myelogram. Because the patient complained of greater leg weakness and stiffness, the neurologist reexamined the patient, performing a detailed history and physical examination. He spent 75 minutes face-to-face with the patient reviewing the medical records and imaging studies, clarifying the patient's problem with further questioning, and explaining the diagnostic and treatment options to the patient. He decided to perform a lumbar puncture on the patient the next day and prescribed for the patient baclofen for spasticity and carbamazepine for neuropathic pain.

   How is the second office visit coded?

8. **Critical Care Services:** A 72-year-old female was seen in the emergency department (ED) of a city hospital within half an hour of a sudden onset of left hemiplegia and atrial fibrillation. The hospital's neurology acute stroke service was paged and the neurologist assumed responsibility for management of the patient. It was necessary for the neurologist to administer critical care services. When the neurologist first evaluated the patient and performed the National Institutes of Health stroke scale in the ED, her blood pressure was 220/110 mm Hg. A computed tomography scan was performed and was normal in the judgment of the neurologist. The patient's blood pressure decreased to 180/110 mm Hg within one and one-half hours after the onset of her stroke. The neurologist reevaluated the patient and ordered administration of a thrombolytic agent in the ED, with an initial 10% bolus and the remainder administered during a one-hour period through an intravenous catheter infusion. The neurologist admitted the patient to the ICU. When the infusion was complete and the neurologist had finished performing subsequent evaluations, the neurologist had spent approximately two and one-half hours managing and performing critical care services for the patient in the ED and the ICU. The ICU nursing staff continued to manage the patient's blood pressure and monitor her vital signs.

   What E/M services code(s) should the neurologist report?

9. **Anticoagulant Management:** A 69-year-old female established patient with atrial fibrillation who was taking long-term warfarin therapy to prevent systemic embolism came to see her physician for

her initial 90 days of anticoagulant management. The physician and his staff accessed her medical record, reviewed the results, and determined whether any dosage adjustment and/or change in care plan was necessary. After this service, the physician made a dosage adjustment and care plan changes to account for acute illness and possible drug interactions, diet changes affecting vitamin K intake, and/or changes to procedures that required withholding or alternative anticoagulation. The physician then made a notation in the medical record, contacted the patient to convey the results/instructions, and arranged repeat testing at the appropriate interval.

How is this service reported?

a. **99363** Anticoagulant management for an outpatient taking warfarin, physician review and interpretation of International Normalized Ratio (INR) testing, patient instructions, dosage adjustment (as needed), and ordering of additional tests; initial 90 days of therapy (must include a minimum of 8 INR measurements)

b. **99377 Physician supervision** of a hospice patient (patient not present) requiring complex and multidisciplinary care modalities involving regular physician development and/or revision of care plans, review of subsequent reports of patient status, review of related laboratory and other studies, communication (including telephone calls) for purposes of assessment or care decisions with health care professional(s), family member(s), surrogate decision maker(s) (eg, legal guardian), and/or key caregiver(s) involved in patient's care, integration of new information into the medical treatment plan and/or adjustment of medical therapy, within a calendar month; 15-29 minutes.

c. **99211 Office or other outpatient visit** for the evaluation and management of an established patient that may not require the presence of a physician. Usually, the presenting problem(s) are minimal. Typically, 5 minutes are spent performing or supervising these services.

10. **Domiciliary, Rest Home (eg, Assisted Living Facility), or Home Care Plan Oversight Services:** A 21-year-old male with Down syndrome was transitioning from home care and public special education to a sheltered work program operated by the community service agency. He was moderately mentally retarded, and ongoing medical problems included hypothyroidism and sensorineural hearing loss. Over the past two months his behavior had become progressively disruptive. His previously developed care plan included the active medical and educational or vocational problems with ongoing adjustments being made based on feedback from the family and other health care professionals and service providers. The primary care physician (internal medicine, family physician, pediatrician) delivered primary care services and managed and coordinated care plan activities. The care plan oversight activities, which were a total time of 15 minutes, included the following:

- Review of reports including a new audiology assessment and endocrine consultation report

- Telephone call to the audiologist about results of the most recent hearing assessment and recommendations to provide hearing amplification to the patient
- Completion of medical forms for the vocational program listing medical problems, general cognitive and physical abilities, and recommendations for behavior management
- Discussion by phone with the family of recent appetite and weight gain noted by the family after beginning a new behavior medication and a subsequent call to the psychiatric nurse practitioner at the mental health center who recommended a dose change and a dietary consultation
- Review of endocrine recommendations to increase the thyroid dosage, with an ensuing telephone call to the family and pharmacy to prescribe a different dose form of Synthroid.

The physician then documented the relevant information in the record that summarized these activities.

How is this procedure reported?

a. **92607** Evaluation for prescription for speech-generating augmentative and alternative communication device, face-to-face with the patient; first hour

b. **99339** Individual physician supervision of a patient (patient not present) in home, domiciliary, or rest home (eg, assisted living facility) requiring complex and multidisciplinary care modalities involving regular physician development and/or revision of care plans, review of subsequent reports of patient status, review of related laboratory and other studies, communication (including telephone calls) for purposes of assessment or care decisions with health care professional(s), family member(s), surrogate decision maker(s) (eg, legal guardian), and/or key caregiver(s) involved in patient's care, integration of new information into the medical treatment plan, and/or adjustment of medical therapy, within a calendar month; 15-29 minutes

c. **99374 Physician supervision** of a patient under care of home health agency (patient not present) in home, domiciliary, or equivalent environment (eg, Alzheimer's facility) requiring complex and multidisciplinary care modalities involving regular physician development and/or revision of care plans, review of subsequent reports of patient status, review of related laboratory and other studies, communication (including telephone calls) for purposes of assessment or care decisions with health care professional(s), family member(s), surrogate decision maker(s) (eg, legal guardian), and/or key caregiver(s) involved in patient's care, integration of new information into the medical treatment plan, and/or adjustment of medical therapy, within a calendar month; 15-29 minutes

Anesthesia

Chapter Objectives

- Describe the types of anesthesia
- Understand the anesthesia guidelines for coding anesthesia services and any additional procedures or services provided
- Explain anesthesia modifiers
- Review the use of codes for reporting qualifying circumstances for anesthesia services
- Understand basic anesthesia administration services

Introduction

Achieving the basic understanding of anesthesia administration services used by an anesthesiologist, anesthetist, or under the responsible supervision of a physician is essential to coding anesthesia services correctly. Although this section may seem straightforward, it is critical to develop an understanding of the anesthesia guidelines, the anesthesia modifiers, and qualifying circumstances codes. This chapter will provide an overview of the Anesthesia codes (**00100-01999**) of the CPT codebook.

Guidelines for Reporting Basic Anesthesia Administration Services

The anesthesia guidelines define items that are necessary to appropriately interpret and report the procedures and services contained in this section. The guidelines also provide explanations regarding terms that apply only to this particular section. For example, in the anesthesia guidelines, a discussion of reporting time is included.

Anesthesia time begins when the anesthesiologist begins to prepare the patient for induction of anesthesia in the operating room (or in an equivalent area). The time continues through the procedure and ends when the anesthesiologist is no longer in personal attendance, that is, when the patient may be safely placed under postoperative supervision.

Basic anesthesia administration services are services provided by or under the responsible supervision of a physician. These services include, but are not limited to, the following:

- Routine preoperative and postoperative visits to evaluate the patient for the planned anesthesia
- Anesthesia care during the procedure and monitoring of the patient's postsurgery recovery from anesthesia
- Administration of fluids and/or blood during the period for anesthesia care
- Interpretation of noninvasive monitoring such as electrocardiography (ECG), body temperature, blood pressure, oximetry (blood oxygen concentration), capnography (blood carbon dioxide concentration), and mass spectrometry.

Invasive forms of monitoring (such as intra-arterial, central venous, pulmonary artery catheters, and transesophageal echocardiography) are not included in basic anesthesia administration services. When these procedures are performed, they should be reported separately according to standard CPT coding guidelines applicable to the given code and the respective section in the CPT codebook in which they are listed.

Generally, a single code is reported for anesthesia administration, whether the operating physician performs one or multiple procedures. When multiple procedures are performed during a single anesthetic administration, usually only the anesthesia procedure code for the **most complex** service and the **total time** for all procedures are reported. However, anesthesia add-on codes are an exception. Codes **01953**, **01968**, and **01969** are anesthesia add-on procedures, which are reported in addition to the primary anesthesia code.

Key Terms

- **Moderate (conscious) sedation**
- **Anesthesia**
- **General anesthesia**
- **Regional anesthesia**
- **Local anesthesia**
- **Monitored Anesthesia Care (MAC)**
- **Anesthesia modifiers**
- **Physical status modifiers**

EXAMPLE

A patient having total knee replacement surgery may receive a regional anesthetic and a postoperative pain management agent through the same epidural catheter, in which case the only code reported would be **01402**.

EXAMPLE

A patient undergoing a thoracotomy might receive an epidural injection of a local anesthetic and/or narcotic (**62318**) for postoperative pain control in addition to the general anesthetic, which is administered through an endotracheal tube (**00540**). In this case, the epidural is not the surgical anesthetic, and it would be reported separately as an independent procedure.

It should be noted that **moderate (conscious) sedation** is *not* an anesthesia service. To report moderate (conscious) sedation provided by a physician also performing the service for which conscious sedation is being provided, see codes **99143-99145**. Moderate sedation does not include minimal sedation (anxiolysis), deep sedation, or monitored anesthesia care (**00100-01999**).

There are certain CPT code descriptors in the CPT codebook that include the phrases "with anesthesia" or "requiring anesthesia." These phrases indicate that the work involved in performing the procedure requires **anesthesia**, whether it is **general anesthesia**, **regional anesthesia**, or **monitored anesthesia care (MAC)**, and the appropriate code is separately reported.

To report regional or general anesthesia provided by a physician who also performs the services for which the anesthesia is being provided, use **modifier 47**, Anesthesia by surgeon, appended to the surgical procedure code, instead of the anesthesia code. (The use of **modifier 47** will be discussed further in Chapter 10.)

Key Terms

Moderate (conscious) sedation: Drug-induced depression of consciousness during which patients respond purposefully to oral commands, either alone or accompanied by light tactile stimulation. No interventions are required to maintain a patent airway, and spontaneous ventilation is adequate. Cardiovascular function is usually maintained.

Anesthesia: Induction or administration of a drug to obtain partial or complete loss of sensation.

General anesthesia: A drug-induced loss of consciousness during which patients are not arousable, even by painful stimulation. Assistance in maintaining a patent airway is usually required. General anesthesia requires the undivided attention of a separate provider who is well trained and appropriately licensed in the monitoring and rescue functions inherently required for the safe provision of general anesthesia.

Regional anesthesia: The use of local anesthetics to temporarily block large groups of sensory nerves or the spinal cord so that the pain signal cannot reach the brain. Regional anesthesia also often results in blockage of motor neurons. This technique is separate and distinct from the use of local anesthesia to numb distal parts of the extremities by numbing nerves that are in proximity to their terminations. Thus, for the purposes of CPT definitions, regional anesthesia does not include use of local anesthesia below the elbow or ankle.

Local anesthesia: The use of local anesthetics to numb sensory nerves that are in proximity to their terminations. This will result in only a small area being numbed, such as a circumscribed area of the integumentary or part of a foot or hand. Motor nerve blockage occurs significantly less frequently with local anesthesia.

Monitored Anesthesia Care (MAC): MAC is a specific anesthesia service for a diagnostic or therapeutic procedure that involves giving sedatives through an intravenous catheter (IV) into the patient's blood stream and is frequently combined with general or regional anesthesia.

Anesthesia modifiers: These are used to indicate the patient's condition at the time anesthesia is administered.

Physical status modifiers: These are used to distinguish among various levels of complexity of the anesthesia service provided, and are represented by the initial letter "P" followed by a single digit from 1 to 6.

✓ Check Your Knowledge

1. List the four different types of anesthesia.
_____, _____, _____ and _____.

Anesthesia Modifiers

Coding Tip

If the anesthesiologist performs other additional procedures, each is separately reportable.

Anesthesia modifiers are used to indicate the patient's condition at the time anesthesia is administered. These services are reported with the anesthesia five-digit procedure codes (**00100-01999**) and two-digit physical status modifiers, as appropriate. It may also be appropriate to report other CPT modifiers when codes for procedural services are reported in addition to basic anesthesia service.

The **physical status modifiers** are found in the anesthesia guidelines and identified with the initial letter "P" followed by a single digit from 1 to 6. The following physical status modifiers are located in the anesthesia guidelines of the CPT codebook and are defined as follows:

P1: A normal healthy patient
P2: A patient with mild systemic disease
P3: A patient with severe systemic disease
P4: A patient with severe systemic disease that is a constant threat to life
P5: A moribund patient who is not expected to survive without the operation
P6: A declared brain-dead patient whose organs are being removed for donor purposes

Qualifying Circumstances

Providing anesthesia services, at times, can be complicated depending on the complexity of the medical condition of the patient. The qualifying circumstances codes (**99100-99140**) represent important qualifying circumstances that significantly affect the character of the anesthesia service provided. These types of cases include:

- Extraordinary condition of the patient
- Notable operative conditions
- Unusual risk factors

Each of these codes are designated as add-on codes and thus must be reported in addition to the procedure number along with the primary anesthesia service provided. More than one qualifying circumstances code may be selected and reported, as appropriate.

EXAMPLE

Induction of anesthesia for a 75-year-old patient during repair of a cleft lip, the coding would be:

00102 Anesthesia for procedures involving plastic repair of cleft lip

✚ 99100 Anesthesia for patient of extreme age, younger than 1 year and older than 70 (List separately in addition to code for primary anesthesia procedure)

However, there is one exception, code **99100**, *Anesthesia for patient of extreme age, younger than 1 year and other than 70 (List separately in addition to code for primary anesthesia procedure)*, should **not** be reported in addition to an anesthesia code that is specific to a very young patient. Note that it is not appropriate to use code **99100** with the anesthesia codes that apply to specific procedures performed on young infants (eg, codes **00834-00836**, anesthesia for hernia repairs; code **00326**, anesthesia for procedures on the larynx and trachea; and code **00561**, pump oxygenator cardiac procedures, all on patients younger than 1 year of age).

✓ Check Your Knowledge

2. Is it appropriate to report codes 00320 and 99100 together? Why or why not?

_____.

Note: As with all add-on codes, these codes are exempt from the use of **modifier 51**. (The use of **modifier 51** will be discussed in Chapter 10.)

✓ Check Your Knowledge Answers

1. General anesthesia, regional anesthesia, local anesthesia, monitored anesthesia care (MAC).

2. No. Both anesthesia code descriptors list the age of the patient as younger than 1 year. Add-on code 99100 should not be reported in addition to an anesthesia code that is specific to a very young patient.

Chapter Exercises

Check your answers in Appendix B.

True or False

1. Anesthesia time begins when the anesthesiologist begins to prepare the patient for induction of anesthesia and ends when the patient is no longer under care of the anesthesiologist. **True or False**

2. Add-on code 99116 may be reported as a stand-alone code. **True or False**

3. The phrase "requiring anesthesia" or "with anesthesia" in a descriptor indicates that the work involved in performing that procedure requires anesthesia and may be reported separately. **True or False**

4. Moderate (conscious) sedation is not an anesthesia service. **True or False**

5. The physical status modifiers are identified with the initial letter "T." **True or False**

6. In some instances, it may be appropriate to append other CPT modifiers with an anesthesia procedure code and a physical status modifier. **True or False**

Fill in the Blank

Select the correct physical status modifiers for the following:

7. Patient with a mild systemic disease.
   Code(s): _____

8. Moribund patient who is not expected to survive without the operation.
   Code(s): _____

9. A normal healthy patient.
   Code(s): _____

10. A declared brain-dead patient whose organs are being removed for donor purposes.
    Code(s): _____

11. A patient with severe systemic disease.
    Code(s): _____

Surgery

Chapter Objectives

- Understand the Current Procedural Terminology (CPT®) Surgical Package definition
- Understand the guidelines for follow-up care for diagnostic and therapeutic surgical procedures
- Become familiar with the Surgery subsections, and understand the guidelines that are unique to reporting codes from the subsections
- Identify when more than one code is necessary to accurately report a procedure
- Become familiar with add-on codes
- Understand the separate procedure concept

The Surgery section is the largest section of the CPT codebook. When using codes from the Surgery section, it is important to be aware of some basic guidelines. Because CPT nomenclature is not a strict classification system, there may be some procedures that do not appear in sections in which you would expect to find them. The code that most accurately describes the service or procedure performed should be selected.

When procedures are evaluated for reporting, reimbursement, or other purposes, it is essential that each procedure be considered on its own merits, not simply on the basis of the location or placement of the code in the CPT codebook. Also, the listing of a service or procedure and its code number in a particular subsection of the Surgery section does not restrict its use to a specific specialty group. Any procedure or service in *any* section of the CPT codebook, or any subsection of service in the Surgery section, may be used to report the services and procedures performed by any qualified physician. The guidelines and definitions that appear at the beginning of the Surgery section and each of the subsections within it are provided so that users have all the information necessary to appropriately interpret and report the procedures and services listed there.

CPT Surgical Package Definition

The definition of the CPT Surgical Package can be found in the Surgery guidelines in the CPT codebook and is restated here, as follows:

> The services provided by the physician to any patient by their very nature are variable. The CPT codes that represent a readily identifiable surgical procedure thereby include, on a procedure-by-procedure basis, a variety of services. In defining the specific services "included" in a given CPT surgical code, the following services are always included in addition to the operation per se:
>
> - Local infiltration, metacarpal/metatarsal/digital block or topical anesthesia
> - Subsequent to the decision for surgery, one related Evaluation and Management (E/M) encounter on the date immediately prior to or on the date of procedure (including history and physical)
> - Immediate postoperative care, including dictating operative notes, talking with the family and other physicians
> - Writing orders
> - Evaluating the patient in the postanesthesia recovery area
> - Typical postoperative follow-up care

This concept is referred to as a *package* for surgical procedures. This definition indicates that when a surgical procedure is reported with a CPT code, the items listed in that guideline are included, if they were performed, and are not reported separately.

Some examples of these variables include:

- The type of procedure performed
- The place where the surgery occurred
- The time (during hospitalization) the surgery was performed
- The insurance contract of each individual patient

Because it is not possible to address all of these variables in a code descriptor, only the preoperative Evaluation and Management (E/M) service related to the procedure performed on the date immediately before the date of the procedure (including the history and physical) is stated as inclusive of the CPT Surgical Package definition.

Also, a specific number of postoperative days is not indicated in the CPT Surgical Package definition. CPT guidelines provide specific instructions regarding follow-up care for diagnostic procedures (eg, endoscopy, arthroscopy, injection procedures for radiography) and follow-up care for therapeutic surgical procedures. However, these guidelines do not designate a set number of days in which this follow-up care may take place. Unfortunately, there is no one standard definition of a global surgical package that is universally accepted. Services that are included in a *global surgical package* may differ for each third-party payer. It is important to be familiar with the reporting and reimbursement policies of the various insurance companies regarding the global surgical package.

Follow-up Care for Diagnostic and Therapeutic Surgical Procedures

CPT guidelines separately address follow-up care for diagnostic procedures and follow-up care for therapeutic surgical procedures. While a specific number of days is not described in the CPT guidelines pertaining to follow-up care, most insurance companies recognize a set number of days in which no separate payment will generally be made for services provided by the surgeon.

Follow-up care for diagnostic procedures (eg, endoscopy, arthroscopy, injection procedures for radiography) includes only that care related to recovery from the diagnostic procedure itself. Care of the condition for which the diagnostic procedure was performed or of other coexisting conditions is not included and may be reported separately.

Follow-up care for therapeutic surgical procedures includes only care that is usually a part of the surgical service. Complications, exacerbations, recurrence, and the presence of other diseases or injuries requiring additional services should be separately reported.

CPT code 99024, located in the Medicine section of the CPT codebook, is available for reporting a postoperative follow-up visit for documentation purposes only. This code is useful to the reporting physician for tracking the number of postoperative visits provided that are included in the package for the procedure performed.

99024 Postoperative follow-up visit, normally included in the surgical package, to indicate that an evaluation and management service was performed during a postoperative period for a reason(s) related to the original procedure.

Add-on Codes

Most of the procedures listed in the CPT nomenclature can be reported by themselves as stand-alone codes because they represent the total procedure that was performed; however, under certain circumstances, it may be necessary to report two or more codes to completely describe the procedures performed. Some of the codes listed in the CPT code set describe procedures or services that must never be reported as stand-alone codes. These codes are referred to as *add-on codes*. Add-on codes describe procedures or services that are always performed in addition to the primary procedure or service. They describe additional intraservice work associated with the primary procedure or service. These additional or supplemental procedures are designated as add-on codes with a ✛ symbol and are listed in Appendix D of the CPT codebook. Add-on codes can also be readily identified by specific language in the code descriptor, which includes phrases such as "each additional" or "(List separately in addition to primary procedure)." The multiple procedure modifier (**51**) is not appended to an add-on code, as these codes are exempt from the multiple procedure concept.

Chapter 4

EXAMPLE

The following is an example of the use of an add-on code for additional lesions.

11100 Biopsy of skin, subcutaneous tissue and/or mucous membrane (including simple closure), unless otherwise listed; single lesion

✚ 11101 each separate/additional lesion (List separately in addition to code for primary procedure)

(Use 11101 in conjunction with code 11100)

Code **11100** is the primary procedure and code **✚11101** is the add-on code. Code **✚11101** would never be reported without first reporting code **11100**. As the code descriptor indicates, code **✚11101** is reported for each separate/additional lesion. The parenthetical note following code **✚11101** instructs the user regarding the code that is considered the primary procedure for that particular add-on code. If biopsy is performed on three separate lesions of the skin, subcutaneous tissue, and/or mucous membrane, then code **11100** would be reported for the first lesion and code **✚11101** would be reported twice, once for the second lesion biopsied, and again for the third lesion biopsied.

Separate Procedure

The separate procedure concept in the CPT codebook is an important one to understand. Some of the codes listed in the CPT nomenclature have been identified by inclusion of the term *separate procedure* in the code descriptor. The separate procedure designation indicates that a certain procedure or service may be:

- Considered an integral component of another procedure or service
- Performed independently
- Unrelated
- Distinct from other procedure(s) or service(s) provided at that time

Codes designated as separate procedures may not be additionally reported when the procedure or service is performed as an integral component of another procedure or service.

EXAMPLE

The following is an example of an integral component of another procedure or service.

58720 Salpingo-oophorectomy, complete or partial, unilateral or bilateral (separate procedure)

58150 Total abdominal hysterectomy (corpus and cervix), with or without removal of tube(s), with or without removal of ovary(s)

When a total abdominal hysterectomy with removal of the tube(s) and ovary(s) is reported, it would not be appropriate to separately report code **58720** in conjunction with code **58150**. The procedure described by code **58720** is considered an integral component of the procedures described by code **58150**.

However, codes designated as separate procedures should be additionally reported when performed independently, unrelated, or distinct from other procedure(s) or service(s) provided.

EXAMPLES

The following is an example of a procedure performed independently from other procedure(s) or service(s).

58720 Salpingo-oophorectomy, complete or partial, unilateral or bilateral (separate procedure)

If removal of the fallopian tubes and ovaries is the only procedure performed, then it would be appropriate to report code **58720** to describe the procedure performed.

The following is an example of unrelated procedures.

56605 Biopsy of vulva or perineum (separate procedure); 1 lesion

49505 Repair initial inguinal hernia, age 5 years or older; reducible

Biopsy of the vulva or perineum is a procedure that is unrelated to repair of an inguinal hernia. In this example, if the same physician performed both of these procedures, then it would be appropriate to report both codes to fully describe the procedures performed. Modifier **59**, *Distinct procedural service*, would be appended to code **56605** to indicate that the procedure was unrelated to the repair of the inguinal hernia. (For more information about the use of modifiers, refer to *Coding with Modifiers: A Guide to Correct CPT® and HCPCS Level II Modifier Usage* published by the American Medical Association.)

When a procedure or service that is designated as a separate procedure is carried out independently or considered to be unrelated or distinct from other procedures or services provided at that time, the procedure or service designated as a separate procedure may be reported by itself, or in addition to other procedures or services by appending modifier **59**, *Distinct procedural service*, to the specific separate procedure code reported. This indicates that the procedure is not considered a component of another procedure, but is a distinct, independent procedure. This may represent any of the following:

- Different session or patient encounter
- Different site or organ system
- Separate incision or excision
- Separate lesion
- Treatment of a separate injury (or area of injury in extensive injuries)

The Surgery chapter is divided into 11 sections to mirror the surgery section in the CPT codebook.

1. Integumentary System
2. Musculoskeletal System
3. Respiratory System
4. Cardiovascular System
5. Digestive System
6. Urinary System
7. Male Genital System
8. Female Genital System
9. Maternity Care and Delivery
10. Nervous System
11. Eye and Ocular Adnexa

Each section contains all the features and chapter exercises pertaining to that section, eg, the Digestive System section contains all of the digestive system codes and guidelines along with the **Key Terms**, **Examples**, questions to **Check Your Knowledge**, and section exercises pertaining to the digestive system. As such, these chapters can be used as individual chapters in a classroom setting or for the self-learner, allowing for a smooth transition from section to section of the CPT codebook.

Surgery: Integumentary System

Section Objectives

- Understand the fundamentals of Skin, Subcutaneous, and Accessory structures
- Distinguish the classification of wound repair closures (simple, intermediate, or complex)
- Know how to measure and code the removal of a lesion
- Understand the different types of skin grafts
- Understand the coding of Mohs micrographic surgery and breast procedures

The Integumentary System subsection of the CPT codebook includes a variety of procedures performed on the integumentary system of the entire body. Because this subsection includes procedures for the whole body, it is important to pay close attention to subheading guidelines, definitions, and the code descriptors to ensure that the appropriate code is chosen, not only for the procedure, but also for the correct anatomic area. Various types of procedure codes involve anatomy such as skin, subcutaneous and accessory structures, nails, and breasts. (See Figures 4-1 and 4-2.)

This chapter will provide an overview of the Integumentary System codes (**10021-19499**) of the CPT codebook. It is important to be familiar

FIGURE 4-1 *CPT Codebook Breakdown for Integumentary System*

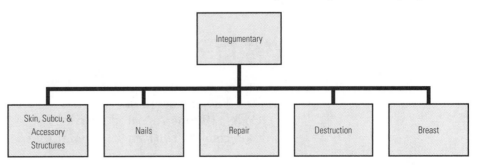

FIGURE 4-2 *The Skin*

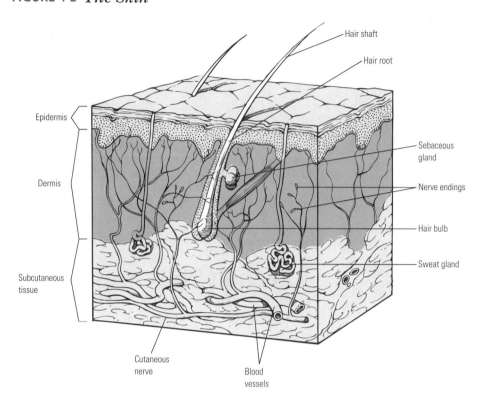

- Hair shaft
- Hair root
- Epidermis
- Dermis
- Subcutaneous tissue
- Sebaceous gland
- Nerve endings
- Hair bulb
- Sweat gland
- Cutaneous nerve
- Blood vessels

with the structure of the skin and medical terms associated with the skin. The CPT codebook should be used in tandem with a medical dictionary to define unfamiliar words. (See Figure 4-2.)

Debridement

The debridement codes in the CPT code set are intended to be used for debridement procedures performed by surgical techniques chosen at the discretion of the physician.

Debridement is the removal of loose, devitalized, necrotic, and/or contaminated tissue, foreign bodies, and other debris on the wound, using mechanical or sharp techniques.

When a physician performs debridement, he or she intends to remove all foreign or dead material, reduce the number of bacteria in the wound, and leave intact the viable tissue. The first set of debridement codes, **11000** and **+11001**, are reported for debridement of extensive eczematous or infected skin.

Coding Tip

When performing debridement of a single wound, report depth using the deepest level of tissue removed. In multiple wounds, sum the surface area of those wounds that are at the same depth, but do not combine sums from different depths.

EXAMPLE

A patient had an infected wound on 15% of his body from a previous injury. The physician debrided the wound.

Code **11000** is reported for the first 10% of body surface and add-on code **+11001** for the remaining 5% (or fraction thereof).

Chapter 4

Coding Tip

Add-on code ✚11008 should not be reported in conjunction with the other debridement procedure codes (11000 and ✚11001, 11010-11044).

Coding Tip

Codes 11042-11047 should not be reported in addition to codes 97597, 97598, and 97602 for active wound care management.

The second set of debridement codes, **11004-11006**, are reported for extensive tissue debridement for necrotizing soft tissue infection performed on specific anatomical areas.

Add-on code ✚11008 is reported for removal of prosthetic material or mesh when performed concurrently with the debridement procedures described by codes **11004-11006**.

The third set of debridement codes, **11010-11012**, describes more extensive debridement procedures performed in preparation for treating an open fracture. It is important to note that codes **11010-11012** address debridement including removal of foreign material at the site of an open fracture and/or an open dislocation (eg, excisional debridement), skin and subcutaneous tissues, muscle fascia, muscle, and bone.

The fourth set of debridement codes, **11042-11047**, are reported by the depth of the tissue that is being removed and by the surface area of the wound. These services may be reported for injuries, infections, wounds, and chronic ulcers, such as stasis ulcers, avascular necrotic tissue, gangrene, and superficial infected wounds.

✓ Check Your Knowledge

1. When performing debridement of wounds of different depths, can you combine the sums? Why or why not?

Removal of Skin Tags

Removal of **skin tags** is defined as the removal by scissoring or any sharp method, ligature strangulation, electrosurgical destruction, or combination of treatment modalities including chemical and electrocauterization. Codes **11200** and ✚**11201** are reported for removal of skin tags from any area of the body. (See Figure 4-3.)

EXAMPLE

A patient had 17 swollen and inflamed skin tags on his back. Because they were of different sizes, the physician cut 10 skin tags off with surgeon's scissors and destroyed 7 skin tags by electrosurgical means.

Code **11200** is reported for up to 15 skin tags and add-on code ✚**11201** for the remaining 2 skin tags, because code ✚**11201** includes any additional lesions up to 10.

Nails

Codes **11720** and **11721** are for debridement of nails. Code **11720** is reported for debridement of one to five nails, and **11721** is for

Key Terms

- **Debridement**
- **Shaving**
- **Skin tags, removal of**

FIGURE 4-3 *Removal of Skin Tags*

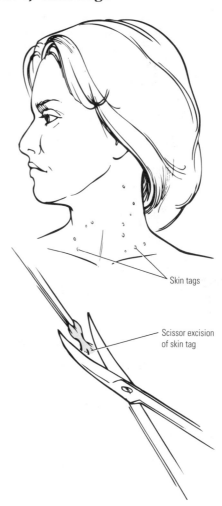

Skin tags

Scissor excision of skin tag

debridement of six or more nails. Only one code should be reported from **11720** and **11721** to describe the number of nails debrided, regardless of which extremity. Code **11721** is not designated as an add-on code. (See Figures 4-4A and 4-4B.)

EXAMPLE

A patient had three painful dystrophic toenails on the left foot and three on the right foot. The physician debrided each of the affected nails.

Code **11721** is reported for the debridement of six toenails, three on the left foot and three on the right foot.

Shaving

The codes for **shaving** of epidermal or dermal lesions (**11300-11313**) are reported for removal of lesions by a shaving technique (sharp

FIGURE 4-4A *Lateral Nail View*

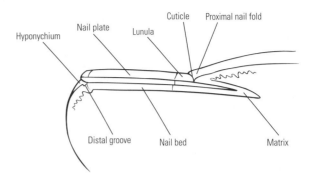

FIGURE 4-4B *Dorsal Nail View*

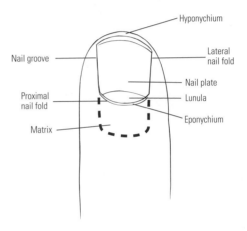

removal by transverse incision or horizontal slicing). This procedure includes local anesthesia, chemical, or electrocauterization of the wound. Suture closure is not required.

Excision of Benign or Malignant Lesions

Key Terms

- Excision
- Lesions
- Benign
- Malignant

The CPT code set includes several different subsections that describe the various techniques used to remove **lesions**. Codes for shaving, excision, and destruction of lesions can be found throughout the Integumentary System subsection. To correctly code the removal of lesions, the group of codes that most accurately describes the technique used by the physician should be chosen. (See Figure 4-5.)

The codes in this subsection describe the excision of **benign** (11400-11471) and **malignant** (11600-11646) lesions. As indicated in the guidelines preceding these code series, an **excision** is defined as full-thickness (through the dermis) removal of a lesion, including

FIGURE 4-5A *Measuring and Coding the Removal of a Lesion*

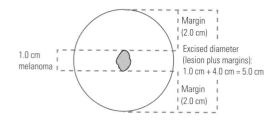

FIGURE 4-5B *Measuring and Coding the Removal of a Lesion*

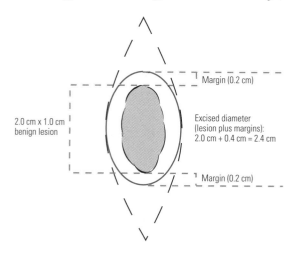

FIGURE 4-5C *Measuring and Coding the Removal of a Lesion*

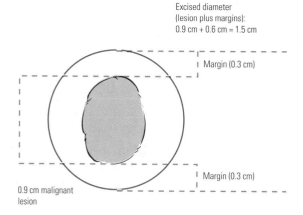

Excision of the lesion is a component of adjacent tissue transfer (**14000-14350**) and should not be reported separately if adjacent tissue transfer is performed.

margins. The guidelines and code descriptors further identify what is included as part of the excision, define what is included as part of the margin, and identify when the measurement is made. Direction for reporting additional excisions and re-excisions(s) is also given. Prior to selecting a code from these series, it is important to carefully review the documentation in the medical record to determine the following:

- Type of lesion (benign vs malignant)
- Site or body part
- Size of lesion (ie, total size of excised area)
- Type of wound closure (eg, simple, intermediate, complex, or reconstructive graft flap)

Excision of Benign Lesions

Each benign lesion excised is reported separately. Code selection is determined by measuring the greatest clinical diameter of the apparent lesion plus that margin required for complete excision (lesion diameter plus the narrowest margins required equals the excised diameter). The margins refer to the narrowest margin required to adequately excise the lesion, based on the physician's judgment. The measurement of lesion plus margins is made before excision. The excised diameter is the same whether the surgical defect is repaired in a linear fashion or reconstructed (eg, with a skin graft). The closure of any defects created by incision, excision, or trauma may require simple, intermediate, or complex closure. Simple repair is included as part of the excision and may not be reported separately. Any repair by intermediate or complex closure should be reported separately with the appropriate repair codes.

Excision of Malignant Lesions

Each malignant lesion excised is reported separately. Code selection is determined by measuring the greatest clinical diameter of the apparent lesion plus the margin required for complete excision (lesion diameter plus the narrowest margins required equals the excised diameter). The margins refer to the narrowest margin required to adequately excise the lesion, based on the physician's judgment. The measurement of lesion plus margins is made before excision. The excised diameter is the same whether the surgical defect is repaired in a linear fashion or reconstructed (eg, with a skin graft). (See Figure 4-5.) The closure of any defects created by incision, excision, or trauma may require simple, intermediate, or complex closure. Simple repair is included as part of the excision and may not be reported separately. Any repair by intermediate or complex closure should be reported separately with the appropriate repair codes.

When frozen section pathology shows the margins of excision were not adequate, an additional excision may be necessary for complete tumor removal. Use only one code to report the additional excision and re-excision(s) based on the final widest excised diameter required for complete tumor removal at the same operative session. To report a re-excision procedure performed to widen margins at a subsequent operative session, codes **11600-11646** are used, as appropriate. Modifier **58** is appended if the re-excision procedure is performed during the postoperative period of the primary excision procedure.

To ensure accurate code selection, the pathology report should also be reviewed. Following are some additional coding tips to consider:

- **Lesions of uncertain morphology:** Code selection is based on the final excised diameter as determined by the physician's judgment of the margins required for adequate excision.
- **Coding a lesion excision with extended margins:** One excision of lesion code is reported on the basis of the final excised diameter of the lesion removed in instances when a lesion is excised and during the operative session the margins are extended after a positive pathologic diagnosis is made.
- **Coding two lesions removed with one excision:** Only one excision of lesion code is reported when two lesions are removed with one excision.
- **Re-excision of lesions:** If the patient returns for a re-excision for positive margins, the re-excision is reported as a malignant lesion even though the pathology report may indicate the re-excision reveals no residual tumor.

✓ Check Your Knowledge

2. What is the formula for determining the size of a lesion?

Key Terms

Debridement: The removal of loose, devitalized, necrotic, and/or contaminated tissue, foreign bodies, and other debris on the wound, using mechanical or sharp techniques.

Skin tags, removal of: The removal by scissoring or any sharp method, ligature strangulation, electrosurgical destruction, or combination of treatment modalities including chemical and electrocauterization.

Excision: Full-thickness (through the dermis) removal of a lesion including margins.

Lesions: A pathological change in the tissues, eg, wound, cyst, abscess, or boil.

Benign: Nonmalignant character of a neoplasm.

Malignant: In reference to a neoplasm, having the property of locally invasive and destructive growth and metastasis.

Shaving: The sharp removal by transverse incision or horizontal slicing to remove epidermal and dermal lesions without a full-thickness dermal excision.

Key Terms

- **Simple repair**
- **Intermediate repair**
- **Complex repair**

Coding Tip

The repair codes are reported by adding the lengths of the repairs. When multiple wounds are repaired, the lengths of those wounds in the same classification (simple, intermediate, or complex) and from those anatomic sites that are grouped together into the same code descriptor should be added together and reported as one code.

Repair

The repair of wounds may be classified as simple, intermediate, or complex.

The **simple repair** codes (**12001-12021**) are typically used for one-layer closure. Simple repair/closure is included in the excision of a benign or malignant lesion and is *not* separately reported. Wound closure using adhesive strips as the sole repair material should be coded by means of the appropriate E/M code.

The **intermediate repair** codes (**12031-12057**) require layered closure of one or more of the deeper layers of subcutaneous tissue and superficial (nonmuscle) fascia, in addition to the skin (epidermal or dermal) closure. These codes are also used for single-layer closure of heavily contaminated wounds that have required extensive cleaning or removal of particulate matter. Intermediate repair does not include excision of benign (**11400-11446**) or malignant (**11600-11646**) lesions. Therefore, the intermediate repair codes may be reported with the excision of benign or malignant lesions.

It should be noted that the layered closure involves one or more of the deeper layers of subcutaneous tissue and superficial (nonmuscle) fascia in addition to the skin (epidermal and dermal closure). If a wound is repaired in two layers but the buried sutures (second layer) do not include at least the deeper layer of subcutaneous tissue, this is not considered an intermediate repair, but rather a simple repair and subject to the simple repair guidelines.

The **complex repair** codes (**13100-13160**) include repair of wounds requiring more than layered closure, such as scar revision, debridement (eg, traumatic lacerations or avulsions), extensive undermining, stents, or retention sutures. Complex repair does not include excision of benign (**11400-11446**) or malignant (**11600-11646**) lesions. Therefore, the complex repair codes may be reported with the excision of benign or malignant lesions.

✓ Check Your Knowledge

> **3.** Is it appropriate to report simple repair when excision of a benign lesion is performed? Why or why not?

It is important to note the following:

- The lengths of repairs from different groupings of anatomic sites (eg, face and extremities) are not added.
- The lengths of repairs from different classifications (eg, intermediate and complex repairs) are not added.

EXAMPLE

A patient required simple repair of a 2-cm laceration of the forehead, intermediate repair of a 3-cm laceration of the neck, simple repair of a 4-cm laceration of the back, simple repair of a 5-cm laceration of the forearm, and complex repair of a 3-cm laceration of the abdomen.

Code **12004** is reported for the simple repair of back and forearm (the two lengths—the back [4 cm] plus the forearm [5 cm]—are included in code **12004**). Code **12011** is reported for the simple repair of the forehead, code **12042** for the intermediate repair of the neck, and code **13101** for the complex repair of the abdomen.

✓ Check Your Knowledge

4. When multiple wounds are repaired, is it appropriate to add the lengths from the anatomic sites that are grouped together into the same code descriptor and report them as one code?

Key Terms

Simple repair: For wounds that are superficial, eg, involving primarily epidermis or dermis, or subcutaneous tissues without significant involvement of deeper structures, and requires simple one layer closure. This includes local anesthesia and chemical or electrocauterization of wounds not closed.

Intermediate repair: Includes the repair of wounds that, in addition to the above, require layered closure of one or more of the deeper layers of subcutaneous tissue and superficial (non-muscle) fascia, in addition to the skin (epidermal and dermal) closure. Single-layer closure of heavily contaminated wounds that have required extensive cleaning or removal of particulate matter also constitutes intermediate repair.

Complex repair: Includes the repair of wounds requiring more than layered closure, namely scar revision, debridement (eg, traumatic lacerations or avulsions), extensive undermining, stents, or retention sutures. Necessary preparation includes creation of a limited defect for repairs or the debridement of complicated lacerations or avulsions. Complex repair does not include excision of benign or malignant lesions, excisional preparation of a wound bed, or debridement of an open fracture or open dislocation.

Defect: An imperfection, malformation, dysfunction, or absence; an attribute of quality, in contrast with deficiency, which is an attribute of quantity.

Key Terms

- **Defect**
- **Skin substitute**
- **Skin replacement**

Adjacent Tissue Transfer or Rearrangement

Codes **14000-14350** identify adjacent tissue transfer or rearrangement procedures (local flaps). The excision of a lesion, whether it is benign or malignant, is included with these codes. Some examples of tissue transfer/rearrangements include the following:

- Z-plasty
- W-plasty
- V-Y plasty
- Rotation flap
- Advancement flap
- Double pedicle flap

Codes **14000-14350** are reported on the basis of the anatomic area and size. The size refers to the defect size, not the lesion size. The term **defect** includes the primary and secondary defects. The primary defect, resulting from the excision, and the secondary defect, resulting from flap design to perform the reconstruction, are measured together to determine the code.

In addition, it is important to note that if a skin graft is necessary to close a secondary defect, then this is considered an additional procedure.

Often the tissue transfer or rearrangement procedure creates an additional defect that must be repaired. For example, if a skin graft or another flap is necessary to close a secondary defect, this should be reported separately.

EXAMPLE

A patient had a lesion of the right cheek removed, resulting in a primary defect of 10 sq cm. After design, elevation, and mobilization of the rotation flap, a 10-sq cm secondary defect was present. The entire defect resulted in a 20-sq cm defect of the right cheek.

The term *defect* includes the primary defect from the excision and the secondary defect from the rotation flap. Code **14041** is reported for a total defect of 20 sq cm.

Skin Replacement Surgery and Skin Substitutes

The Skin Replacement Surgery and Skin Substitutes subsection includes services describing harvesting of the graft, caring for the donor site, the application of the **skin replacement or substitute** by location and incremental units, and the application ("surgical fixation") of the skin substitute or graft.

Skin grafts differ by their origin and, for autografts, by their anatomic source. Skin grafts, by origin, are as follows:

Autograft: Tissue transplanted from one part of the body to another in the same patient

Allograft (homograft): Tissue transplanted from one individual to another of the same species

Xenograft (heterograft): Tissue transplanted from one species to an unlike species (eg, baboon to human)

There are four types of autografts defined by anatomic source:

Epidermal: Grafts composed of the epidermis, the outermost layer of the two layers that make up the skin; the epidermis and dermis.
Dermal: Grafts composed of the dermis, the second layer of skin immediately below the epidermis.
Split-thickness skin grafts: Grafts composed of the full layer of epidermis and part of the dermis.
Full-thickness skin grafts: Grafts composed of the full layer of both the epidermis and dermis.

Key Terms

Skin replacement: A tissue or graft that permanently replaces lost skin with healthy skin.

Skin substitute: A biomaterial, engineered tissue, or combination of materials and cells or tissues that can be substituted for skin autograft or allograft in a clinical procedure.

Temporary wound closure: Not the final resurfacing material but provides closure of the wound surface until the skin surface can be permanently replaced.

Tissue cultured autograft: Cultured first in the laboratory from skin cells harvested from the patient and then, once grown into sheets of graft material, are shipped in sterile containers by the laboratory to arrive in the operating room where they are applied to the recipient site(s).

Mohs micrographic surgery: A technique for the removal of skin cancer in a critical location, recurrent tumors, ill-defined skin cancer, and large or aggressive tumors with histologic examination of 100% of the surgical margins, all of the peripheral and deep margins are examined.

The first step in selecting the appropriate code to report is to identify the size and location of the defect (recipient area) and the type of graft or skin substitute. Simple debridement of granulation tissue or recent avulsion is included in the graft or skin substitute codes. However, when a primary procedure such as orbitectomy, radical mastectomy, or deep tumor removal requires skin graft for definitive closure, see the appropriate anatomical subsection for the primary procedure and this section for skin graft or skin substitute.

It should be noted that these codes are not intended to report simple graft application alone or application stabilized with dressings (eg, by simple gauze wrap) without surgical fixation of the skin substitute or graft. However, the skin substitute or graft is anchored using the surgeon's choice of fixation. While routine dressing supplies are not reported separately, the supply of the skin substitute or graft is reported separately when services are performed in the office setting.

Surgical Preparation

Codes **15002-15005** describe the services related to preparing a clean and viable wound surface for placement of a graft, flap, skin replacement, skin substitute, or negative pressure wound therapy. In some cases, closure may be possible using adjacent tissue transfer (**14000-14061**) or complex repair (**13100-13153**). In all cases, appreciable nonviable tissue is removed to treat a burn, traumatic wound, or a necrotizing infection. The intent is to heal the wound by primary intention, or by the use of negative pressure wound therapy. Patient conditions may require the closure or application of graft, flap, skin replacement, or skin substitute to be delayed, but in all cases the intent is to include these treatments or negative pressure wound therapy to heal the wound. These codes are differentiated by anatomical site. Codes **15002** and **15004** are reported for the first 100 sq cm or 1% of body area of infants and children. Codes **+15003** and **15005** are add-on codes reported for each additional 100 sq cm or each additional 1% of body area of infants and children. These codes are used for initial wound recipient site preparation.

Key Terms

Coding Tip

Do not report **15002-15005** for removal of nonviable tissue or debris in a chronic wound (eg, venous or diabetic) when the wound is left to heal by secondary intention. Instead, see active wound management codes (**97597-97598**) and debridement codes (**11042-11047**) for this service.

> ### EXAMPLE
>
> A 27-year-old patient with burns on the shoulder was admitted to the burn center.
>
> After the induction of anesthesia, the subcutaneous tissue beneath the full-thickness burn is infiltrated with crystalloid solution containing epinephrine in order to minimize blood loss. The eschar is excised down to viable subcutaneous tissue. Hemostasis is obtained with electrocautery, epinephrine-soaked laparotomy pads, and/or a topical hemostatic agent. A total of 200 sq cm is excised in preparation for immediate or staged skin grafting and/or application of a skin substitute or replacement.
>
> Code **15002** is reported for the surgical preparation of the first 100 sq cm. Add-on code **+15003** is reported for the additional 100 sq cm.

Grafts

Autograft/Tissue-Cultured Autograft

Codes **15040-15157** are used to report autografts and tissue-cultured autografts. Codes **15050** and **15100-15136** are used to report autografts other than those that are tissue cultured. Codes **15040** and **15150-15157** are used to report tissue-cultured autografts. A **tissue-cultured autograft** is one that has been first cultured in the laboratory from skin cells harvested from the patient and then, once grown into sheets of graft material, are shipped in sterile containers by the laboratory to arrive in the operating room where they are applied to the recipient site(s).

Coding Tip

When square centimeters are indicated, this refers to 1 sq cm up to the stated amount.

Acellular Dermal Replacement Codes

Codes **15170** and **15175** describe acellular dermal replacement for the first 100 sq cm or less, or 1% of body area of infants and children. Add-on codes **15171** and **15176** have been established to report each additional 100 sq cm, or each additional 1% of body area of infants and children or part thereof.

Allograft/Tissue-Cultured Allogeneic Skin Substitute

Codes **15300-15366** are used to report the application of a nonautologous human skin graft (ie, homograft) from a donor to a part of the recipient's body to resurface an area damaged by burns, traumatic injury, soft tissue infection, and/or tissue necrosis or surgery. (See Figure 4-6.)

Specific guidelines apply to codes **15330-15336** for application of acellular dermal allograft. Acellular dermal allograft is a product that may require immediate, concurrent coverage with autologous tissue such as split-thickness autograft or a tissue flap. Report the appropriate acellular dermal autograft code and the appropriate code for application of the autologous tissue graft from the **15100-15261** code set.

Xenograft

Codes **15400-15431** are used to report the application of a nonhuman skin graft or biologic wound dressing (eg, porcine tissue or pigskin) to a part of the recipient's body following debridement of the burn wound or area of traumatic injury, soft tissue infection and/or tissue necrosis, or surgery. See Figure 4-7 below.

FIGURE 4-6 *Allograft, Skin*

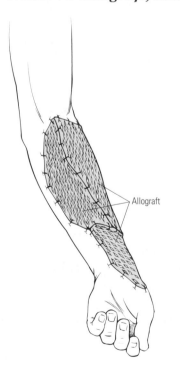

Allograft

FIGURE 4-7 *Xenograft, Skin*

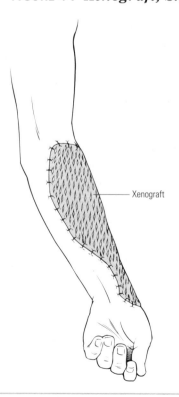

Xenograft

Selecting the Appropriate Code

Table 4-1 is provided to assist in the selection of the appropriate code and not the brand name of the material. This table represents examples only. Codes are based on the anatomic source and type of graft, not on the brand name of the material.

TABLE 4-1 *Selecting the Appropriate Code*

Code Range	Type of Graft	Definition and Product Examples
15150-15157	Tissue-cultured epidermal autograft	Cultured autologous skin with only an epidermal layer (eg, CEA, Epicel®, EpiDex®)
15170-15176	Acellular dermal replacement	A tissue-derived or manufactured device that provides immediate, temporary wound closure and that incorporates into the wound and promotes the generation of a neodermis that can support epidermal tissue (eg, Integra®)
15300-15321	Allograft skin	Cadaveric human skin allograft (eg, homograft—from skin banks)
15330-15336	Acellular dermal allograft	Decellularized allogeneic dermis may require immediate concurrent coverage with autologous tissue (eg, Alloderm®, Graft Jacket®)
15340-15341	Tissue-cultured allogeneic skin substitute	Cultured allogeneic skin with both a dermal and epidermal layer (eg, Apligraf®, Orcel™)
15360-15366	Tissue-cultured allogeneic dermal substitute	Cultured allogeneic neonatal dermal fibroblasts (eg, Transcyte®, Dermagraft®)
15400-15421	Xenogeneic dermis	Nonhuman dermis for temporary wound closure (eg, EZ Derm™, Mediskin®)
15430-15431	Acellular xenogeneic implant	Decellularized nonhuman connective tissue (eg, Oasis®, Surgisis®, PriMatrix®, etc)

Note: This table represents examples only. Codes are based on the anatomic source and type of graft, not on the brand name of the material.

✓ Check Your Knowledge

5. How would you code a full-thickness graft of the forehead 18 sq cm and excisional preparation of the recipient site with excision of extensive scarring?

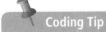

Coding Tip

A repair of a donor site requiring a skin graft or local flaps is considered an additional separate procedure.

Flaps (Skin and/or Deep Tissues)

The regions listed for Flaps codes **15570-15738** refer to the recipient area (not the donor site) when a flap is being attached in a transfer or to a final site. The regions listed also refer to a donor site when a tube is formed for later transfer or when a "delay" of flap occurs prior to the transfer. Codes **15732-15738** are described by donor site of the muscle, myocutaneous, or fasciocutaneous flap. (See Figure 4-8.)

Key Terms

- **Destruction**
- **Curettement (curettage)**
- **Electrosurgery**
- **Cryosurgery**
- **Cryotherapy**

FIGURE 4-8 *Axial Pattern Forehead Flap*

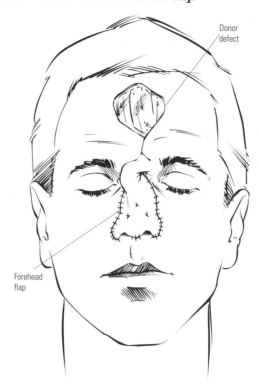

Donor defect

Forehead flap

Destruction

The **destruction** of lesions codes (**17000-17286**) are reported for destruction of lesions (ablation or obliteration of benign, premalignant, or malignant tissues) by any method, with or without **curettement**, including local anesthesia and generally not requiring closure. As indicated in the guidelines preceding this series of codes, "any method" includes **electrosurgery, cryosurgery**, laser, and chemical treatment. Codes **17000-17004** are used only for premalignant lesions. (See Figure 4-9.) Codes **17106-17108** are used for vascular proliferative lesions. Code **17110** (up to 14 lesions) and code **17111** (15 or more lesions) are stand-alone codes used for benign lesions other than skin tags or cutaneous vascular proliferative lesions.

Codes **17260-17268** are used for destruction of malignant lesions.

For further clarification on the appropriate code selection of excisions and destruction of lesions, see Figure 4-10.

EXAMPLES

Five actinic keratoses on the hands are destroyed by **cryotherapy**.

Code **17000** would be reported for the first lesion, and add-on code **17003** would be reported with a 4 in the units column for the second through the fifth lesion because code **17003** is an add-on code reported for each second through 14th lesion.

Five warts on the hands are destroyed by cryotherapy. Code **17110** once. Seventeen warts on the hands are destroyed by laser. Code **17111** once.

FIGURE 4-9 *Destruction, Premalignant Lesions*

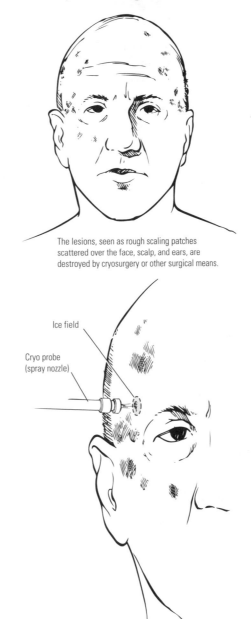

The lesions, seen as rough scaling patches scattered over the face, scalp, and ears, are destroyed by cryosurgery or other surgical means.

Ice field

Cryo probe (spray nozzle)

Key Terms

Destruction: The ablation of benign, premalignant, or malignant issues by any method, with or without curettement, including local anesthesia and not usually requiring closure.

Curettement (curettage): Scraping, usually of the interior of a cavity or tract, for the removal of new growth or other abnormal tissues, or to obtain material for tissue diagnosis.

Electrosurgery: The division of tissues by high-frequency current applied locally with a metal instrument or needle.

Cryosurgery: An operation using freezing temperature (achieved by liquid nitrogen or carbon dioxide) as an independent agent or in an instrument to destroy tissue.

Cryotherapy: The use of cold in the treatment of disease.

FIGURE 4-10 *Lesion Excision or Destruction*

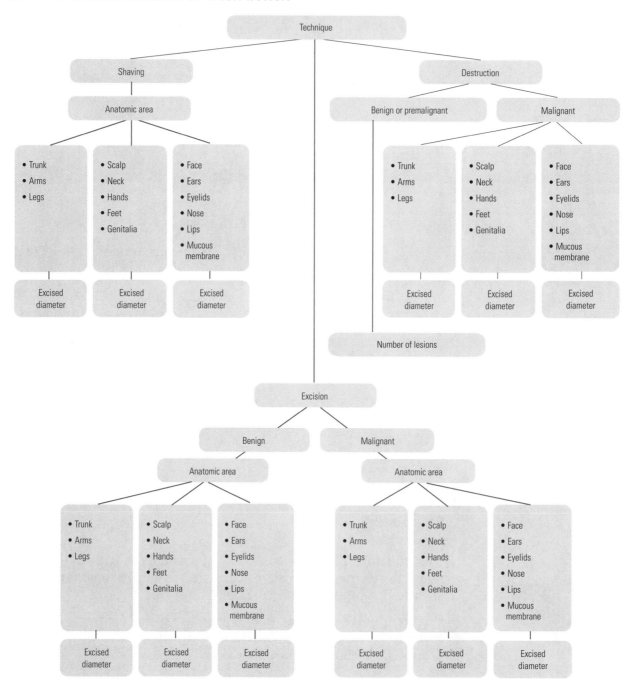

Mohs Micrographic Surgery

Mohs micrographic surgery is a technique for the removal of skin cancer in a critical location (ie, periorbital, perioral, periauricular, perinasal, hands and feet, genitalia), recurrent tumors (ie, tumors that have recurred after prior treatment), ill-defined skin cancer (eg, tumor has ill-defined margins), and large (ie, greater than 2 cm) or aggressive tumors with histologic examination of 100% of the surgical margins (all of the peripheral and deep margins are examined). This technique has the highest cure rate (97%–99% for primary tumors and 94% for recurrent tumors) and spares healthy tissue. Mohs surgery is the only CPT procedure for which the surgeon and the pathologist are one and the same person. The Mohs surgeon removes the tumor tissue and maps and divides the tumor specimen into pieces. Each piece is embedded into an individual tissue block for histopathologic examination. In the context of Mohs surgery, a *tissue block* is defined as an individual tissue piece embedded in a mounting medium for sectioning. This tissue block more accurately describes the unit of service.

Codes **17311-17315** describe Mohs surgery procedures based on anatomic site and the unit of service. To more accurately reflect the unit of service, these codes describe the unit of service as blocks rather than as specimens. Codes **17311** and **17313** describe the first stage of Mohs surgery with up to five tissue blocks. Code **17311** describes the work involved for treating tumors of the head, neck, hands, feet, genitalia, or any location with surgery directly involving muscle, cartilage, bone, tendon, major nerves, or vessels. Code **17313** describes the work involved in treating tumors on the trunk, arms, or legs. Codes **17312** and **17314** are add-on codes reported for each additional stage of up to five tissue blocks, whereas code **17315** is an add-on code reported for each additional block beyond the first five tissue blocks at any given stage. Code **17315** is reported once per additional tissue block. The parenthetical notes instruct users to report code **17312** in conjunction with code **17311**, code **17314** in conjunction with code **17313**, and code **17315** in conjunction with codes **17311-17314**.

EXAMPLES

Cancers of the nose and left ear are treated with one stage of Mohs surgery. Code **17311** would be reported two times.

A tumor of the nose required a first and second stage of Mohs surgery. Code **17311** would be reported for the first stage. Add-on code **17312** would be reported for the second stage.

Breast Procedures

Codes **19100-19499** describe surgical procedures performed on the breast. It is important to note that these procedures are considered unilateral procedures. When these procedures are performed bilaterally, modifier **50**, *Bilateral procedure,* should be appended.

Coding Tip

Mohs surgery requires a single physician to act in two integrated but separate and distinct capacities: surgeon and pathologist. If either of these responsibilities is delegated to another physician who reports the services separately, these codes should not be reported.

A first-stage code, either **17311** or **17313** is reported only one time for each lesion treated by Mohs surgery at the same treatment session.

Breast biopsies are reported with codes **19100-19103**. There are two types of breast biopsies:

1. percutaneous, and
2. open.

Percutaneous needle core biopsy, which is aspiration or removal of tissue, is reported with codes **19100** and **19102** using imaging guidance. Open incisional biopsy, which is surgical removal of part of the lesion into the skin and exposure of the lesion, is reported with code **19101**.

Code **19105** describes cryosurgical ablation of a fibroadenoma using ultrasound guidance. Each fibroadenoma that is ablated is reported separately. Code **19105** includes ultrasound guidance; therefore, a separate code for ultrasound guidance should not be reported. A parenthetical note following code **19105** instructs users not to report codes **76940** or **76942** in conjunction with **19105**. (See Figure 4-11.)

Codes **19125** and **19126** describe excision of a breast lesion performed after being identified by preoperative placement of a radiological marker. Codes **19300-19307** describe various mastectomy procedures. It is important to review the documentation in the medical record prior to selecting the appropriate mastectomy code. A partial mastectomy, also referred to as *lumpectomy, tylectomy, quadrantectomy,* and/or *segmentectomy,* is reported with codes **19301** and **19302**. Total mastectomy

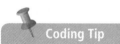
Coding Tip

In some instances, two adjacent fibroadenomas are treated with one insertion of the cryoprobe. In such circumstances, code **19105** should be reported only one time.

FIGURE 4-11 *Percutaneous Needle Core Breast Biopsy*

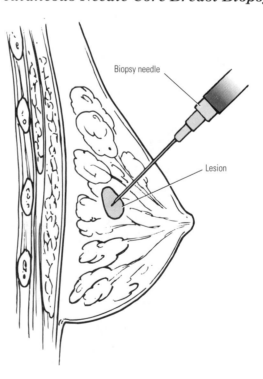

Biopsy needle

Lesion

is described with various codes ranging from **19303-19307**, depending upon the structures being removed.

✓ Check Your Knowledge Answers

1. No, when performing debridement of a single wound, report depth using the deepest level of tissue removed. In multiple wounds, sum the surface area of those wounds that are at the same depth, but do not combine sums from different depths.

2. Lesion diameter plus the most narrow margins required equals the excised diameter.

3. No, it is not appropriate to report simple repair separately. Simple repair is included as part of the excision and may not be reported separately.

4. Yes, when multiple wounds are repaired, the lengths of those wounds in the same classification (simple, intermediate, or complex) and from those anatomic sites that are grouped together into the same code descriptor should be added together and reported as one code.

5. Code(s) **15240, 15004**

Integumentary System Exercises

Check your answers in Appendix B.

True or False

1. The complex repair codes include repair of wounds requiring more than layered closure. **True or False**
2. When an excision is being performed, the margins refer to the widest diameter required to adequately excise the lesion based on the physician's judgment. **True or False**
3. Removal of lesions by a shaving technique includes local anesthesia, chemical, or electrocauterization of the wound. **True or False**
4. If a skin graft is necessary to close a secondary defect, then this is considered an additional procedure. **True or False**
5. Codes **19100-19499** are considered bilateral procedures. **True or False**

Matching

6. Tissue transplanted from one part of the body to another in the same patient. _____
7. Tissue transplanted from one individual to another of the same species. _____
8. Tissue transplanted from one species to an unlike species (eg, non-human, baboon to human). _____

9. A tissue or graft that permanently replaces lost skin with healthy skin. _____

10. A biomaterial, engineered tissue, or combination of materials and cells or tissues that can be substituted for skin autograft or allograft in a clinical procedure. _____

11. Not the final resurfacing material but provides closure of the wound surface until the skin surface can be permanently replaced. _____

    a. skin replacement
    b. temporary wound closure
    c. autograft
    d. xenograft (heterograft)
    e. allograft (homograft)
    f. skin substitute

Multiple Choice

12. A patient had five corns pared by a physician. These were all located on the patient's feet.

    a. 11055
    b. 11057
    c. 11056
    d. None of the above

13. Code the excision of a 2.6-cm benign lesion of the arm with closure of the excision site.

    a. 11403
    b. 11422
    c. 11603
    d. None of the above

14. Fine needle aspiration of a breast cyst with imaging guidance.

    a. 19000
    b. 76942
    c. 10022
    d. None of the above

15. Decubitus heel ulcer, diameter 6.5 cm requiring debridement of skin and subcutaneous tissue.

    a. 11043
    b. 11044
    c. 11042
    d. None of the above

16. Wide local excision of a basal cell carcinoma (15.4 cm) of the leg with an adjacent tissue transfer of a skin flap.
    a. 14020
    b. 14021
    c. 14040
    d. None of the above

Surgery: Musculoskeletal System

Section Objectives

- Distinguish when to report excisions from the Musculoskeletal System
- Understand the spine (vertebrae column)
- Differentiate the various types of fracture treatments
- Understand the reporting for Application of Casts and Strapping
- Review the use of Endoscopy/Arthroscopy services
- Assess various techniques for bunions and associated deformities

The Musculoskeletal System subsection of the Surgery section of the CPT codebook is organized by musculoskeletal anatomy. The subsection is further divided by a consistent theme of procedures: incision; excision; introduction or removal; repair, revision, and/or reconstruction; fracture and/or dislocation; arthrodesis; and amputation. This format is repeated throughout the subsection by anatomy (see Figure 4-12). The codes in the Musculoskeletal System subsection are for the reporting of procedures involving tendons, muscles, fractures and dislocations, spine surgery, bunions, and casting and strapping. Procedures performed via an arthroscope are specifically addressed at the end of the subsection, and terms related to the treatment of fractures are included in the introductory language of the Musculoskeletal System subsection in the CPT codebook.

Sections of the Musculoskeletal System subsection are highlighted in this chapter along with a review of some basic coding guidelines

FIGURE 4-12 *CPT Codebook Surgery Categories Regarding the Musculoskeletal System*

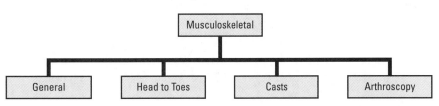

Key Terms

- **Subcutaneous soft tissue tumors, removal of**

- **Fascial or subfascial soft tissue tumors, removal of**

- **Radical resection of soft tissue tumors, removal of**

- **Radical resection of bone tumors, removal of**

associated with reporting excisions, fractures and dislocations, spine surgery, bunion procedures, and casting and strapping procedures. This chapter will provide an overview of the Musculoskeletal System codes (**20005-29999**) of the CPT codebook. (See Figures 4-13A and 4-13B.)

Musculoskeletal Lesion Excisions

There is often confusion in determining whether the excision of soft tissue tumors is reported with codes from the Integumentary system or the Musculoskeletal system. Musculoskeletal lesion excision codes pertain to subcutaneous, superficial, or deep soft tissues under the skin, which may include subcutaneous fat, fascia, muscle, and bone. Soft tissue excision codes are dispersed throughout the musculoskeletal section of the CPT codebook and are categorized by anatomic site. Be sure to review and understand the guidelines in this section. When coding musculoskeletal procedures, it is important to note that the excision must meet the criteria listed in the code descriptor. For example, in order to report code **26116**, *Excision, tumor, soft tissue, or vascular malformation, of hand or finger; subfascial (eg, intramuscular); less than 1.5 cm,* the tumor must be down to the muscle (ie, located between the fascia and muscle) or be intramuscular, such as a muscle sarcoma. There are different musculoskeletal tumors listed throughout this section, such as **subcutaneous soft tissue tumors, fascial or subfascial soft tissue tumors, radical resection of soft tissue tumors,** and **radical resection of bone tumors.**

FIGURE 4-13A *Muscular System, Front*

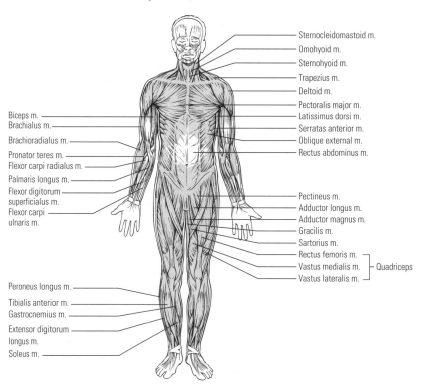

FIGURE 4-13B *Muscular System, Back*

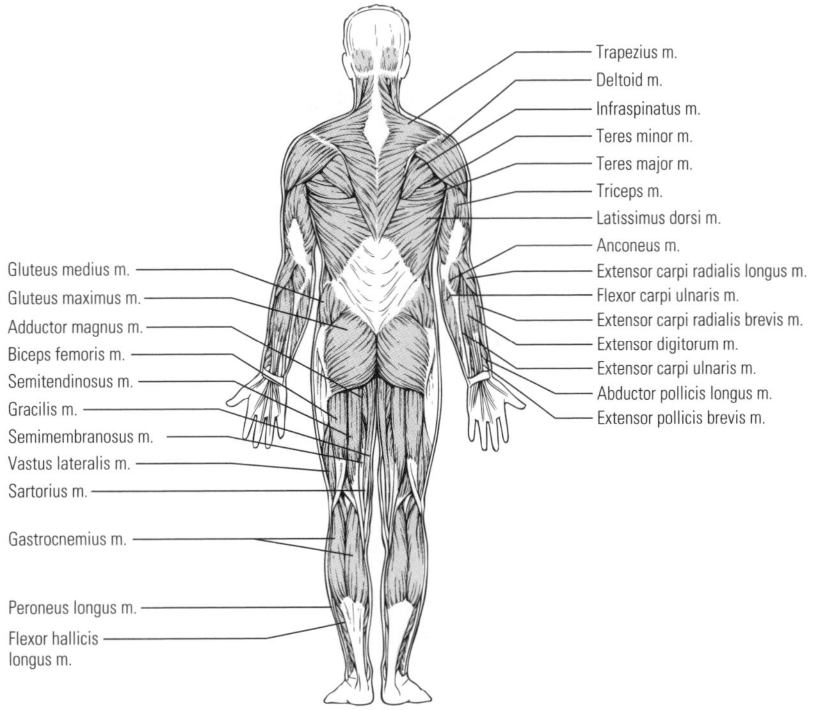

Trapezius m.
Deltoid m.
Infraspinatus m.
Teres minor m.
Teres major m.
Triceps m.
Latissimus dorsi m.
Anconeus m.
Extensor carpi radialis longus m.
Flexor carpi ulnaris m.
Extensor carpi radialis brevis m.
Extensor digitorum m.
Extensor carpi ulnaris m.
Abductor pollicis longus m.
Extensor pollicis brevis m.

Gluteus medius m.
Gluteus maximus m.
Adductor magnus m.
Biceps femoris m.
Semitendinosus m.
Gracilis m.
Semimembranosus m.
Vastus lateralis m.
Sartorius m.
Gastrocnemius m.
Peroneus longus m.
Flexor hallicis longus m.

Key Terms

Subcutaneous soft tissue tumors, removal of: These involve the simple or marginal resection of tumors confined to subcutaneous fatty tissue below the skin, but above the deep fascia.

Fascial or subfascial soft tissue tumors, removal of: These involve the resection of tumors confined to the tissue within or below the deep fascia, but not involving the muscle or bone. Included are digital (ie, fingers and toes) subfascial tumors that involve the tendons, tendon sheaths, or joints of the digit.

Radical resection of soft tissue tumors, removal of: These involve the resection of a tumor, usually malignant, with wide margins of normal tissue.

Radical resection of bone tumors, removal of: These involve the resection of the tumor with wide margins of normal tissue. Radical resection of bone tumors is usually performed for malignant tumors or very aggressive tumors.

Similar to the guidelines for the Integumentary System, the code selection for musculoskeletal lesion excisions is determined by measuring the greatest diameter of the tumor, in addition to the narrowest margin required for the complete excision of the tumor, based on the physician's judgment, at the time of the excision. The radical resection of soft tissue tumors may be confined to a specific layer, for instance, the subcutaneous or subfascial tissue, or it may involve the removal of tissue from one or more layers. Radical resection of soft tissue tumors is most commonly used for malignant or very aggressive benign tumors.

✓ Check Your Knowledge

1. List the different musculoskeletal tumors.

Fractures and Dislocations

When fractures and dislocations are reported, it is important to have a clear understanding of the various types of treatment, as well as the anatomy. See Figures 4-14 through 4-16. In addition, before selecting the appropriate fracture/dislocation CPT code, it is important to note the following information in the medical record:

- The site of the fracture
- Type of treatment (eg, open, percutaneous skeletal fixation)
- With or without manipulation
- Whether traction or internal or external fixation is performed

FIGURE 4-14A *Skeletal System*

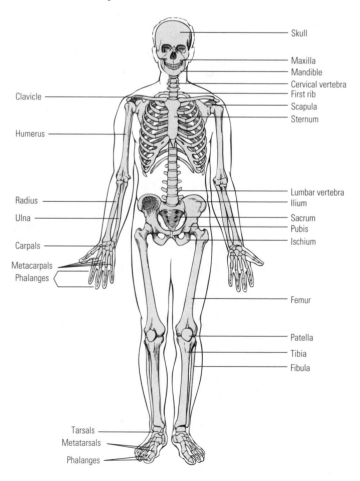

FIGURE 4-14B *Skull*

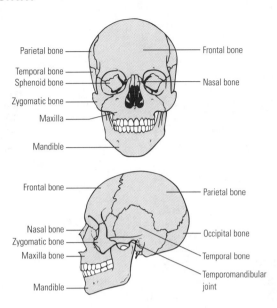

Parietal bone — Frontal bone
Temporal bone —
Sphenoid bone — Nasal bone
Zygomatic bone —
Maxilla —
Mandible —

Frontal bone — Parietal bone
Nasal bone — Occipital bone
Zygomatic bone —
Maxilla bone — Temporal bone
Mandible — Temporomandibular joint

Closed vs Open Treatment

Closed treatment of a fracture or dislocation specifically means that the fracture or dislocation site is not surgically opened. This treatment is used to describe procedures that treat fractures by one of the following three methods:

- Without manipulation
- With manipulation
- With or without traction

Open treatment means that the fracture is surgically opened and visualized to allow internal fixation, or as noted in the musculoskeletal

FIGURE 4-15A *Bones of Hand*

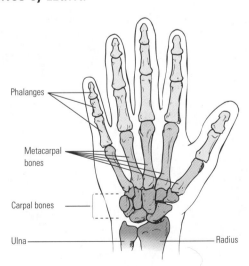

Phalanges

Metacarpal bones

Carpal bones

Ulna — Radius

FIGURE 4-15B *Tendons of Hand*

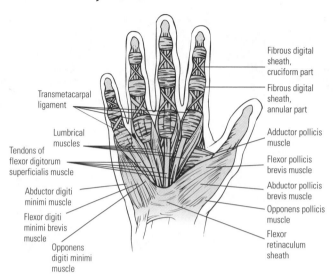

system guidelines of the CPT codebook, an intramedullary fixation of a fracture is also considered an open procedure, unlike percutaneous fixation. An incision remote to the fracture is required for insertion of the intramedullary rod, and the fracture site is often not visualized directly. This requires more work and skill in correct placement of the incision and accurate distal rod positioning compared with percutaneous insertion of a pin.

FIGURE 4-16A *Bones of Foot*

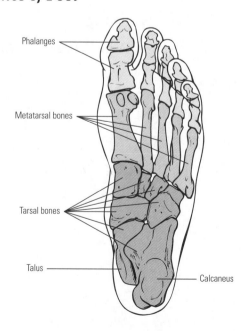

Key Terms

- **Closed treatment**
- **Open treatment**
- **Percutaneous skeletal fixation**
- **Manipulation**
- **Sheaths**
- **Ligament**
- **Trigger point**

FIGURE 4-16B *Muscles of Foot*

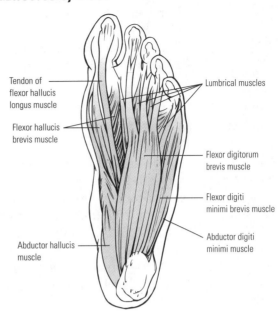

Tendon of flexor hallucis longus muscle

Flexor hallucis brevis muscle

Abductor hallucis muscle

Lumbrical muscles

Flexor digitorum brevis muscle

Flexor digiti minimi brevis muscle

Abductor digiti minimi muscle

Percutaneous Skeletal Fixation

This type of treatment is neither open nor closed. In this procedure, the fracture fragments are not visualized, but fixation (eg, with pins) is placed across the fracture site, usually under X-ray imaging.

Manipulation

The term **manipulation** is used in many sections of the CPT codebook. The definition used here applies to codes in the Musculoskeletal System section. Manipulation is the attempted reduction or restoration of a fracture or joint dislocation to its normal anatomic alignment by applying forces.

✓ Check Your Knowledge

2. How many types of fracture treatments are there? Briefly describe each.

3. List the different methods of closed treatment.

Injections

The Musculoskeletal System section includes codes to report injections into tendon sheaths, ligaments, muscles, and trigger points. Code **20550**, *Injection(s); single tendon sheath, or ligament, aponeurosis (eg, plantar "fascia"),* is used to report single or multiple injections per single anatomic tendon sheath, ligament, or aponeurosis. Code **20551**, *Injection(s); single tendon origin/insertion,* is used to report single or

Coding Tip

The codes for trigger point injections, **20552** and **20553**, are intended to be reported once per session, regardless of the number of trigger points or muscles injected. Whenever radiological imaging guidance is performed in addition to the injection procedures, the appropriate radiology code **76942** should be reported in addition to the injection codes to describe the imaging guidance.

multiple injections per single tendon origin or insertion. When **multiple** injections to the same tendon are performed, they are reported only **once**. When injections to **multiple** tendon sheaths, ligaments, tendon origins, or tendon insertions are performed, they are reported **one** time for **each** injection. See Figure 4-17.

EXAMPLES

A 40-year-old female presents with stenosing tenosynovitis of the right index finger. She is treated with two steroid injections into the flexor tendon sheath.

Code **20550** is reported one time for the two steroid injections because multiple injections to the same tendon would be reported only once.

A 60-year-old male presents with a three-month history of pain in the low left back above the posterior iliac crest with radiation of pain

FIGURE 4-17 *Trigger Point Injection*

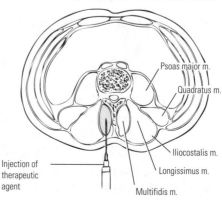

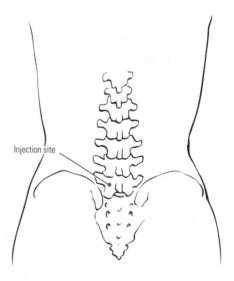

Injection site

Cross section through the body wall at level of lumbar vertebra

Psoas major m.

Quadratus m.

Iliocostalis m.

Injection of therapeutic agent

Longissimus m.

Multifidis m.

into the left buttock. He undergoes injection of the trigger point in the multifidus muscle left of the L5 spinous process and an injection in the gluteus medius muscle.

Code **20552** is reported for the two injections because this code is intended to be reported once per session.

Key Terms

Closed treatment: The fracture or dislocation site is not surgically opened.

Open treatment: The fracture is surgically opened and visualized to allow internal fixation.

Percutaneous skeletal fixation: Utilizes a type of treatment that holds the position of a fracture by the use of external pins inserted across the skin into bone.

Manipulation: The attempted reduction or restoration of a fracture or joint dislocation to its normal anatomic alignment by applying forces. Please note that this definition applies to codes in the Musculoskeletal System section.

Sheaths: Any enveloping structure, such as the membranous covering of a muscle, nerve, or blood vessel; any sheathlike structure.

Ligament: A band or sheet of fibrous tissue connecting two or more bones, cartilages, or other structures or serving as support for fasciae or muscles.

Trigger point: A specific point or area where stimulation by touch, pain, or pressure induces a painful response.

When an arthrocentesis, aspiration, or injection of a major joint or bursa (**20610**) is performed, the insertion of needle into major joint or bursa for the injection of therapeutic or diagnostic agent, aspiration, or arthrocentesis is included in the procedure, and should not be reported separately. (See Figure 4-18.)

When performing the halo application for a thin skull osteology (**20664**), a cranial halo is placed on the head of a child whose skull is unusually thin due to congenital or developmental problems. (See Figures 4-19A and 4-19B.)

Figures 4-20 and 4-21 are examples of types of stabilization devices. Codes **20690** and **20692** describe the placement of types of external fixation devices. The method of stabilization depends upon fracture grade (degree of soft tissue injury or skin integrity disruption), type (eg, comminuted, spiral, impacted), and location (eg, extremity, pelvis).

Spine Surgery

When coding for spine surgery, the coder must consider and apply various guidelines that are included in the beginning of the Spine

FIGURE 4-18 *Arthrocentesis, Aspiration, or Injection of Major Joint or Bursa*

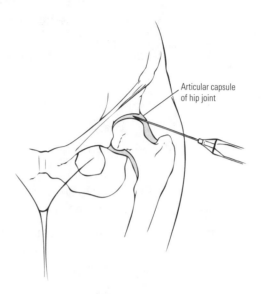

Articular capsule
of hip joint

FIGURE 4-19A *Halo Application for Thin Skull Osteology*

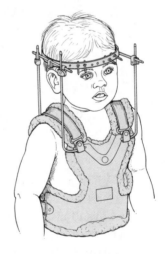

FIGURE 4-19B *Halo Application for Thin Skull Osteology*

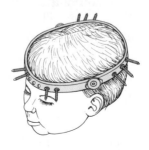

Chapter 4

Key Terms

- **Interspace**
- **Segment**
- **Vertebral components**
- **Arthrodesis**
- **Segmental instrumentation**
- **Nonsegmental instrumentation**

FIGURE 4-20A *Uniplane External Fixation System*

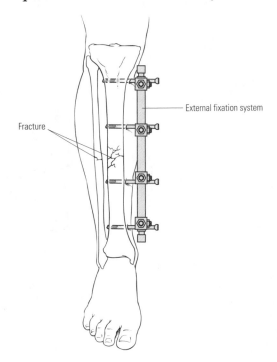

External fixation system

Fracture

FIGURE 4-20B *Uniplane External Fixation System*

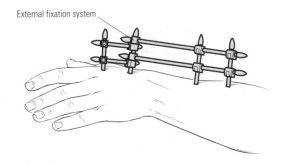

External fixation system

subsection in the CPT codebook. These guidelines include various coding components such as bone grafting, arthrodesis, and spinal instrumentation. Careful review of these instructions along with each code descriptor is also imperative to ensure that the correct codes are selected.

It is important to understand various anatomic terms when spine surgeries are coded. (See Figure 4-22.) The Key Terms on p. 98 offer further definitions for spine surgery. The spine (vertebral column) consists of a series of bones known as *vertebrae*. There are 33 vertebrae in an adult human, which are divided into the following five types:

- Cervical vertebrae (C1-7): neck area
- Thoracic vertebrae (T1-12): upper back area
- Lumbar vertebrae (L1-5): lower back
- Sacral vertebrae (S1-5): the sacrum
- Coccygeal vertebrae (coccyx): the tailbone

FIGURE 4-21 *Multiplane External Fixation System*

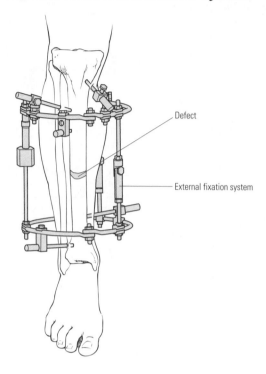

Defect

External fixation system

Key Terms

Interspace: The nonbony compartment between two adjacent vertebral bodies that contains the intervertebral disc and includes the nucleus pulposus, annulus fibrosus, and two cartilaginous endplates.

Segment: The basic constituent part into which the spine may be divided. It represents a single complete vertebral bone with its associated articular processes and laminae.

Vertebral components: The vertebral body, spinous process, laminae, facets, and intervertebral disc.

Arthrodesis: The surgical fusion or fixation of a joint.

Segmental instrumentation: The fixation at each end of the construct and at least one additional interposed bony attachment.

Nonsegmental instrumentation: The fixation at each end of the construct, possibly spanning several vertebral segments without attachment to the intervening segments.

FIGURE 4-22A *Thoracic Vertebra, Superior View*

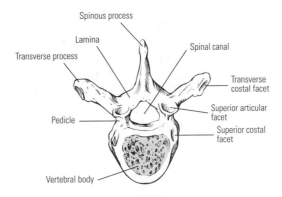

FIGURE 4-22B *Lumbar Vertebra, Superior View*

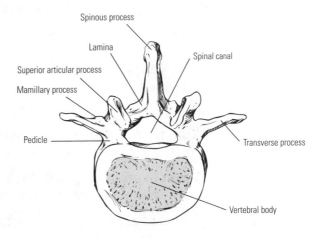

FIGURE 4-22C *Lumbar Vertebrae, Lateral View*

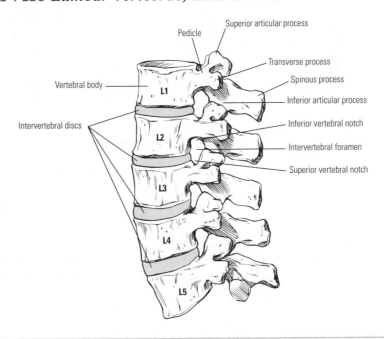

Sometimes spinal procedures include reporting codes from the Nervous System subsection in addition to codes from the Musculo-skeletal System subsection for reporting various procedures such as laminectomy and spinal cord decompression.

When multiple surgeons act as primary surgeons on the basis of the complexity of the procedure(s), modifier **62** can be appended to certain appropriate codes to reflect that surgeons worked together as primary surgeons. Modifier **62** may not be appended to the spinal instrumentation codes and spinal bone graft codes.

Grafts (or Implants)

Codes **20930-20938**, located under the Grafts (or Implants) subsection of the Musculoskeletal procedures of the CPT codebook, describe various types of bone graft procedures used for spine surgery (ie, allograft, autograft, structural, morselized). It is imperative to understand the terms used in the bone graft code descriptors before selecting the correct code.

Key Terms

Allograft: A donor bone obtained from a bone bank.

Autograft: Cancellous or bone cortex surgically removed from another area of the patient's own body.

Morselized bone graft: Small pieces of bone obtained either from a bone bank or from the patient's own body.

Structural bone graft: A whole piece of cancellous and/or bone cortex obtained from a bone bank or removed from the patient's own body.

When performing the reconstruction of the mandibular rami (**21196**), the mandibular ramus is reconstructed to lengthen, set back, or rotate the mandible. (See Figure 4-23.)

When performing percutaneous vertebroplasty (**22520**), augmentation of a vertebral fracture is achieved by percutaneous injections of polymethylmethacrylate under fluoroscopic guidance. (See Figure 4-24.)

Vertebral Body, Embolization, or Injection

Percutaneous vertebroplasty describes a procedure in which a sterile biomaterial such as polymethylmethacrylate is injected from one side or both sides into the damaged vertebral body to act as a bone cement to reinforce the fractured or collapsed vertebra. Various polymethylmethacrylate cements are commonly used; however, a cement indicated for craniofacial defect repair mixed with commercially available barium sulfate may be used.

- **Allograft**
- **Autograft**
- **Morselized bone graft**
- **Structural bone graft**

FIGURE 4-23 *Reconstruction of Mandibular Rami*

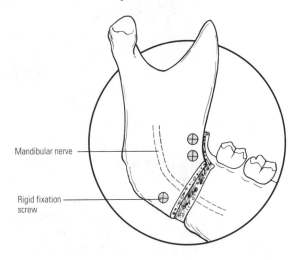

Mandibular nerve

Rigid fixation
screw

FIGURE 4-24 *Percutaneous Vertebroplasty*

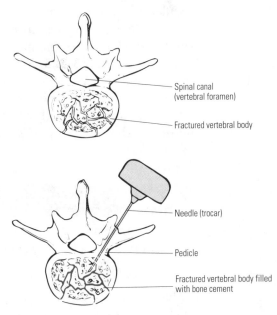

Spinal canal
(vertebral foramen)

Fractured vertebral body

Needle (trocar)

Pedicle

Fractured vertebral body filled
with bone cement

Chapter 4

This procedure is indicated primarily for relief of pain related to vertebral compression fractures secondary to osteoporosis. However, other conditions such as aneurysmal bone cysts, hemangioma, giant-cell tumor, or metastatic malignancy may also result in vertebral compression fractures. It is important to note, however, that these conditions are merely provided as examples. The percutaneous vertebroplasty code set, **22520-22522**, is intended to report a unilateral or bilateral injection and is delineated based upon spinal level (ie, thoracic or lumbar).

Key Terms

- **Percutaneous vertebroplasty**
- **Kyphoplasty**

EXAMPLE

Vertebroplasty is performed on T3, T4, and T5. Code **22520** is reported one time for the first level (T3). Code **22522** is reported twice, one time for each additional level (T4 and T5).

Kyphoplasty

Percutaneous vertebral augmentation **(kyphoplasty)** is a minimally invasive surgical technique for treating fractures of the spine that occur because of osteoporosis, usually in postmenopausal women. Mechanical devices (miniature expandable jacks, curved tamps, expandable balloon tamps, etc) were developed to provide physicians with new tools and options to treat vertebral body compression fractures. Codes **22523-22525** describe vertebral fracture augmentation and injection of polymethylmethacrylate (bone cement).

It is important to note that cavity creation using a mechanical device at a single thoracic and lumbar vertebral body is included in codes **22523** and **22524**. In addition, fracture reduction and bone biopsy are incidental to the procedure and should not be reported separately. An exclusionary parenthetical note following **22525** instructs to preclude the use of the deep bone biopsy code **20225** with the vertebral augmentation codes **22523-22525**.

Add-on code **22525** describes each additional thoracic or lumbar vertebral body on which percutaneous vertebral augmentation is performed. A parenthetical note following this code instructs users to delineate the reporting of **22525** in conjunction with **22523** and **22524**, as appropriate.

✓ Check Your Knowledge

4. Is it appropriate to report deep bone biopsy (code **20225**) in addition to a vertebral augmentation procedure?

The radiological supervision and interpretation (RS&I) portions of the percutaneous vertebroplasty and percutaneous vertebral augmentation procedures are reported separately based upon the type of guidance used: fluoroscopic guidance (**72291**) or computed tomographic (CT) guidance (**72292**).

Code **22526** and add-on code **22527** describe the performance of intradiscal electrothermal annuloplasty. This procedure is performed by inserting a needle or catheter, which is subsequently heated, into a disc to effect a thermal change in the annular tissue. This modulates the nerve fibers in a disrupted disc's annulus and stabilizes the collagen of the annulus as a treatment for back pain. Code **22526** is reported one time only when performed bilaterally. Code **22527** is also reported one time for electrothermal annuloplasty of additional levels, regardless of the number of additional levels treated in a single session. As indicated in the code descriptor, fluoroscopic guidance is included in codes **22526** and **22527**. Therefore, codes **77002** and **77003** should not be reported separately in addition to the electrothermal annuloplasty codes.

Key Terms

Percutaneous vertebroplasty: A procedure in which a sterile biomaterial such as methylmethacrylate is injected from one side or both sides into the damaged vertebral body to act as a bone cement to reinforce the fractured or collapsed vertebra.

Kyphoplasty: A new, minimally invasive surgical technique for treating fractures of the spine that occur because of osteoporosis, usually in postmenopausal women.

Arthrodesis

Spinal arthrodesis is performed on vertebral segments of the spine to firmly join joint surfaces by promoting the proliferation of bone cells and new bone. Codes **22800-22819** describe arthrodesis procedures performed for scoliosis or kyphosis. Codes **22532-22632** describe arthrodesis procedures performed for a reason other than to correct a spinal deformity and are categorized by the anatomic approach (anterior, posterior, or lateral). See Figure 4-25 for the arthrodesis by anterior approach.

Figure 4-26 shows an example of an exposure technique used to reach anterior cervical vertebrae for spinal procedures (eg, discectomy, arthrodesis, spinal instrumentation) (**22554**), while Figure 4-27 shows an example of an exposure technique used to reach anterior lumbar vertebrae for spinal procedures (eg, discectomy, arthrodesis, spinal instrumentation) (**22558**).

FIGURE 4-25 *Arthrodesis (Anterior Transoral Technique)*

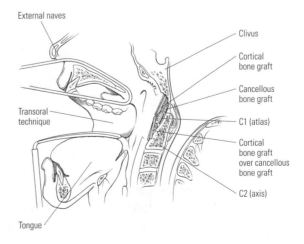

Chapter 4

FIGURE 4-26 *Anterior Approach for Cervical Fusion*

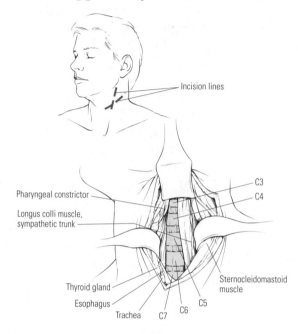

FIGURE 4-27 *Anterior Approach for Lumbar Fusion (Anterior Retroperitoneal Exposure)*

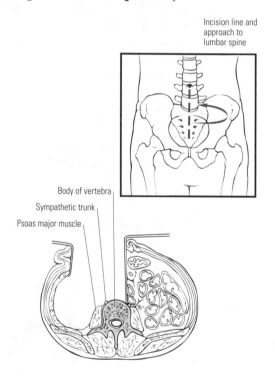

Spinal Instrumentation

Insertion of spinal instrumentation is reported with codes **22840-22848** and **22851**. The insertion of spinal instrumentation is separately reported in addition to the arthrodesis procedure and any definitive

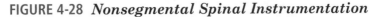

procedure(s) performed. These codes are categorized as follows by the type of instrumentation performed:

- Posterior nonsegmental instrumentation (fixation at each end of the construct and may span several vertebral segments without attachment to the intervening segments): **22840** (See Figure 4-28.).
- Posterior segmental instrumentation (posterior approach fixation at each end of the construct and at least one additional interposed bony attachment): **22842-22844** (See Figure 4-29.).

FIGURE 4-28 *Nonsegmental Spinal Instrumentation*

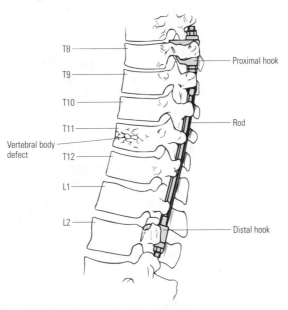

FIGURE 4-29 *Segmental Spinal Instrumentation*

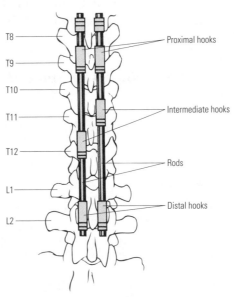

Coding Tip

Code **22849** should not be reported in conjunction with codes **22850, 22852,** and **22855** at the same spinal levels.

- Anterior instrumentation (anterior approach fixation at each end of the construct and at least one additional interposed bony attachment): **22845-22847**
- Pelvic fixation: **22848**

Code **22849** describes reinsertion of a spinal fixation device. This code may be used for all types of devices, as the type of instrumentation is not specified in the code descriptor.

Code **22851** describes application of intervertebral biomechanical device(s) to a vertebral defect or interspace. This code is reported only **one** time per interspace, regardless of the number of devices placed at that same interspace. There are occasions when metal cages are placed at two different vertebral interspaces. In these instances, code **22851** may be reported once for each interspace. (See Figure 4-30.) Codes **22850, 22852,** and **22855** describe the various procedures associated with removal of instrumentation.

It is important to note that codes **22849, 22850, 22852,** and **22855** may be appended with modifier **51** if reported with other definitive procedure(s) including arthrodesis, decompression, and exploration of fusion.

Codes **22857, 22862,** and **22865** are used to report the variations of lumbar disc replacement surgery. The placement of an artificial disc requires anchoring plates to the vertebral end plates on the vertebrae above and below the intradiscal space. The artificial disc is sandwiched between these plates. These codes describe an anterior approach through the abdomen to access the anterior portion of the spine without disruption of the spinal cord area. Code **22857** describes initial placement of a lumbar artificial disc in a single interspace. The placement of one or more additional discs in additional interspaces is reported with Category III add-on code **0163T**.

Code **22862** describes the revision and replacement of an existing lumbar artificial disc at a single level. Category III code **0165T** is reported for revision of other previously placed discs at other interspaces.

Code **22865** describes the removal of an existing lumbar artificial disc at a single level. The removal of lumbar artificial discs at additional levels is reported with Category III add-on code **0164T**.

FIGURE 4-30 *Spinal Prosthetic Devices*

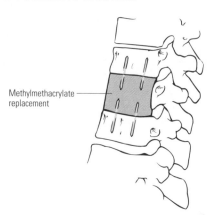

Methylmethacrylate replacement

When performing a partial hip replacement with or without bipolar prosthesis (**27125**), the femoral neck is excised so the physician can measure and then replace the femoral stem. (See Figure 4-31.)

When performing a total hip replacement (**27130**), the femoral head is excised, osteophytes are removed, and acetabulum is reamed out before replacement is inserted in the femoral shaft. (See Figure 4-32.)

When performing a percutaneous treatment of a femoral fracture (**27235**), the femoral fracture is treated without fracture exposure. (See Figure 4-33.) With an open treatment of a femoral fracture (**27236**), the femoral fracture is treated by internal fixation device (with fracture exposure). (See Figure 4-34.)

FIGURE 4-31 *Partial Hip Replacement With or Without Bipolar Prosthesis*

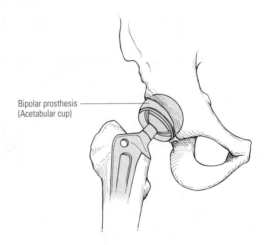

Bipolar prosthesis
(Acetabular cup)

FIGURE 4-32 *Total Hip Replacement*

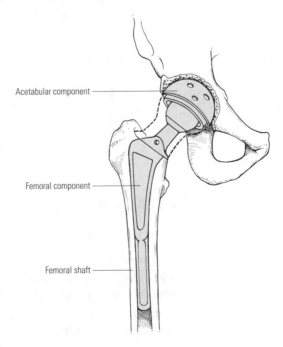

Acetabular component

Femoral component

Femoral shaft

FIGURE 4-33 *Percutaneous Treatment of Femoral Fracture*

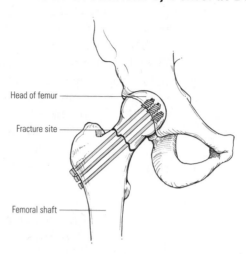

Head of femur

Fracture site

Femoral shaft

FIGURE 4-34A *Open Treatment of Femoral Fracture*   FIGURE 4-34B *Open Treatment of Femoral Fracture*

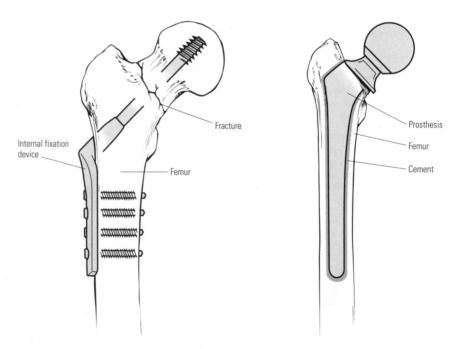

Fracture

Internal fixation device

Femur

Prosthesis

Femur

Cement

Foot and Toes

Bunion Procedures

Coding for the correction of a bunion and its associated deformities can be challenging. Not all bunion deformities are the same, and different techniques are needed to repair different levels of deformity. A common deformity of the first metatarsophalangeal (MTP) joint is a hallux valgus (bunion). The CPT code set includes codes for reporting various techniques used to correct bunion deformities. Figures 4-35 through 4-42 illustrate the various techniques, such as:

- Hallux Valgus correction (**28290**), which is the simple resection of the medial eminence (Silver-type procedure).

FIGURE 4-35 *Hallux Valgus Correction*

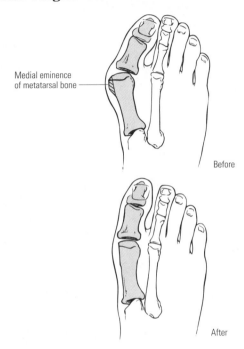

Medial eminence of metatarsal bone

Before

After

- Keller-type procedure (**28292**), which is the simple resection of the base of the proximal phalanx with removal of the medial eminence. A hemi implant is optional.

FIGURE 4-36 *Keller-Type Procedure*

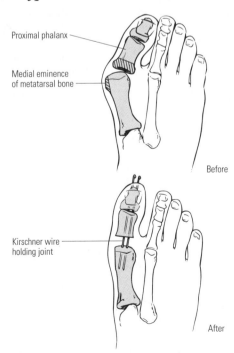

Proximal phalanx

Medial eminence of metatarsal bone

Before

Kirschner wire holding joint

After

Chapter 4

- Keller-Mayo procedure with Implant (**28293**), which is a total double stem implant, is usually used.

FIGURE 4-37 *Keller-Mayo Procedure with Implant*

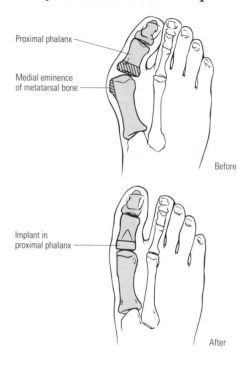

- Joplin procedure (**28294**), in which a tendon transplant is an important part of the procedure.

FIGURE 4-38 *Joplin Procedure*

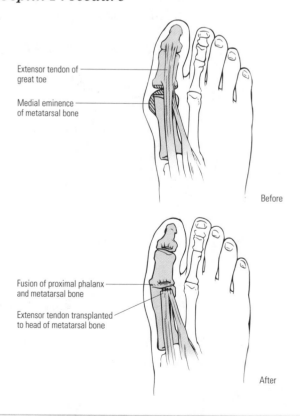

- Mitchell procedure (**28296**), which is a complex, biplanar, double step-cut osteotomy through the neck of the first metatarsal. Also called Mitchell Chevron (Austin) procedure.

FIGURE 4-39 *Mitchell Procedure*

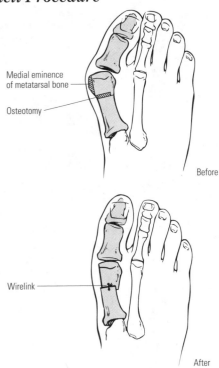

- Lapidus-Type procedure (**28297**), in which a metatarsocuneiform fusion of bones and a distal bunion repair are performed to correct a valgus deformity.

FIGURE 4-40 *Lapidus-Type Procedure*

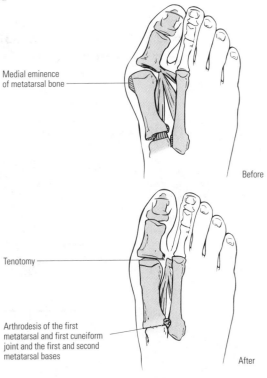

- Phalanx osteotomy (**28298**), which is the Akin procedure that involves removal of a bony wedge from the base of the proximal phalanx to reorient the axis.

FIGURE 4-41 *Phalanx Osteotomy*

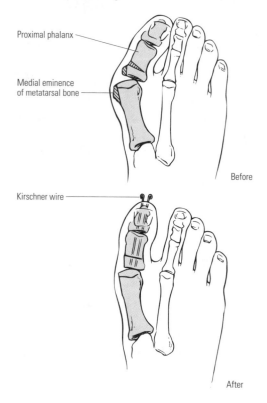

- Double osteotomy (**28299**), which is a technique that depicts both a medial resection of the first metatarsal with correction of the hallux valgus, and also a hallux valgus correction.

FIGURE 4-42A *Double Osteotomy*

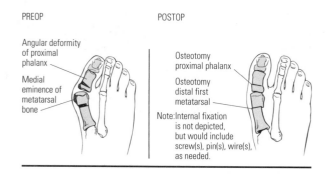

FIGURE 4-42B *Double Osteotomy*

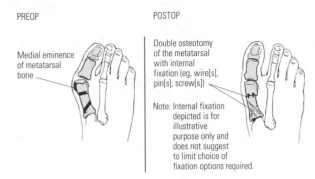

PREOP

POSTOP

Medial eminence of metatarsal bone

Double osteotomy of the metatarsal with internal fixation (eg, wire[s], pin[s], screw[s])

Note: Internal fixation depicted is for illustrative purpose only and does not suggest to limit choice of fixation options required.

All the codes in the **28290-28299** series include integral components when performed at the first MTP joint. The following procedures, therefore, are not reported separately:

- Capsulotomy
- Arthrotomy
- Synovial biopsy
- Neuroplasty
- Synovectomy
- Tendon release
- Tenotomy
- Tenolysis
- Excision of medial eminence
- Excision of associated osteophytes
- Placement of internal fixation
- Scar revision
- Articular shaving
- Removal of bursal tissue

Application of Casts and Strapping

The guidelines at the beginning of the Musculoskeletal System section in the CPT codebook indicate that the services listed include the application and removal of the first cast or traction device only. Subsequent replacement of a cast and/or traction device may require an additional listing with the **29000-29799** series of codes from the Application of Casts and Strapping subsection. These codes have specific guidelines pertaining to their use. It is important to develop a good understanding of these guidelines to appropriately code for the application of casts and strapping. Application of casts and strapping may be reported for the following:

- A replacement cast or strapping procedure during or after the period of normal follow-up care
- An initial service performed without restorative treatment or procedures to stabilize or protect a fracture, injury, or dislocation and/or to relieve pain

- An initial cast or strapping service when no other treatment or procedure is performed or expected to be performed by the same physician
- An initial cast or strapping service when another physician provides a restorative treatment or procedure(s)

The following are two questions to consider before reporting an initial cast or strapping with a casting and strapping code:

1. Will any restorative treatment or procedure(s) (eg, surgical repair, closed or open reduction of a fracture or joint dislocation) be performed, or is treatment expected to be performed?
2. Will the same physician assume all subsequent fracture, dislocation, or injury care?

Answering these questions will assist in establishing a good basis for deciding whether the casts and strapping codes should be reported.

> ### ✓ Check Your Knowledge
>
> **5.** What questions should you ask yourself when trying to establish whether the casts and strapping codes should be reported?

Endoscopy/Arthroscopy

Codes **29800-29999** are used to report endoscopic and arthroscopic musculoskeletal procedures. (See Figure 4-43) The guidelines at the beginning of this category of codes in the CPT codebook indicate that surgical arthroscopy always includes a diagnostic arthroscopy, as the diagnostic arthroscopy is considered an integral component of surgical arthroscopy.

When an arthroscopy of the knee (**29870-29887**) is performed, the portal incisions are made on either side of the patellar tendon and compartments of the knee are examined using the arthroscope and a probe. Additional treatment is performed as needed. (See Figure 4-44.) When an arthroscopy of the ankle (**29894-29899**) is performed, incisions are made allowing the ankle to be examined using the arthroscope and a probe. Additional treatment is performed as needed. (See Figure 4-45.)

General guidelines for coding endoscopic and arthroscopic procedures are as follows:

- The coder should look up *endoscopy, arthroscopy,* or *laparoscopy* in the index and locate the organ or system being examined or treated with a scope.
- The codes in that system or organ section should be reviewed to find an endoscopy, arthroscopy, or laparoscopy heading.
- If there is no endoscopy, arthroscopy, or laparoscopy heading in that section, a code with a descriptor that includes the suffix "-oscopy" and describes the procedure performed should be selected.

FIGURE 4-43 *Arthroscopy, Shoulder, Distal Claviculectomy (Mumford Procedure)*

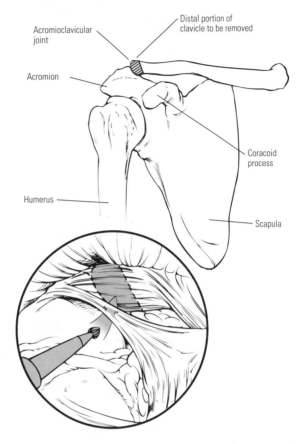

Acromioclavicular joint

Distal portion of clavicle to be removed

Acromion

Coracoid process

Humerus

Scapula

FIGURE 4-44 *Arthroscopy of the Knee*

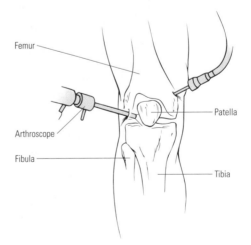

Femur

Patella

Arthroscope

Fibula

Tibia

FIGURE 4-45 *Arthroscopy of the Ankle*

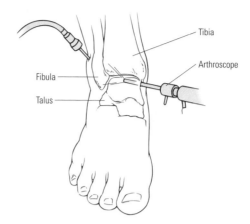

- If there is no heading for endoscopy, arthroscopy, or laparoscopy or there is no specific code mentioning the use of an endoscope in its descriptor, the codes described in that section are for open surgical procedures and should not be used to report a procedure using an endoscopic approach.
- The physician should be asked to clarify that the procedure was performed with an endoscope or laparoscope.
- If there is no specific code for the endoscopy/arthroscopy/laparoscopy procedure in question, the unlisted procedure code in the Endoscopy/Arthroscopy subsection is used to report the procedure. When an unlisted code is reported, a copy of the operative report should be submitted to the insurance company when the claim is filed.

✓ Check Your Knowledge Answers

1. subcutaneous soft tissue tumors, fascial or subfascial soft tissue tumors, radical resection of soft tissue tumors, and radical resection of bone tumors

2. There are three types of fracture treatments.

   i. Closed treatment of a fracture or dislocation specifically means that the fracture or dislocation site is not surgically opened.

   ii. Open treatment means that the fracture is surgically opened and visualized to allow internal fixation.

   iii. *Percutaneous Skeletal Fixation* is neither open nor closed. The fracture fragments are not visualized, but fixation (eg, with pins) is placed across the fracture site, usually under X-ray imaging.

3. • Without manipulation
   • With manipulation
   • With or without traction

4. No, the intraoperative services includes deep bone biopsy (code **20225**). An exclusionary parenthetical note following **22525** instructs to preclude the use of the deep bone biopsy code **20225** with the vertebral augmentation codes **22523-22525**.

5. **a.** Will any restorative treatment or procedure(s) (eg, surgical repair, closed or open reduction of a fracture or joint dislocation) be performed, or is treatment expected to be performed?

   b. Will the same physician assume all subsequent fracture, dislocation, or injury care?

Musculoskeletal System Exercises

Check your answers in Appendix B.

True or False

1. It would be appropriate to report code **20552**, *Injection(s); single or multiple trigger point(s), 1 or 2 muscle(s),* for each injection if four injections were performed. **True or False**
2. The codes in the Musculoskeletal System subsection are for the reporting of procedures involving tendons, muscles, fractures and dislocations, spine surgery, bunions, and casting and strapping. **True or False**
3. Surgical endoscopy/arthroscopy always includes a diagnostic endoscopy/arthroscopy. **True or False**
4. When reporting code **22523**, *Percutaneous vertebral augmentation, including cavity creation (fracture reduction and bone biopsy included when performed) using mechanical device, 1 vertebral body, unilateral or bilateral cannulation (eg, kyphoplasty); thoracic,* it is appropriate to report fracture reduction and bone biopsy separately. **True or False**
5. It would not be appropriate to report tenotomy separately when performing codes **28290-28299** at the first metatarsophalangeal (MTP). **True or False**

Matching

6. Cervical vertebrae (C1-7) _____
7. Sacral vertebrae (S1-5) _____
8. Thoracic vertebrae (T1-12) _____
9. Coccygeal vertebrae (coccyx) _____
10. Lumbar vertebrae (L1-5) _____
    a. the sacrum
    b. lower back
    c. neck area
    d. upper back area
    e. the tailbone

Multiple Choice: How Are the Following Procedures Coded?

11. Arthroscopic lateral and medial meniscectomy on the right knee.
    a. 29870
    b. 29871
    c. 29880
    d. None of the above

12. A patient had surgery that involved a posterior approach for a thoracic spinal arthrodesis with a local bone graft.
    a. 20931, 22614
    b. 20936, 22610
    c. 22600, 20936
    d. None of the above

13. Closed treatment of a fractured great toe, without manipulation.
    a. 28510
    b. 28490
    c. 28415
    d. None of the above

14. Open reduction and internal fixation of the right calcaneus.
    a. 28300
    b. 28292
    c. 28285
    d. None of the above

15. A diagnostic arthroscopy of the right elbow was performed.
    a. 24363
    b. 24100
    c. 29830
    d. None of the above

16. Reconstruction of webbed toe with skin graft.
    a. 28345
    b. 26551
    c. 20973
    d. None of the above

17. Fracture of the shaft of femur repair with screws.
    a. 27244
    b. 27507
    c. 27514
    d. None of the above

18. Open osteochondral autograft of knee.
    a. 29866
    b. 28966
    c. 27416
    d. None of the above

19. Surgical treatment is performed for a patient who has sustained a humeral shaft fracture. The orthopedic surgeon performs open treatment of the fracture by using an intramedullary implant and locking screws. After the surgical procedure, a cast is applied. Assign the appropriate code(s).

    a. 25526

    b. 24516

    c. 23600

    d. None of the above

Surgery: Respiratory System

Section Objectives

- Recognize the differences in the Respiratory subsection
- Understand the Respiratory System guidelines

The Respiratory System subsection is divided into the following five anatomic sites (See Figures 4-46 and 4-47):

1. Nose
2. Accessory Sinuses
3. Larynx
4. Trachea and Bronchi
5. Lungs and Pleura

Consistent with other subsections of the CPT codebook, the Respiratory System also includes an Endoscopy subsection for each anatomic site where an endoscopic approach is applicable. It is important to note that surgical endoscopy **always** includes diagnostic endoscopy when performed by the same physician.

FIGURE 4-46 *Paranasal Sinuses*

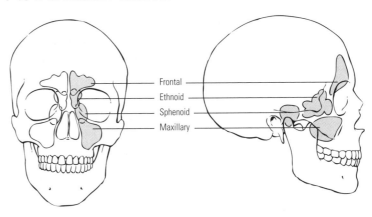

Frontal
Ethnoid
Sphenoid
Maxillary

FIGURE 4-47 *Respiratory System*

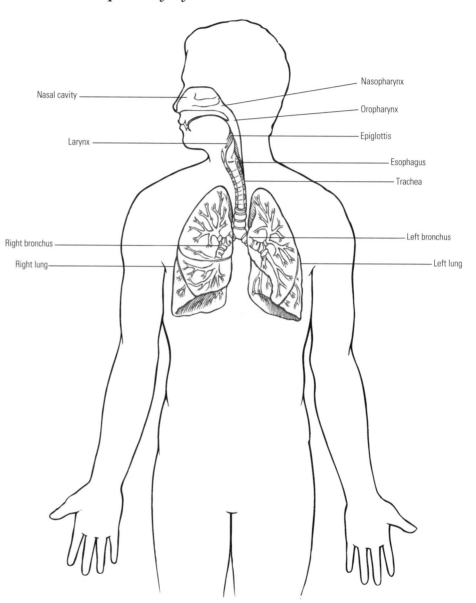

Nose

Within each of the five anatomic sites, there are subsections that organize the codes further. For example, under the first anatomic site, Nose, the following subheadings are categorized by the type of procedure performed:

- Incision
- Excision
- Introduction
- Removal of Foreign Body
- Repair
- Destruction
- Other Procedures

When selecting a code, look for the type of procedure performed under the correct anatomic site. For example, the treatment of inferior turbinate hypertrophy may be performed by excision (**30130**, **30140**) or by destruction (**30801**, **30802**). These are in different subsections of the anatomic site of the nose. In other words, if only looking under the subheading Excision for the term inferior turnibate, coders would miss the other inferior turbinate codes for the nose listed under the Destruction subheading. These codes clarify widespread usage specific to inferior turbinates. Code **30130** describes excision of partial or complete inferior turbinate only, whereas code **30140** describes submucous resection of inferior turbinate. The excision or submucous resection of the superior and middle turbinate is reported with the unlisted code **30999**. Codes **30801** and **30802** are reported for destruction procedures on the inferior turbinate mucosa via cautery and/or ablation. For cautery and ablation of superior or middle turbinates, report the unlisted code **30999** as well.

Coding Tip

Codes **30130** and **30140** are unilateral, so if these procedures are performed bilaterally, the modifier **50** would be appended. Codes **30801** and **30802** are bilateral and would not have the modifier **50** appended.

Coding Tip

Code **30465** is reported for a bilateral procedure. If a unilateral procedure is performed, Modifier **52**, *Reduced Services,* should be appended. (See Figure 4-48.)

✓ Check Your Knowledge

1. When selecting the correct code for the nose, look for the _____, under the correct anatomic site.

Accessory Sinuses

Codes **31231-31297** are reported for nasal sinus endoscopy procedures. The physician uses a nasal/sinus endoscope to visualize the interior of the nasal cavity and the middle and superior meatus, the turbinates,

FIGURE 4-48 *Surgical Repair of Vestibular Stenosis*

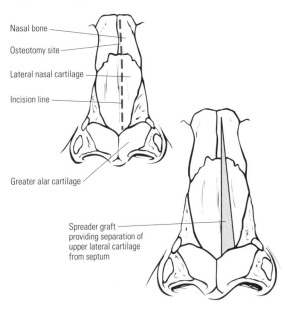

Nasal bone

Osteotomy site

Lateral nasal cartilage

Incision line

Greater alar cartilage

Spreader graft providing separation of upper lateral cartilage from septum

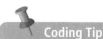

Key Terms

- Indirect laryngoscopy
- Direct laryngoscopy
- Flexible laryngoscopy

Coding Tip

Sinus endoscopy codes **31233-31297** are used to report unilateral procedures, unless otherwise specified, and if performed bilaterally would be appended with the modifier **50**.

A separate code should not be assigned when diagnostic evaluation is performed on different areas.

and the spheno-ethmoid recess. The procedure may either be diagnostic (**31231-31235**) or surgical (**31237-31297**). The documentation in the medical record should be carefully reviewed to determine the extent of the procedure before selecting the CPT code.

It is important to note that a surgical sinus endoscopy **includes** a sinusotomy (when appropriate) and diagnostic endoscopy. The codes **31231-31235** for diagnostic evaluation refer to employing a nasal/ sinus endoscope to inspect the interior of the nasal cavity and the middle and superior meatus, the turbinates, and the spheno-ethmoid recess. Any time a diagnostic evaluation is performed, all of these areas would be inspected and a separate code would not be reported for each area. Codes **31295-31297** describe dilation of sinus ostia by displacement of tissue, any method, and include fluoroscopy if performed. (See Figure 4-49.)

Larynx

Codes **31505-31579** describe laryngoscopy procedures. These procedures allow the physician to visualize the larynx, or voice box, for any abnormalities. The laryngoscopy can be performed for diagnostic purposes (**31505, 31520-31526, 31575,** and **31579**) or surgical/therapeutic purposes (**31510-31515, 31527-31571,** and **31576-31578**).

When selecting the appropriate laryngoscopy code to report, it is also important to distinguish between the type of laryngoscope used (indirect, direct, or flexible). **Indirect laryngoscopy** involves the use

FIGURE 4-49 *Sinus Endoscopy*

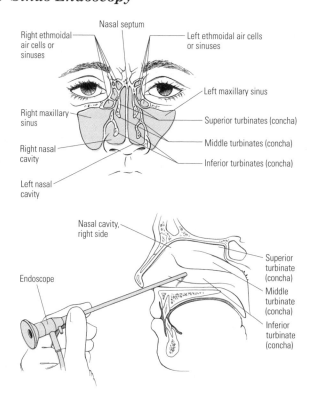

of a mirror to visualize the larynx (meaning the larynx is not directly visualized) or the use of a rigid telescope, if used indirectly. Indirect laryngoscopy is reported with codes **31505-31513**. **Direct laryngoscopy** is performed with a lighted scope placed into the larynx to allow direct visualization of the larynx. Magnification may be performed with a telescope or by operating a microscope through this scope. Direct laryngoscopy is reported with codes **31515-31571**. Laryngoscopy performed with a flexible fiberoptic laryngoscope is reported with codes in the **31575-31578** series. Whereas laryngeal stroboscopy, code **31579**, may be performed with either a rigid **or** flexible laryngoscope.

Key Terms

Indirect laryngoscopy: A procedure in which a mirror is used to visualize the larynx or the use of a rigid telescope.

Direct laryngoscopy: A procedure in which a lighted scope is placed into the larynx to allow direct visualization of the larynx. Magnification may be performed with a telescope or by operating a microscope through this scope.

Flexible laryngoscopy: A procedure in which a flexible fiberoptic laryngoscope is used.

Coding Tip

Surgical laryngoscopy includes diagnostic laryngoscopy. Therefore, when both are performed, only the surgical laryngoscopy should be reported.

Trachea and Bronchi

A bronchoscopy consists of a rigid or flexible bronchoscope being inserted through the oropharynx, vocal cords, and beyond the trachea into the right/left bronchi. Bronchoscopies are reported with codes in the **31622-31656** series. Bronchoscopy is considered an inherently bilateral procedure, and would not be appended with the modifier **50**. All of the codes in the **31622-31656** series include fluoroscopic guidance during the procedure. Therefore, a separate code would not be reported for fluoroscopy in conjunction with bronchoscopy. Different codes are available to describe various procedures performed using bronchoscopy. These include the following three distinctly different types of biopsies:

1. Bronchial mucosal biopsies (**31625**), which are taken by direct vision and can be reported only once, even if performed at different anatomic sites.
2. Transbronchial lung biopsies (**31628**), which are lung biopsies taken peripherally with fluoroscopic guidance of the biopsy forceps and should be reported only once regardless of how many transbronchial lung biopsies are performed in a lobe. However, when the biopsies are taken from different lobes, this represents new procedures with independent risk factors including biopsy forceps location of the lesion, bleeding, pneumothorax, air embolism, etc.

Coding Tip

It is important to note that bronchoscopy codes **31615-31629, 31634, 31635,** and **31645-31656** include conscious sedation as an inherent component of the procedure, and therefore, conscious sedation would not be reported separately. These codes are identified in the CPT codebook with the conscious sedation symbol (⊙) and can be found in Appendix G of the CPT codebook. For additional information on Appendix G, please refer to Chapter 11.

3. Transbronchial needle aspiration biopsies (**31629**), which are taken centrally by penetration of a large airway with a specially designed biopsy needle and aspiration of a lymph node or central mass lesion. This represents a less invasive approach than an open procedure for a surgical biopsy.

Add-on code ✚**31632** is intended to describe performance of transbronchial lung biopsy in each additional lobe, and **31633** describes the needle aspiration biopsies in each additional lobe after the initial lobar needle aspiration procedure. While these add-on codes may be reported for each biopsy in a separate lobe, parenthetical instructions direct coders that it would be inappropriate to report multiple biopsies or aspirations within the same lobe, as codes ✚**31632** and ✚**31633** should be reported only once regardless of how many transbronchial needle aspiration lung biopsies are performed in a lobe. Some possible sites for a bronchoscopic biopsy include the upper airway, which extends from the vocal cords to the lobar bronchi; each of the five lobes of the lungs and their bronchi; the right upper, middle, and lower lobes; and the left upper and lower lobes. (See Figure 4-50.)

✓ Check Your Knowledge

2. When performing numerous transbronchial needle aspiration lung biopsies in the same lobe, how many times may the add-on codes ✚**31622** and ✚**31633** be reported?

FIGURE 4-50 *Bronchoscopy*

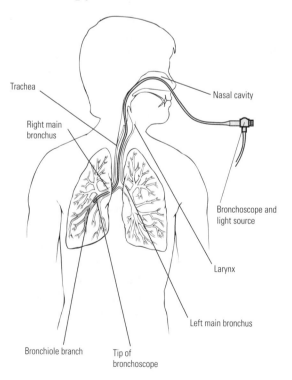

Lungs and Pleura

Thoracentesis is a procedure where accumulated fluid or air is removed from the pleural space by puncturing space between the ribs and is reported with codes **32421** and **32422**. Code **32422** represents a component procedure of the larger procedure and therefore should not be reported separately in addition to the chest wall codes (**19260**, **19271**, and **19272**) and apical tumor resection codes (**32503** and **32504**). If imaging guidance is performed with thoracentesis codes, then it would be appropriate to report one of the Radiology codes for fluoroscopic guidance in addition (eg, **76942**, **77002**, **77012**). (See Figure 4-51.)

Lung Transplantation (32850-32856)

The Lung Transplantation guidelines describe the three distinct components of physician work involved in **lung allotransplantation**, which are cadaver donor pneumonectomy, backbench work, and recipient lung allotransplantation.

1. **Cadaver donor pneumonectomy(s)**, which include(s) harvesting the allograft and cold preservation of the allograft (perfusing with cold preservation solution and cold maintenance) (**32850**).
2. **Backbench work**:
   a. Preparation of a cadaver donor single lung allograft prior to transplantation, including dissection of the allograft from surrounding soft tissues to prepare the pulmonary venous/atrial cuff, pulmonary artery, and bronchus unilaterally (**32855**).
   b. Preparation of a cadaver donor double lung allograft prior to transplantation, including dissection of the allograft from surrounding soft tissues to prepare the pulmonary venous/atrial cuff, pulmonary artery, and bronchus bilaterally (**32856**).
3. **Recipient lung allotransplantation**, which includes transplantation of a single or double lung allograft and care of the recipient (**32851-32854**).

Code **32855** is reported for a unilateral procedure, so if performed bilaterally, modifier **50** would be appended to it. Code **32856** is reported

FIGURE 4-51 *Thoracentesis*

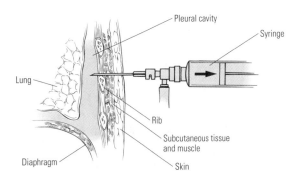

for a bilateral procedure, and would not require the appending of modifier **50**.

Code **32850** does not include the preparation and maintenance of cadaver allograft, as this work is separately reportable with the two new backbench preparation codes (**32855**, **32856**). The parenthetical note following bilateral backbench code **32856** instructs that for repair or resection procedures on the donor lung, use codes **32491**, **32500**, **35216**, or **35276**.

> ## ✓ Check Your Knowledge Answers
>
> 1. type of procedure performed
> 2. Add-on codes **+31632** and **+31633** should be reported only once regardless of how many transbronchial needle aspiration lung biopsies are performed in a lobe.

Respiratory System Exercises

Check your answers in Appendix B.

True or False

1. Surgical sinus endoscopy does not include sinusotomy and diagnostic endoscopy. **True or False**
2. When diagnostic endoscopy code **31231** is performed bilaterally, it is appended with the modifier **50**. **True or False**
3. Trachea and Bronchi Endoscopy codes **31615-31629** may be reported with the anesthesia codes for conscious sedation. **True or False**
4. If a backbench preparation procedure for lung transplantation is performed unilaterally, code **32856** may be reported with the modifier **52**, *Reduced services*. **True or False**. Explain why.

Short Answer

5. When surgical endoscopy code **31237** is performed bilaterally, how is it reported?
6. When performing direct diagnostic larynoscopy, would code **31505** be reported? Indicate either yes or no and why.

Choose the Correct Code for the Following Procedure Report

7. **History:** A 68-year-old female had peripheral alveolar infiltrates in the right lower lobes that had been unchanged for six weeks. **Procedure:** Once the patient was properly sedated and locally anesthetized, the oxygen was turned up to 5 L/min. A fiberoptic bronchoscope was inserted through the nostril, visualizing the upper airways to the vocal cords. The vocal cords were visualized and observed for function. The bronchoscope was advanced into the

trachea, and all the airways were inspected. Forceps were advanced through the suction channel of the bronchoscope into the right lower-lobe bronchus, leading to the infiltrate.

A fluoroscope was activated, and the biopsy forceps were advanced into the infiltrate, then backed off by 1 to 2 cm. Under fluoroscopic guidance, the forceps were opened, a transbronchial biopsy was obtained on expiration, and the forceps were removed. Three to six biopsies were obtained in one lobe with fluoroscopic guidance. The bronchoscope was withdrawn from the airways, carefully visualizing the trachea, and then withdrawn from the patient. The chest was inspected for a pneumothorax with the fluoroscope. The biopsies were placed in formalin and sent to pathology. How is this procedure reported?

8. **History:** A 50-year-old female with Stage IV (metastatic) adenocarcinoma of the left lower lobe developed shortness of breath and left lower lobe atelectasis from progressive endobronchial tumor growth seen on serial CT scans. At bronchoscopy, following dilation a stent was placed in the left lower lobe bronchus.

Procedure: A rigid bronchoscope was advanced to the stenotic area. A dilation catheter was placed through the bronchoscope into the small opening in the tumor mass and was threaded distally to just beyond the tumor mass under fluoroscopy. The dilating catheter was removed, and a guidewire was inserted through the bronchoscope into the now patent trachea. The bronchoscope was removed, leaving the guidewire in place, and the stent catheter was manipulated over the guidewire into the previously stenotic area. The bronchoscope was again inserted, and the area was visualized both through the bronchoscope and by fluoroscopy. Two metal markers were taped to the external chest wall under fluoroscopy. The stent was then deployed using both the markers for fluoroscopic guides and under direct vision by the physician using the bronchoscope. How is this procedure reported?

Surgery: Cardiovascular System*

Section Objectives

- Understand the Cardiovascular System guidelines
- Understand coding for different pacemaker systems
- Understand coding for coronary artery bypass procedures

The Cardiovascular System section of the CPT codebook contains codes for reporting procedures of the heart and pericardium, arteries, and veins. (See Figures 4-52 and 4-53.)

The focus of this chapter is on guidelines associated with certain techniques (eg, epicardial, transcatheter, thoracotomy, sternotomy, open, endovascular) and technology (eg, endovascular modular grafts, pacing cardioverter defibrillators, permanent pacemakers) used to perform diagnostic and therapeutic procedures of the heart and lungs and peripheral and coronary vascular systems. (See Figures 4-54 and 4-55.)

FIGURE 4-52 *Basic Vascular Anatomy of the Heart*

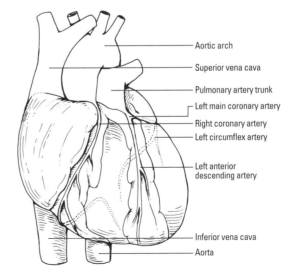

- Aortic arch
- Superior vena cava
- Pulmonary artery trunk
- Left main coronary artery
- Right coronary artery
- Left circumflex artery
- Left anterior descending artery
- Inferior vena cava
- Aorta

*Please see *CPT 2012* codebook for updates on codes and/or code descriptors.

FIGURE 4-53 *Basic Anatomical Structures of the Heart*

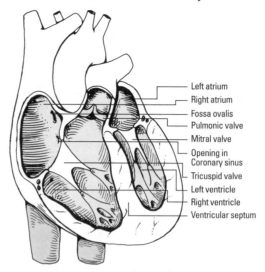

- Left atrium
- Right atrium
- Fossa ovalis
- Pulmonic valve
- Mitral valve
- Opening in Coronary sinus
- Tricuspid valve
- Left ventricle
- Right ventricle
- Ventricular septum

FIGURE 4-54 *Blood Flow Through the Heart and Lungs*

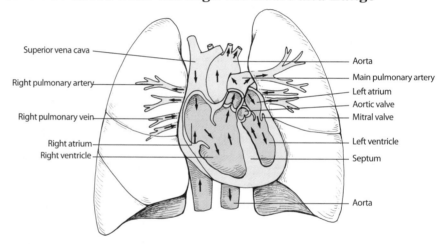

- Superior vena cava
- Right pulmonary artery
- Right pulmonary vein
- Right atrium
- Right ventricle
- Aorta
- Main pulmonary artery
- Left atrium
- Aortic valve
- Mitral valve
- Left ventricle
- Septum
- Aorta

FIGURE 4-55 *Anterior View of the Heart*

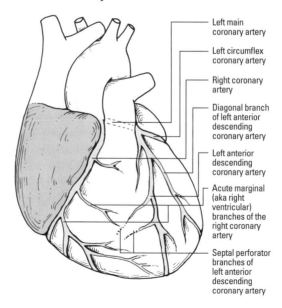

- Left main coronary artery
- Left circumflex coronary artery
- Right coronary artery
- Diagonal branch of left anterior descending coronary artery
- Left anterior descending coronary artery
- Acute marginal (aka right ventricular) branches of the right coronary artery
- Septal perforator branches of left anterior descending coronary artery

Pacemaker Systems

A pacemaker system includes a pulse generator (containing electronics and a battery) and one or more electrodes (leads). The pulse generator is placed in a subcutaneous pocket created either in an infraclavicular site or underneath the abdominal muscles just below the ribcage. Electrodes (leads) may be inserted through a vein (transvenous) or placed on the surface of the heart (epicardial). Epicardial placement of electrodes requires a thoracotomy or sternotomy.

In addition to the various placement methods, different types of systems may also be inserted. A single-chamber pacemaker system includes a pulse generator and one electrode inserted in either the atrium or the right ventricle. A dual-chamber pacemaker system involves the insertion of electrodes into both the atrium and the right ventricle that are then connected to a pulse generator capable of pacing and sensing both the atrium and the ventricle. (See Figures 4-56 and 4-57.)

In certain circumstances, an additional electrode may be required to achieve pacing of the left ventricle (bi-ventricular pacing).

Coding Tip

For single- and dual-chamber pacemaker systems, epicardial placement of the electrode should be separately reported using **33202** and **33203**.

FIGURE 4-56 *Implanted Pacemaker (33212)*

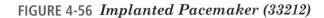

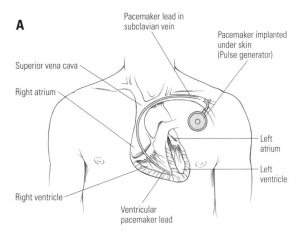

FIGURE 4-57 *Implanted Pacemaker (33213-33214)*

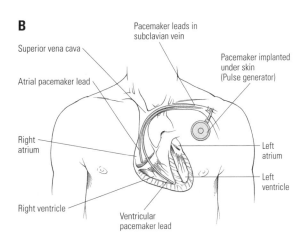

Chapter 4

Biventricular pacing systems (see Figure 4-58) are used when pacing of the left ventricle is required in addition to pacing of the right ventricle. The implant procedure for the biventricular system is similar to that of a single- or dual-chamber system, with the additional complexity of the transvenous placement of the lead in a cardiac vein to reach the left ventricle. Implantation of a biventricular system requires a coronary guide catheter and the use of venography to guide the lead through the coronary sinus and into a cardiac vein for placement in the left ventricle. In this event, transvenous (cardiac vein) placement of the electrode should be separately reported using code **33224** or code **33225**.

EXAMPLE

A permanent pacemaker system (generator and electrode[s]) is removed, and a pacing cardioverter-defibrillator system is replaced (at the same operation). (See Figure 4-58.)

In the instance in which a permanent pacemaker system (pulse generator and electrode[s]) is removed and replaced with a pacing cardioverter-defibrillator system (at the same operation), codes **33233**, **33234**, or **33235** would be reported in addition to code **33249**. The assessment and reassessment of the pacing cardioverter-defibrillator electrodes related to sensing, pacing and electrode impedance characteristics at the time of insertion, repair, revision, or replacement is additionally reported using codes **93640** and **93641**.

✓ Check Your Knowledge

1. Describe what a pacemaker system is.

FIGURE 4-58 *Biventricular Pacing*

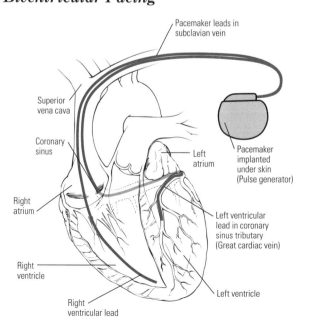

Pacemaker leads in subclavian vein

Superior vena cava

Coronary sinus

Left atrium

Pacemaker implanted under skin (Pulse generator)

Right atrium

Left ventricular lead in coronary sinus tributary (Great cardiac vein)

Right ventricle

Left ventricle

Right ventricular lead

Coding Tip

The assessment and reassessment of the pacing cardioverter-defibrillator electrodes related to sensing, pacing, and electrode impedance character-istics at the time of insertion, repair, revi-sion, or replacement are additionally reported using codes **93640** and **93641**.

Coding Tip

For pacing cardioverter-defibrillator systems, epicardial placement of the electrode should be separately reported using **33202** and **33203**.

Pacing Cardioverter-Defibrillator Systems

The combination pacing cardioverter-defibrillator ICD (system) is designed to recognize and provide antitachycardia pacing, low-energy cardioversion or defibrillating shocks to treat ventricular tachycardia or ventricular fibrillation. A pacing cardioverter-defibrillator system includes a pulse generator and electrodes, although pacing cardioverter-defibrillators may require multiple leads, even when only a single chamber is being paced. A pacing cardioverter-defibrillator sys-tem may be inserted in a single chamber (pacing in the ventricle) or in dual chambers (pacing in the atrium and ventricle). Pacing cardioverter-defibrillator pulse generators may be implanted in a subcutaneous infraclavicular pocket or in an abdominal pocket. Removal of a pacing cardioverter-defibrillator pulse generator requires opening of the exist-ing subcutaneous pocket and disconnecting the pulse generator from its electrode(s). A thoracotomy (or laparotomy in the case of abdominally placed generators) is not required to remove the pulse generator.

The electrodes (leads) of a pacing cardioverter-defibrillator system are positioned in the heart via the venous system (transvenously) in most circumstances. However, in certain circumstances an additional electrode may be required to achieve pacing of the left ventricle (biven-tricular pacing). In this event, transvenous (cardiac vein) placement of the electrode should be separately reported using code **33224** or **33225**. Epicardial placement of the electrode should be separately reported using code **33202-33203.**

The appropriate codes should be used in addition to the thoracotomy or endoscopic epicardial lead placement codes to report the insertion of the generator if done by the same physician during the same session.

Epicardial Lead Placement

Electrode positioning on the epicardial surface of the heart requires thoracotomy, or thoracoscopic placement of the leads. Removal of electrode(s) may first be attempted by transvenous extraction. However, if transvenous extraction is unsuccessful, a thoracotomy may be required to remove the electrodes. Use the appropriate codes in addi-tion to the thoracotomy or endoscopic epicardial lead placement codes to report the insertion of the generator if done by the same physician during the same session.

EXAMPLE

Removal of a permanent epicardial pacemaker and electrodes is performed via thoracotomy.

Codes **33236-33238** describe the removal of a pacemaker pulse generator and pacing electrodes via thoracotomy for epicardial single-chamber systems, epicardial dual-chamber systems, or per-manent transvenous electrode systems. Removal of a single-lead system (**33236**) requires exposure of a small area of the heart. Removal of a dual-lead system (**33237**) usually requires more extensive exposure. The procedure described by code **33238** is used

Chapter 4

in cases in which an infected transvenous lead has to be removed but attempts to remove it by the usual mechanisms (ie, **33234**) are unsuccessful. For a failed attempt at transvenous extraction, it would be appropriate to use **33244 52** in addition to code **33238**.

Electrophysiologic Operative Procedures

Supraventricular arrhythmias originate above the bundle of His. Surgical treatment of atrial fibrillation or flutter may be performed by either open incision (**33254-33256**) or endoscopic approach (**33265-33266**). These families of codes describe the surgical treatment of supraventricular dysrhythmias (no rhythm). Tissue ablation, disruption, and reconstruction can be accomplished by many methods including surgical incision or through the use of a variety of energy sources (eg, radiofrequency, cryotherapy, microwave, ultrasound, laser). If excision or isolation of the left atrial appendage by any method including stapling, oversewing, ligation, or plication is performed in conjunction with any of the atrial tissue ablation and reconstruction (maze) procedures (**33254-33259**, **33265**, and **33266**), it is considered part of the procedure and not reported separately.

Limited operative ablation and reconstruction (**33254** and **33265**) is the surgical isolation of triggers of supraventricular dysrhythmias by operative ablation that isolates the pulmonary veins or other anatomically defined triggers in the left or right atrium. Code **33254** describes a closed-heart operation for paroxysmal or short-duration atrial fibrillation/flutter using atrial incision(s) and adjunctive ablation techniques that are limited to the left atrium or do not extend to the atrioventricular annulus. Code **33265** describes a closed-heart endoscopic operation for paroxysmal or short-duration atrial fibrillation/flutter using atrial incision(s) and adjunctive ablation techniques that are limited to the left atrium or do not extend to the atrioventricular annulus.

Extensive operative ablation and reconstruction (**33255**, **33259**, and **33266**) includes both those services included in the limited service description and any additional ablation of atrial tissue to eliminate sustained supraventricular dysrhythmias. To be considered extensive, the procedure must include operative ablation that involves the right atrium, atrial septum, or left atrium in continuity with the atrioventricular annulus.

Coronary Artery Bypass Procedures

Coronary artery bypass graft procedures may be reported in three ways, depending upon the type of operation performed. The first two reporting methods require only a single code as follows:

Venous Grafting or Arterial Grafting

- A bypass operation performed with only venous grafts. This is reported with a single code from the **33510-33516** series, reflecting the number of distal anastomoses performed.
- A bypass operation performed with arterial grafts. This is reported with a single code from the **33533-33536** series, with code selection

again reflecting the number of distal anastomoses performed. The codes in this series are also used to report coronary artery bypass procedures with a combination of arterial and venous grafts.

Combined Arterial-Venous Grafting

- Bypass operations performed with a combination of venous and arterial grafts for distal anastomoses.

The third reporting method requires the use of two codes:

- A code to indicate that both arteries and veins were used (from the **33517-33523** series; the appropriate add-on code should describe the number of distal venous anastomoses used for the bypass)
- An arterial graft code to indicate the number of distal arterial anastomoses required for the bypass procedure (from the **33533-33536** series)

Codes in the combined arterial-venous grafting for coronary bypass series are not to be reported alone. The appropriate vein graft code from this series is used in conjunction with a code from the arterial grafting series to completely describe combined arterial-venous grafting for coronary bypass. As indicated by the symbol placed before each code, codes **33517-33523** are add-on codes and exempt from the use of modifier **51**.

Open Procurement of Graft Material

Open procurement of the saphenous vein graft is included in the description of work for the venous grafting and combined arterial-venous grafting for coronary artery bypass codes and should not be reported as a separate service or cosurgery. Additionally, arterial graft procurement is included in the description of work for the arterial grafting for coronary artery bypass codes and should not be reported as a separate service or cosurgery.

Open procurement of these three types of graft material is reported separately as follows:

Upper extremity vein: **+35500**
Femoropopliteal vein: **+35572**
Upper extremity artery: **35600**

Redo Operations

CPT code **33530** is an add-on code used to report coronary artery bypass or valve reoperation procedures performed more than one month after the original operation. It is not reported alone but is reported in addition to the appropriate code(s) to describe the bypass or valve procedure performed.

Component Coding

Many of the procedures in the Cardiovascular System subsection represent vascular interventions using "component coding." It is impossible to discuss all aspects of vascular services reporting in this chapter, but offered here are fundamental explanations for coding vascular interventional procedures.

To facilitate accurate coding, component coding was introduced to the CPT code set. The component system provides flexibility by allowing the freedom to appropriately combine procedural and imaging codes in a variety of ways to accurately describe the actual service rendered without requiring multiple duplicative codes. The proper use of the procedure codes for vascular interventions, both diagnostic and therapeutic, requires knowledge of vascular anatomy, the types of services performed, what is included in each code, and the coding conventions necessary when codes are used in combination.

Component coding is differentiated by vascular and nonvascular interventional procedures and allows for the proper description of image-guided procedures. It allows for the following:

- Accurate reporting when one or multiple providers perform different services to provide the total service
- Accurate tracking of professional services for outcome analysis, utilization review, and billing purposes
- Tracking and reporting of interventional radiological hospital services in a manner identical to that of other surgical and radiological services
- Fair relative valuation of similar types of services without regard to the specialty of the provider

Interventional Coding Conventions

For procedures reported using component codes, the surgical components of the service are described by the codes listed outside the **70000** series. The radiological or imaging services are described by **70000** series RS&I codes or the **90000** vascular ultrasound codes. Typically, one physician performs the entire interventional procedure, providing both the surgical component(s) and the imaging RS&I component(s). To completely describe the services rendered, the physician would report both the codes describing the surgical service and the imaging RS&I. Frequently, one provider performs the surgical component(s) and another performs the imaging RS&I component(s). In these instances, the physician performing the surgical component(s) reports the code(s) outside the **70000** series, whereas the physician responsible for the imaging RS&I reports the appropriate procedure code(s) from the **70000** series.

Vascular Injection Procedures

All vascular procedures, whether diagnostic or therapeutic, begin with establishing vascular access (vascular catheterization). The codes available for reporting the catheterization portion of the procedure are found in the Vascular Injection Procedures series of codes (**36000** series).

To code catheterization procedures correctly, it is necessary to become familiar with the anatomy of the vascular system. Primary vessels branch off the aorta. When the primary vessels branch out, these branches are secondary branches, and as the secondary branches split, there are tertiary branches, etc. In the arterial system, catheter placement in a primary branch is described as a *first order*

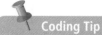

Coding Tip

Component coding allows for the flexibility of combining a diagnostic and a therapeutic examination on the same occasion without overstating or understating the services provided.

Coding Tip

To properly code catheterizations, the puncture site(s), vascular family or families, and final catheter position(s) must be known.

catheterization. The first order vessel is defined as selective catheterization of the first major branch off the main vessel (aorta).

Selective catheterization of a secondary branch is a *second order* catheterization, etc. A second order vessel is defined as a catheterization of the first major branch off a first order vessel. Likewise, a third order branch is the catheterization of a first major branch off a second order vessel. Each artery belongs to a *vascular family,* which is defined as a group of vessels (arteries) fed by a primary branch of the aorta or a primary branch of the vessel punctured. The five vascular systems considered for component coding are as follows:

- Systemic arterial
- Systemic venous
- Pulmonary
- Portal
- Lymphatic

Noncoronary vascular catheterization procedures are reported either using *selective* or *nonselective* catheter placement codes. *Selective* catheter placement involves more physician work and effort than nonselective catheterizations and increases complication risk to the target vessels. Selective catheterization typically involves the exchange of the catheter to a more flexible device that can be moved, manipulated, or guided into a part of the arterial system other than the aorta or the vessel punctured (usually under fluoroscopic guidance), most often using a guidewire. *Nonselective* catheter placement means the catheter or needle is placed directly into the major arterial conduit (not moved or manipulated farther into a branch) or is delivered only into the aorta (thoracic and abdominal) from any approach (puncture site).

A nonselective catheter placement is *not* coded in addition to a selective catheter placement when a single access (puncture) is used. Even if a nonselective catheter placement is performed first, the highest selective placement with each vascular family is the determining factor for the level of coding. This vessel may or may not be the most distal in absolute distance from the puncture site or the origin of the primary vessel. All lesser-order catheter placements in the same vascular family performed for the most selective catheter position to be achieved are included in the higher-order catheterization code.

Coding Tip

Nonselective arterial catheterization codes include **36100, 36120, 36140, 36147, 36148, 36160,** and **36200.** Selective arterial catheterization codes include **36215, 36216, 36217, ✚36218, 36245, 36246, 36247,** and **✚36248.**

Coding Tip

Even if a nonselective catheter placement is performed first, the highest selective placement with each vascular family is the determining factor for the level of coding.

✓ Check Your Knowledge

2. Which range of codes are selective and which are nonselective catherizations?

Frequently Asked Questions

What is the highest-order selective catheterization when a left middle cerebral catheterization is performed from a femoral artery approach?

Only the highest-order (third-order selective) code **36217** is reported for this scenario. The primary branch of the thoracic aorta is the left common carotid, the secondary branch is the left internal carotid, and

Chapter 4

the tertiary branch is the middle cerebral artery. If the catheter is pulled back into the common carotid or the proximal internal carotid and proximal internal carotid and the cervical left carotid is studied, the first- or second-order code is not used because the work of getting the catheter to this point would be included in the third-order selective code.

What if additional second- or third-order arterial catheterizations are performed in the same vascular family?

If more than one second- or third-order branch in a given vascular family is catheterized, the additional branch catheterization should be described by the use of add-on code **36218** (each additional second-, third-, or higher-order artery, thoracic or brachiocephalic branch) or add-on code **36248** (each additional second-, third-, or higher-order abdominal, pelvic, or lower extremity artery branch). If multiple selective catheterizations are performed in *different* vascular families, the highest level of selectivity is reported for each vascular family.

In the example given in the previous question, if the catheter was positioned into the left middle cerebral artery, **36217** is coded as described above. If the catheter is pulled back and then used to select the left external carotid artery and a selective external carotid arteriogram is performed, **36218** is coded as well, denoting an additional second-order selective catheterization in the same vascular family (left common carotid vascular family).

What if an additional vascular family is catheterized (ie, the left common carotid artery)?

If either the right internal carotid artery or middle cerebral artery is catheterized, then **36217** is used. This includes the more proximal arteries for the middle cerebral (including the common carotid and internal carotid). However, if the left common carotid artery is catheterized (an additional vascular family), a separate code with the highest-order catheter location in the additional family is reported. Code **36216** is also reported for this scenario.

What if more than one puncture site access is performed?

If two separate access procedures (two different punctures) are performed, each is treated separately for coding purposes. For example, if a nonselective catheter placement from one femoral artery puncture (ie, for an abdominal aortogram) and then a third-order selective catheterization from the contralateral femoral artery puncture are performed, then the nonselective code **36200** should be reported for the aortic catheter and **36247** for the third-order abdominal selective catheterization from the other puncture. (The second puncture should be clearly documented.) It is appropriate to add a modifier (eg, **59**) to **36200** to indicate that a separate access/distinct procedure was performed.

Are venous catheterizations described as selective and nonselective?

Yes. Venous catheterizations can be described as *selective* (requiring additional movement or manipulation of the catheter) or *nonselective* (direct placement of a catheter). The same vascular family concept as arterial procedures is used to describe venous catheterizations. Determination of first or second order is dependent upon the vein punctured. A venous vascular family includes a first-order vein and all of its secondary branches.

Coding Tip

Additional second-, third-, and higher-order arterial catheterizations within the same vascular family include ➕**36218** and ➕**36248**.

There are no codes for each additional second-, third-, or higher-order catheterization in the venous system. Therefore, the codes may be reported again to describe the total number of separate catheterizations performed (eg, **36011** with two units).

How is pulmonary angiography reported in the absence of diagnostic cardiac catheterization?

Pulmonary catheterization procedures may be performed independent of right heart catheterizations and the pulmonary angiography performed at that time (eg, **93501**, **93541**). There are only two vascular families: the right and left pulmonary arteries. Code **36014** or **36015** would be reported with modifier **50** appended to most correctly describe right and left pulmonary angiograms performed, because catheter placements were performed in both the right and left pulmonary arteries.

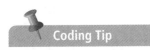

Coding Tip

Pulmonary angiography codes include **36013**, **36014**, and **36015**.

Aneurysm Repair Procedures

The Cardiovascular System subsection of Surgery in the CPT codebook includes four families of codes describing the various techniques for aneurysmal repair. An *aneurysm* is an abnormal bulging of a vessel, usually due to a weakness or thinning of the vessel wall at that location, caused by congenital or acquired weakness of the vessel wall. Because emergent treatment of ruptured aneurysms carries a very high morbidity and mortality rate, the obvious solution is to treat them electively before rupture.

Open Aneurysm Repair

Codes **35001-35152** describe the traditional method for treating aneurysms by direct (open surgical) repair of an aneurysm, pseudo-aneurysm, ruptured aneurysm, and associated occlusive disease directly at the aneurysm site (eg, abdominal aorta, hepatic, celiac, renal, iliac, subclavian artery).

EXAMPLE

Codes **35001-35152** are reported in the absence of any aneurysmal dilation in the presence of occlusive disease (ie, atherosclerotic plaque) causing diminished blood flow.

For direct vessel repairs associated with occlusive disease only, codes **35201-35286** should be reported. Code choice is dependent upon the anatomic site of the vessel and the type of repair performed.

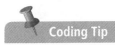

Coding Tip

The *target zone* is the region within the vessel where the endoprosthesis is intended to be deployed.

Endovascular Aneurysm Repair

Different methods now exist that do not require open dissection of the abdominal aorta to accomplish the repair. Endovascular aneurysm repair involves placing a prosthetic graft within the aneurysm to completely exclude the aneurysm sac from the general circulation. Placement involves the use of both surgical and catheter-based skills and technologies. Compared with conventional repair, the endoluminal approach is less invasive because it eliminates the need for laparotomy and cross-clamping of the aorta and iliac artery.

Although the end product of traditional and endovascular abdominal aortic aneurysm (AAA) repair is the same, the devices and techniques are entirely dissimilar.

EXAMPLE

This example describes application of component coding for endovascular aneurysm repair.

The CPT codes for endovascular repair of abdominal and thoracic aortic and iliac artery aneurysms reflect the various stages or steps in the procedure with device-specific codes for prosthesis placement. Often, a team approach is used in performing these procedures. Step-by-step coding allows for accurate coding in which skills of multiple physicians may be necessary, allowing each physician to report those services he or she performed. Whereas a single operator within the team may perform all aspects of a distinct portion of the procedure, other components of the procedure may be performed with the operators working in concert as co-surgeons.

To assist in understanding how multiple codes are required to report endovascular aneurysm repair, Figure 4-59 is provided as an example of the steps typically involved in abdominal aneurysm repair (under normal circumstances).

FIGURE 4-59 *Typical Steps of AAA Repair*

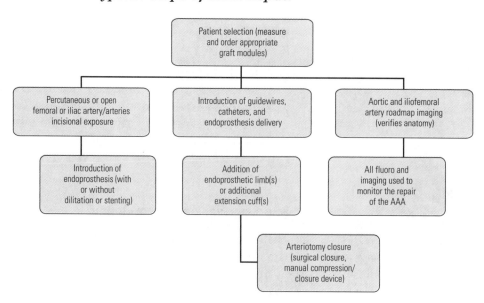

Endovascular Abdominal Aneurysm Repair

The codes for endovascular repair of AAA are intended to be used as component codes (to identify the specific services provided for the repair performed). (See Figure 4-60.) These codes can be separated into the following seven groups:

- Codes for open surgical exposure of the femoral arteries (less often the iliac arteries)
- Codes for RS&I
- Introduction of catheters/guidewires
- Primary repair codes
- Codes for extension prostheses
- Codes that identify less commonly performed but separately reportable maneuvers/interventional procedures
- Codes that identify "conversion" surgery

FIGURE 4-60 *Endovascular Repair of AAA*

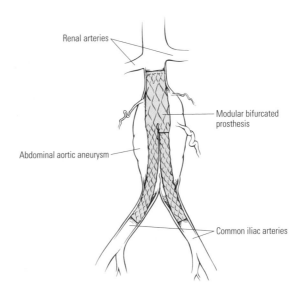

Renal arteries

Modular bifurcated prosthesis

Abdominal aortic aneurysm

Common iliac arteries

Coding Tip

All balloon angioplasty and/or stent deployment within the target treatment zone for the endoprosthesis, either before or after endograft deployment, for any reason, are not separately reportable.

EXAMPLE

This example describes catheter introduction into the aorta or an aortic branch (renal artery).

The introduction of catheters is reported separately in addition to device placement and should be reported according to regular coding conventions for catheterization procedures (see guidelines included in the CPT codebook for vascular injection procedures for more information regarding use of catheterization codes). Examples of catheterization codes may include the following:

- Aorta alone (no selective catheterization): **36200**
- Aorta bilateral (identifies accessing aorta via both legs): **36200** with modifier **50** appended
- Aorta and renal artery via different access points (both legs): **36200** and **36245**

Coding Tip

If the procedure requires extensive repair or replacement of an artery, this should also be reported separately (eg, **35226**, **35286**).

EXAMPLE

How to differentiate the types of prostheses placed in the procedures described by codes **34802** and **34803**?

The primary differences between the procedures described are the configuration, length, and shape of the prosthesis required for effective aneurysm treatment. To compare the procedures described by **34802** and **34803**, both procedures use modular components that attain an inverted-Y–shape following complete deployment. The primary difference between the procedures is the number of modular components that make up the device. The prosthesis repair procedure described by code **34802** involves two separate pieces that are joined inside the patient's body during placement, with the main body prosthesis component extending into the ipsilateral iliac artery and creating a distal seal. Code **34803** involves three components that are joined inside the patient during the procedure.

Other Procedures

In some circumstances, in addition to placing endovascular graft component(s), the repair provided may require placement of an occlusion device to close an iliac artery. This procedure is identified by the add-on code **34808**. In addition, to provide revascularization of the leg vessels that arise from the occluded iliac limb, a femoral-femoral bypass may be performed. When performed as part of an endorepair, the code for a femoral-femoral bypass graft is unique (**34813**). This additional bypass is separately reported using the add-on code **34813**. Because these are add-on codes, they should only be reported in addition to other repair services.

Endovascular Repair of Descending Thoracic Aorta

Codes **33880-33891** represent a family of procedures to report placement of an endovascular graft for repair of the descending thoracic aorta differentiated by the coverage (**33880**) or noncoverage (**33881**) of the subclavian artery. Endovascular prostheses for the descending aorta are obtained in modules. The first component of the endovascular repair is deployed such that the leading edge arrives in a nearly normal segment of the proximal aorta, allowing firm fixation. Subsequently, components are deployed through the diseased portion of aorta such that each partially overlaps the preceding one to prevent any leaks between the modules. The components are "tiled" in this fashion until the diseased portion of aorta is completely covered, and the distal-most component lies in normal aorta. Repairs may require one, two, three, or more modules, depending on the diseased descending thoracic aorta. These codes include all device introduction, manipulation, positioning, deployment, and ballooning/stenting done within the endograft.

The codes for endovascular repair of an aneurysm of the descending thoracic aorta are also intended to be used as component codes (to identify the specific services provided for the repair performed). These codes can be separated into the following six groups:

Coding Tip

Codes **33880** and **33881** include placement of all distal extensions, if required, in the distal thoracic aorta, whereas proximal extensions, if needed, are reported separately.

Coding Tip

Balloon angioplasty and/or stent deployment performed within the target zone of the endoprosthesis is not reported separately, regardless of whether performed before or after endograft deployment.

- Open surgical exposure of the femoral, iliac, or brachial arteries or abdominal aorta
- RS&I
- Introduction of catheters/guidewires
- Primary repair codes
- Extension prostheses
- Other interventional procedures separately reportable

Endovascular Repair of Iliac Aneurysm

In many cases, an AAA extends into the iliac artery. Isolated iliac artery aneurysms are less common than aortic aneurysms. In the absence of aortic aneurysm, endovascular repair of iliac artery aneurysm (IAA) involves a minimally invasive technique that eliminates the need for a large abdominal or retroperitoneal incision to expose the aneurysm.

The endovascular repair technique involves the access of femoral arteries either percutaneously or with open exposure, with introduction and advancement of a collapsed prosthesis through the iliac artery or arteries in the pelvis. The endograft is then positioned to cover the aneurysm using fluoroscopic guidance. Once in the correct location, positioned exactly across the aneurysm, the device is deployed, expanding the prosthesis to full size. The services that are inherent components of the endovascular IAA repair include balloon dilatation within the endoprosthesis to achieve full expansion of the graft and complete contact of the attachment devices necessary to properly secure the prosthesis.

The codes for endovascular repair of an IAA are also intended to be used as component codes (to identify the specific services provided for the repair performed). These codes can be separated into the following six groups:

- Open surgical exposure of the femoral or iliac arteries
- RS&I
- Introduction of catheters/guidewires
- Primary repair codes
- Extension prostheses
- Other interventional procedures separately reportable

How to Code Aneurysm Repair

Because a number of methods now exist to perform aneurysm repair, it is important to identify the codes that accurately describe the procedures performed. To address this, it may help to ask the following questions:

- Is the procedure an open "direct" aneurysm repair, or is it an endovascular repair?
- If an endovascular repair, was there open surgical exposure of an artery?
- What catheters were introduced into the aorta or aortic branches for the endovascular repair?
- What type of device was used for the endovascular repair?
- What RS&I was performed?

Chapter 4

- Were other separately reportable services provided?
- Which physician performed each component, and were some components of the procedure accomplished as cosurgeons or assistant surgeons?

Arteries and Veins: Thromboendarterectomy

Thromboendarterectomy is performed for treatment of severe stenosis of arteries, typically because of atherosclerosis. Severity of disease is related to gender, age, lipid status, family history, presence of diabetes, and tobacco abuse. Codes **35301-35381** describe open thromboendarterectomy procedures. Codes **35301-35306** describe thromboendarterectomy of the distinct vessels of the lower extremities, including the superficial femoral artery, the popliteal artery, the tibioperoneal trunk artery, and the tibial and peroneal arteries. In addition to code **35305** for the initial endarterectomy procedure of the tibial or peroneal branch artery, add-on code **35306** is used to report thromboendarterectomy of each additional tibial or peroneal artery in addition to the initial procedure.

It is not appropriate to report code **35500**, *Harvest of upper extremity vein, 1 segment, for lower extremity or coronary artery bypass procedure,* in addition to **35302-35306**, because harvest of a vein graft may be necessary to complete the procedure with a patch graft following the removal of plaque and the diseased portions of the artery and is included in this procedure.

EXAMPLE

Vein harvest, if performed, includes the following intraprocedural steps, thus precluding the additional reporting of code **35500**:

- Shift attention to the vein harvest site—usually predetermined and previously prepped.
- Incise the skin over the vein.
- Dissect through the soft tissue to find the vein.
- Carefully dissect out the vein, tying and dividing all side branches.
- Check the original operative site to ensure that a sufficient length of vein is exposed.
- Clamp the vein and excise the segment to be used for the patch.
- Ligate the transected ends of the vein that remain in the patient.
- Open and examine the removed segment of the vein on the back table to ensure suitability.
- Crop the vein to the shape required to serve as a patch.
- Preserve the vein patch in heparinized saline until it is time to be used.

Bypass Graft

Bypass grafts are traditionally described by including the inflow artery and the outflow target artery. Some clinical indications for performing bypass grafts are trauma or severe stenosis of arteries, typically

Chapter 4

because of atherosclerosis. Severity of disease is related to gender, age, lipid status, family history, presence of diabetes, and tobacco use.

Vein

Bypass grafts are traditionally described by including the inflow artery and the outflow target artery. Some clinical indications for performing bypass grafts are trauma or severe stenosis of arteries, typically because of atherosclerosis. Severity of disease is related to gender, age, lipid status, family history, presence of diabetes, and tobacco use. Codes **35501-35571** describe open surgical procedures that involve the use of venous material alone. Certain bypass graft codes from this family are discussed.

Code **35501** is reported for performance of bypass graft from the common carotid to the internal carotid on the same side of a person's neck (ie, a common carotid to ipsilateral internal carotid bypass graft). Code **35509** is intended to report bypass graft carotid bypass on the opposite side of the neck (ie, carotid-contralateral carotid bypass graft).

Code **35506** describes a carotid-subclavian bypass procedure using vein conduit. Aortoiliac bypass graft with vein (**35537**) and aortobi-iliac bypass graft with vein (**35538**) distinguish the effort required to perform each of these procedures.

Aortofemoral bypass with vein (**35539**) and aortobifemoral bypass graft with vein (**35540**) distinguish the effort required to perform each of these procedures.

✓ Check Your Knowledge Answers

1. A pacemaker system includes a pulse generator (containing electronics and a battery) and one or more electrodes (leads). The pulse generator is placed in a subcutaneous pocket created either in an infraclavicular site or underneath the abdominal muscles just below the ribcage.

2. Nonselective arterial catheterization codes include **36100**, **36120**, **36140**, **36147**, **36148**, **36160**, and **36200**. Selective arterial catheterization codes include **36215**, **36216**, **36217**, **✚36218**, **36245**, **36246**, **36247**, and **✚36248**.

Cardiovascular System Exercises

Check your answers in Appendix B.

True or False

1. Removal of an existing pacing cardioverter-defibrillator device is not included in the replacement code and should be separately reported. **True or False**
2. The procurement of an upper extremity vein is included when a coronary artery or lower extremity bypass procedure is reported. **True or False**

Short Answer

3. How is replacement of a dual-chamber permanent pacemaker and transvenous electrodes with a new dual-chamber permanent pacemaker and electrodes reported?

4. Harvesting of the radial artery for coronary artery bypass procedure is reported with which code(s)?

5. A redo coronary artery bypass graft was performed on a patient involving the left internal mammary artery to the left anterior descending artery and a saphenous vein graft to the right coronary artery. The original coronary artery bypass graft was two years ago. How is this reported?

6. Abdominal aortogram (by catheter in aorta, femoral approach). How is this reported?

7. Bilateral main (R) and (L) pulmonary arteriograms. How is this reported?

8. For endovascular AAA repair, Physician A performed bilateral femoral artery open exposures. Physician B placed catheters/sheaths into the aorta bilaterally. (Both physicians placed the modular bifurcated prosthesis with two docking limbs.) Physician A closed the cutdowns. Physician B performed RS&I for the procedure. How is this reported?

9. A 54-year-old male underwent aortoiliofemoral arteriography to evaluate an endoleak detected 10 months subsequent to an endovascular aortic aneurysm repair. The angiogram was performed from a left common femoral percutaneous puncture. The diagnostic study confirmed an endoleak, which was a Type I leak from the distal anastomosis in the left common iliac artery. Initially, this was treated with balloon angioplasty to try to achieve a seal at the distal anastomosis, but despite multiple attempts to close the leak with the balloon, the endoleak persisted. To resolve the leak, an extension into the external iliac was required. The hypogastric artery was patent, and selective angiography of the hypogastric artery was done. Based on the findings, it was determined that coil embolization of the hypogastric artery would also be necessary to resolve the leak, so this was done. Final angiography after embolization confirmed good position of the coils with closure of the main trunk of the hypogastric artery. A covered stent extension was then placed from the left limb of the graft into the external iliac, and the anastomoses were secured with balloon angioplasty. Final angiography confirmed that the left limb was now widely patent with no persistent endoleak. Collateral filling was seen into the distal branches of the hypogastric artery, but no retrograde filling was seen into the common iliac artery. The arteriotomy was closed with a percutaneous closure device. How is this reported?

10. A 73-year-old male with hypertension (55-pack-a-year smoking habit and prior myocardial infarction) underwent endovascular repair of the descending thoracic aortic aneurysm nine months ago. On the follow-up CT scan, he was found to have a distal endoleak. Placement of a distal extension was undertaken to seal the leak. How is this procedure reported?

Surgery: Digestive System

Section Objectives

- Familiarize yourself with the digestive system terminology and subsections
- Understand how to accurately report digestive system services and procedures

In the Digestive System subsection of the CPT codebook, codes exist for reporting services and procedures performed on the gastrointestinal tract and the accessory digestive organs. These structures include the lips, mouth, tongue, dentoalveolar structures, palate and uvula, salivary gland and ducts, pharynx, adenoids and tonsils, esophagus, stomach, intestines, appendix, rectum, anus, liver, biliary tract, pancreas, abdomen, peritoneum, and omentum. (See Figure 4-61.) This chapter includes information and guidelines on the more common endoscopy procedures, bariatric surgery, and hernia repair procedures.

Coding Tip

When the endoscopy procedures are reported, it is important to remember that surgical endoscopy always includes diagnostic endoscopy. Also, when two distinct endoscopic procedures are performed on the same day or at the same session, it is appropriate to report these procedures separately.

✓ Check Your Knowledge

1. Name three of the structures included in the digestive system.

Endoscopic Procedures

Endoscopy is a method of exploration and treatment for conditions and diseases that allows viewing of the site without requiring an open surgical incision. See Table 4-2 for the endoscopic code ranges. The types of endoscopy procedures include the following:

- **Esophagoscopy.** Limited study of the esophagus. When the endoscope passes the diaphragm into the stomach, the procedure is an esophagogastroscopy.
- **Esophagogastroduodenoscopy.** When the pyloric channel is traversed.

FIGURE 4-61 *Digestive System*

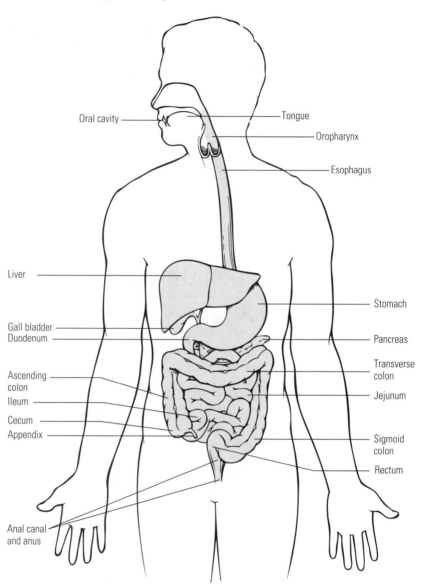

TABLE 4-2 *Endoscopy Types and Code Ranges*

Type of Endoscopy	Code Range
Esophagoscopy	43200-43232
Esophagogastroduodenoscopy (EGD)	43234-43259
Proctosigmoidoscopy	45300-45327
Sigmoidoscopy	45330-45345
Colonoscopy	45378-45392
Anoscopy	46600-46615

- **Endoscopic retrograde cholangiopancreatography.** The examination of the hepatobiliary system and gallbladder.
- **Enteroscopy** (or small intestinal endoscopy). The examination of the small intestine beyond the second portion of the duodenum.
- **Proctosigmoidoscopy.** The examination of the rectum and sigmoid colon.
- **Sigmoidoscopy.** The examination of the entire rectum and sigmoid colon and may include examination of a portion of the descending colon.
- **Colonoscopy.** An endoscopy in which a colonoscope is inserted in the anus and moved through the colon proximally past the splenic flexure (meaning the examiner is able to advance the colonoscope beyond the splenic flexure) to visualize the lumen of the transverse and ascending colon (right side) to the cecum and/or terminal ileum.
- **Anoscopy.** The examination of the anal canal and lower rectum.

✓ Check Your Knowledge

2. List and describe five types of endoscopy procedures.

Key Term

Endoscopy: A method of exploration and treatment for conditions and diseases that allows viewing of the site without requiring an open surgical incision.

An upper gastrointestinal endoscopy with or without collection of specimen(s) by brushing or washing is reported with code **43235**, *Upper gastrointestinal endoscopy including esophagus, stomach, and either the duodenum and/or jejunum as appropriate; diagnostic, with or without collection of specimen(s) by brushing or washing (separate procedure).* (See Figure 4-62.)

When an endoscopic retrograde cholangiopancreatography (ERCP) **(43260)** is performed, an examination of the hepatobiliary system (pancreatic ducts, hepatic ducts, common bile ducts, duodenal papilla [ampulla of Vater], and gallbladder [if present]) is performed through a side-viewing flexible fiberoptic endoscope. (See Figure 4-63.)

EXAMPLE

An esophagogastroduodenoscopy with biopsy **(43239)** and an esophagogastroduodenoscopy with dilation of gastric outlet for obstruction **(43245)** are performed. The physician reports the codes as follows:

43245 Upper gastrointestinal endoscopy including esophagus, stomach, and either the duodenum and/or jejunum as appropriate; with dilation of gastric outlet for obstruction (eg, balloon, guidewire, bougie)

43239 51 Upper gastrointestinal endoscopy including esophagus, stomach, and either the duodenum and/or jejunum as appropriate; with biopsy, single or multiple

In this case, both codes are reported to completely describe the procedures performed. The primary procedure is reported without the use of a modifier. Modifier **51** is appended to the secondary procedure performed. Modifier **51** is also used to report multiple procedures (other than E/M services) performed at the same session by the same provider.

A 62-year-old male with progressive dysphagia has been identified to have an exophytic mass lesion in the mid and distal esophagus that on prior biopsy is proven to be an adenocarcinoma. A CT examination of the chest and abdomen demonstrates thickening of the mid and distal esophagus without evidence of distant metastases. The physician is requested to further stage the tumor with endoscopic ultrasound. A small-caliber gastroscope is inserted per ora into the esophagus and, with some difficulty, is negotiated past the tumor into the stomach and duodenum. An esophagogastroduodenoscope (EGD) examination is performed that identifies an esophageal tumor that extends into the proximal stomach. The gastroscope is removed, and the radial scanning echoendoscope is advanced per ora into the esophagus. The echoendoscope is able to traverse approximately one third of the length of the tumor but because of tumor stenosis (and the larger caliber of the echoendoscope compared to the standard EGD) further advancement of the echoendoscope is precluded. On imaging, transmural infiltration of the tumor is appreciated and abutment vs invasion of the posterior trachea is identified. Several malignant-appearing peritumoral lymph nodes are identified. No suspicious lymphadenopathy is seen in the peri-esophageal space proximal to the tumor. The echoendoscope is withdrawn. The patient is taken to the recovery suite where postprocedure vital signs are monitored. The physician records a postprocedure note, prepares postprocedure orders, dictates a note to the referring physician, and discusses the findings with the family and patient. The patient is discharged when vital signs are stable. The physician reports the procedure as follows:

43237 Upper gastrointestinal endoscopy including esophagus, stomach, and either the duodenum and/or jejunum as appropriate; with endoscopicultrasound examination limited to the esophagus

Laparoscopy

When a laparoscopic fundoplasty (**43280**) is performed, the esophagus and fundus are held aside, sutures are placed in both crus diaphragmatis muscles below the esophagus to bring them together to close the hiatal hernia, and the anterior and posterior walls of the fundus are wrapped and stitched around the esophagus to complete the laparoscopic fundoplasty. (See Figure 4-64.)

FIGURE 4-62 *Upper Gastrointestinal Endoscopy*

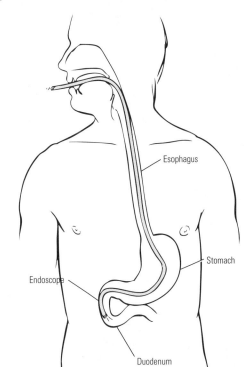

Esophagus

Stomach

Endoscope

Duodenum

FIGURE 4-63 *Endoscopic Retrograde Cholangiopancreatography*

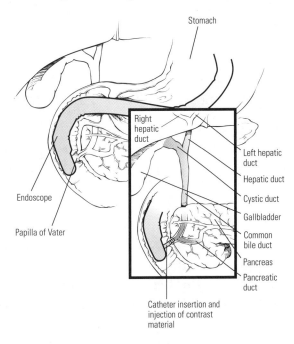

Stomach

Right hepatic duct

Left hepatic duct

Hepatic duct

Cystic duct

Gallbladder

Common bile duct

Pancreas

Pancreatic duct

Endoscope

Papilla of Vater

Catheter insertion and injection of contrast material

FIGURE 4-64 *Laparoscopic Fundoplasty*

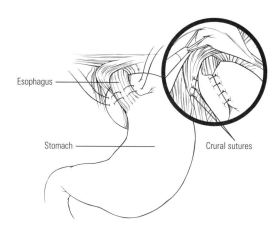

When performing a Nissen fundoplasty (**43327**, **53328**), the lower eshogus is accessed through an upper abdominal or lower thoracic incision. The fundus of the stomach is mobilized and wrapped around the lower esophageal sphincter, and the wrap is sutured into place. (See Figure 4-65.)

FIGURE 4-65 *Nissen Fundoplasty*

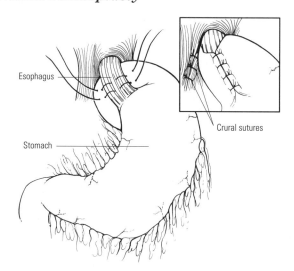

When performing a gastric intubation (**43753**), a large-bore gastric lavage tube is inserted orally through the esophagus into the stomach for expedient lavage and evacuation of stomach contents (eg, poisionings, hemorrhage). (See Figure 4-66.)

FIGURE 4-66 *Gastric Intubation*

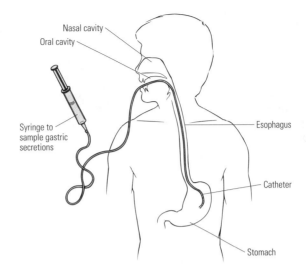

Bariatric Surgery

Bariatrics is the branch of medicine concerned with the management (prevention or control) of obesity and allied diseases. When conservative means of weight reduction such as dieting, exercise, behavioral modification, and pharmacological therapy have been unsuccessful for individuals suffering from clinically severe obesity, surgical treatment based on established principles for weight control are considered. These procedures involve the stomach, duodenum, jejunum, and/or ileum.

Types of Bariatric Surgery

Surgeries that use laparoscopic techniques to perform gastric restrictive procedures for morbid obesity include:

- Roux-en-Y gastric bypass (**43644**), which is the most frequently performed bariatric procedure in the United States;
- Small bowel reconstruction to limit absorption (**43645**);
- Gastric restrictive procedures, which identify laparoscopic placement of the adjustable band (**43770**);
- Laparoscopic revision of the band (**43771**);
- Laparoscopic removal of the band (**43772**);
- Laparoscopic removal and replacement of the band component (**43773**); and
- Laparoscopic removal of the band and subcutaneous port components (**43774**).

Open procedures of a related nature include:

- Gastric restrictive procedure with partial gastrectomy, pyloruspreserving duodenoileostomy, and ileoileostomy (**43845**);
- Gastric restrictive procedure with gastric bypass; short limb Roux-en-Y gastroenterostomy (**43846**) (See Figure 4-67.);

Chapter 4

FIGURE 4-67 *Gastric Bypass for Morbid Obesity*

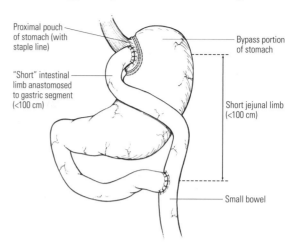

Proximal pouch of stomach (with staple line)

Bypass portion of stomach

"Short" intestinal limb anastomosed to gastric segment (<100 cm)

Short jejunal limb (<100 cm)

Small bowel

• Revision, open, of gastric restrictive procedure for morbid obesity other than adjustable gastric band (**43848**);
• Revision of the subcutaneous port component (**43886**);
• Open removal of the subcutaneous port component (**43887**); and
• Open removal and replacement of the subcutaneous port (**43888**).

EXAMPLE

In a gastric bypass for morbid obesity (**43846**), the stomach is partitioned with a staple line on the lesser curvature (no band, no gastric transection). A short limb of small bowel (less than 100 cm) is divided and anastomosed to the small upper stomach pouch.

Intestines (Except Rectum)

The enterectomy, resection for congenital atresia is reported with code **44127**, *Enterectomy, resection of small intestine for congenital atresia, single resection and anastomosis of proximal segment of intestine; Enterectomy, resection of small intestine for congenital atresia, single resection and anastomosis of proximal segment of intestine; with tapering.* (See Figure 4-68.)

When a partial colectomy (code **44140**) is performed, a segment of the colon is resected and an anastomosis is performed between the remaining ends of the colon. (See Figure 4-69.)

When a colectomy is performed with the removal of the terminal ileum and ileocolostomy (**44160**), a segment of the colon and terminal ileum is removed and an anastomosis is performed between the remaining ileum and colon. (See Figure 4-70.)

Rectum

The illustration in Figure 4-71 is a rectal tumor excised via transanal approach. This is reported with codes **45171-45172**.

FIGURE 4-68 *Enterectomy, Resection for Congenital Atresia*

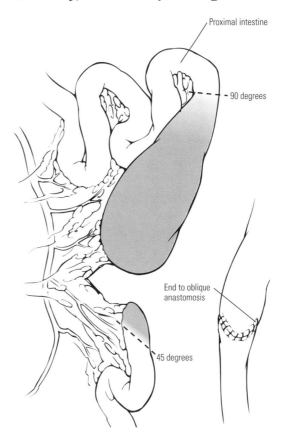

Proximal intestine

90 degrees

End to oblique
anastomosis

45 degrees

FIGURE 4-69 *Colectomy, Partial*

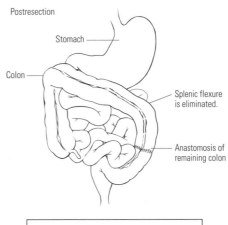

Postresection

Stomach

Colon

Splenic flexure
is eliminated.

Anastomosis of
remaining colon

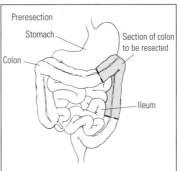

Preresection

Stomach

Colon

Section of colon
to be resected

Ileum

Chapter 4

FIGURE 4-70 *Colectomy with Removal of Terminal Ileum and Ileocolostomy*

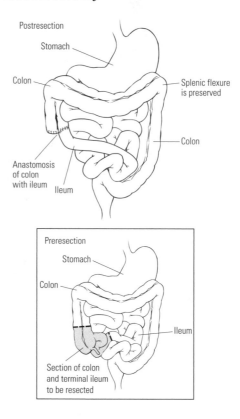

FIGURE 4-71 *Rectal Tumor Excision*

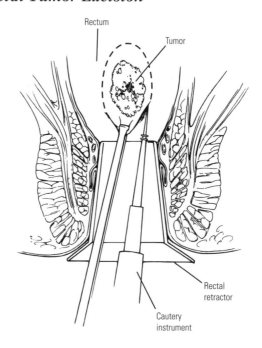

Key Terms

Bariatrics: The branch of medicine concerned with the management (prevention or control) of obesity and allied diseases.

Proctosigmoidoscopy: The examination of the rectum and sigmoid colon.

Sigmoidoscopy: The examination of the entire rectum, sigmoid colon, and may include examination of a portion of the descending colon.

Colonoscopy: The examination of the entire colon, from the rectum to the cecum, and may include the examination of the terminal ileum.

With a colonoscopy (**45378**), a colonoscope is inserted in the anus and moved through the colon past the splenic flexure in order to visualize the lumen of the rectum and colon. (See Figure 4-72.)

FIGURE 4-72 *Colonoscopy*

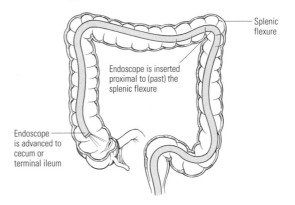

Splenic flexure

Endoscope is inserted proximal to (past) the splenic flexure

Endoscope is advanced to cecum or terminal ileum

A colonoscopy with lesion ablation or removal (**45383, 45385**) is performed with the insertion and advancement of a colonoscope through the colon and past the splenic flexure for ablation (**45383**) or removal (**45385**) of tumors, polyps, or other lesions. (See Figure 4-73.)

FIGURE 4-73 *Colonoscopy With Lesion Ablation or Removal*

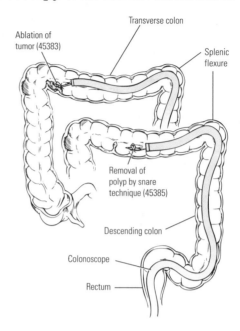

Anus

For the placement of seton, use code **46020**. (See Figure 4-74.) For the incision of thrombosed external hemorrhoid, use code **46083**. For ligation of internal hemorrhoid(s), see **46221**, **46945**, **46946**. For excision of internal and/or external hemorrhoid(s), see **46250-46262**, **46320**. (See Figure 4-75.) For injection of hemorrhoid(s), use **46500**. For destruction of internal hemorrhoid(s) by thermal energy, use **46930**. For destruction of hemorrhoid(s) by cryosurgery, use **46999**. For hemorrhoidopexy, use **46947**.

FIGURE 4-74 *Placement of Seton*

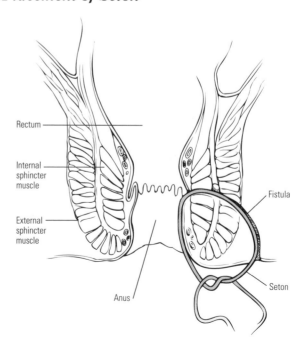

FIGURE 4-75 *Hemorrhoidectomy of Internal Prolapsed Hemorrhoid Columns*

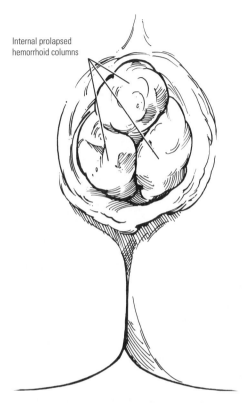

Hemorrhoidectomy of Internal Prolapsed Hemorrhoid
Columns 46250-46262

Internal prolapsed
hemorrhoid columns

Anal column is considered to be an internal hemorrhoid
with 3 major areas in the anal canal: right posterior
(1 o'clock), right anterior (5 o'clock), and left lateral
(9 o'clock) positions of the anus

Biliary Tract

When performing a laparoscopic cholecystectomy (code **47562**), the gall-bladder is dissected and removed from the liver bed under laparoscopic guidance. (See Figure 4-76.)

Abdomen, Peritoneum, and Omentum

The code series **49203-49205** describes open excision, ablation, or destruction of intra-abdominal tumors, cysts, or endometriomas in the peritoneum, mesentery, or retroperitoneum. These codes differentiate according to the size of the tumor(s) removed at a single session. If multiple tumors within the same size range are excised, then the code reflecting that size is reported only once. If multiple tumors are in different size ranges, then the codes reflecting the size of the tumors are reported. For exploratory laparotomy, use code **49000**, *Exploratory*

Introduction to CPT® Coding

FIGURE 4-76 *Laparoscopic Cholecystectomy*

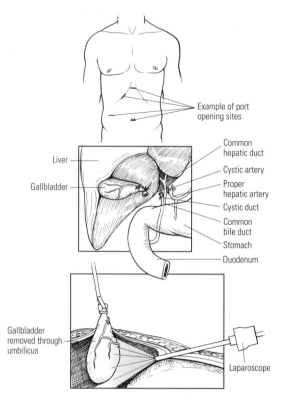

laparotomy, exploratory celiotomy with or without biopsy(s) (separate procedure). (See Figure 4-77.)

When performing a laparoscopy (code **49320**), the physician inserts a fiberoptic laparoscope to observe the necessary organs in these procedures. (See Figure 4-78.)

Chapter 4

162

FIGURE 4-77 *Exploratory Laparotomy*

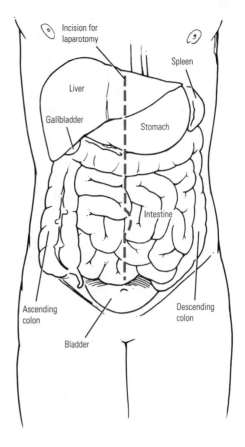

FIGURE 4-78 *Laparoscopy*

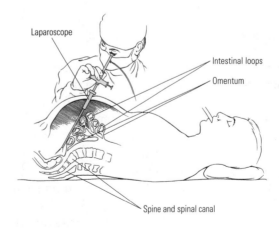

Key Terms

- Incarcerated
- Indirect
- Initial
- Nonreducible hernia
- Recurrent
- Reducible
- Strangulated

Hernia Repair

In the hernia repair section of codes, a hernia is commonly the protrusion of abdominal contents through a gap in the abdominal wall. A hernia develops when the outer layers of the abdominal wall weaken, bulge, or tear. The opening in this outer layer allows the inner lining of the cavity to protrude and to form a sac. A hernia can develop in any part of the abdominal wall.

The hernia repair section includes codes that describe hernioplasty (surgical correction of a hernia), herniorrhaphy (surgical repair of a hernia), and herniotomy (surgical division of the constriction or strangulation of a hernia, often followed by herniorrhaphy). Hernia repair codes are categorized primarily by the type of hernia. See Table 4-3 for the hernia repair code ranges.

TABLE 4-3 *Types of Hernias and Code Ranges*

Type of Hernia	Code Ranges
Inguinal	49491-49525; 49650, 49651
Lumbar	49540
Femoral	49550-49557
Incisional or ventral	49560-49566
Epigastric	49570-49572
Umbilical	49580-49587
Spigelian	49590
Omphalocele	49600-49611

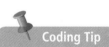

Coding Tip

Medical reduction of a hernia is performed as part of an E/M service and is not reported separately. When manual reduction is the only service performed, unlisted code **49999** should be reported.

Types of Hernias

Inguinal hernia (49491-49525, 49650, 49651): A hernia that occurs in the groin (the area between the abdomen and thigh). It is called *inguinal* because the intestines push through a weak spot in the inguinal canal. Obesity, pregnancy, heavy lifting, or straining to pass stool can cause the intestine to push against the inguinal canal.

Lumbar hernia (49540): A protrusion between the last rib and the iliac crest where the transverse muscle is covered by the latissimus dorsi. Lumbar hernias rarely result in strangulation, and hence the prognosis is good.

Femoral hernia (49550-49557): A hernia through the femoral ring.

Incisional or ventral hernia (49560-49566, 49568): Ventral or incisional hernias occur in the area of a prior abdominal incision. They develop as the result of a thinning, separation, or tear in the muscle or tendon closure from prior surgery.

Epigastric hernia (49570-49572): A hernia through the linea alba above the navel.

Umbilical hernia (49580-49587): A protrusion of the intestine and omentum through a hernia in the abdominal wall near the navel; usually self-correcting after birth.

Spigelian hernia (49590): A rare lateral ventral hernia.

Omphalocele/gastroschisis (49600-49611): Presence of congenital outpouching of the umbilicus containing internal organs in the fetus or newborn infant.

Codes **49491-49611** describe open surgical repair procedures. Codes **49650-49659** describe various laparoscopic hernia repairs. Code **49659** is used to report unlisted laparoscopy procedures for hernioplasty, herniorrhaphy, or herniotomy.

Key Terms

Incarcerated: The abnormal entrapment of a part (ie, a hernia that is nonreducible).

Indirect: An inguinal hernia that leaves the abdomen, protrudes through the inguinal ring, and passes down obliquely through the inguinal canal, lateral to the inferior epigastric artery.

Initial: The hernia has not required previous repair(s).

Nonreducible hernia: A hernia that cannot be reduced by manipulation. In these types of hernias, the hernial contents are fixed in the hernial sac.

Recurrent: The hernia has required previous repair(s).

Reducible: A hernia that can be corrected by manual manipulation; there is free mobility of the hernia contents through the hernial orifice.

Strangulated: The most serious complication related to the hernia. Congestion or strangulation at the hernial ring impairs the blood supply to the herniated part. Once the vessels are obstructed, a simple incarceration becomes a strangulation.

Coding Tip

Repair of diaphragmatic or hiatal hernia is reported with CPT codes **39502-39541** from the Mediastinum and Diaphragm subsection of Surgery.

✓ Check Your Knowledge Answers

1. lips, mouth, tongue

2. i. **Esophagoscopy.** *Esophagoscopy* is limited to study of the esophagus. When the endoscope passes the diaphragm into the stomach, the procedure is an esophagogastroscopy.

    ii. **Esophagogastroduodenoscopy.** When the pyloric channel is traversed, it is described as an *esophagogastroduodenoscopy.*

    iii. **Endoscopic retrograde cholangiopancreatography.** *Endoscopic retrograde cholangiopancreatography* is the examination of the hepatobiliary system and gallbladder.

> iv. **Enteroscopy.** *Enteroscopy,* or small intestinal endoscopy, is the examination of the small intestine beyond the second portion of the duodenum.
>
> v. **Proctosigmoidoscopy.** *Proctosigmoidoscopy* is the examination of the rectum and sigmoid colon.

Digestive System Exercises

Check your answers in Appendix B.

Match the following hernia terms to the correct definitions:

1. An inguinal hernia that leaves the abdomen, protrudes through the inguinal ring, and passes down obliquely through the inguinal canal, lateral to the inferior epigastric artery. _____
2. The hernia has required previous repair(s). _____
3. The hernia has not required previous repair(s). _____
   a. recurrent
   b. indirect
   c. initial

True or False

4. When the endoscopy procedures are reported, the surgical endoscopy does not include the diagnostic endoscopy. **True or False**
5. When two distinct endoscopic procedures are performed on the same day or at the same session, it is appropriate to report these procedures separately. **True or False**

Surgery: Urinary System

Section Objectives

- Understand the reporting procedures in the Urinary System subsection
- Understand the various endoscopic procedures performed in the Urinary System

The Urinary System subsection of the CPT codebook (**50010-53899**) contains codes for reporting procedures of the kidneys, ureters, bladder, and urethra. Generally, under each anatomic heading, codes can be found for reporting procedures involving incision, excision, introduction, repair, and endoscopy procedures. Procedures and guidelines associated with reporting renal pelvis catheter procedures, endoscopy procedures, and prostate procedures are detailed below. (See Figure 4-79.)

Renal Pelvis Catheter Procedures

Renal pelvic catheter procedures are most often performed for the treatment of ureteral strictures and obstructions. They are differentiated by approach (percutaneous and transurethral) and type (internally dwelling and externally dwelling). When the drainage of a renal abscess (**50020**) is performed, an incision is made to the abscess cavity, and the site is irrigated and drained. (See Figure 4-80.) When a nephrolithotomy is performed with calculus removal (**50060-50075**), a kidney stone (calculus) is removed by an incision in the kidney. Use **50070** if complicated by a congenital kidney abnormality. (See Figure 4-81.) Use codes **50382-50389** to report the removal of ureteral stents.

Ureteral stents are thin catheters threaded into the ureter for diversion of the urine either internally into the bladder or externally into a collection system. These stents must be monitored while in place and removed when no longer needed. They are required to be periodically changed, especially when they are chronically indwelling.

Code **50382** is used to report a percutaneous approach for the removal and replacement of an internally dwelling ureteral stent.

FIGURE 4-79 *Urinary System*

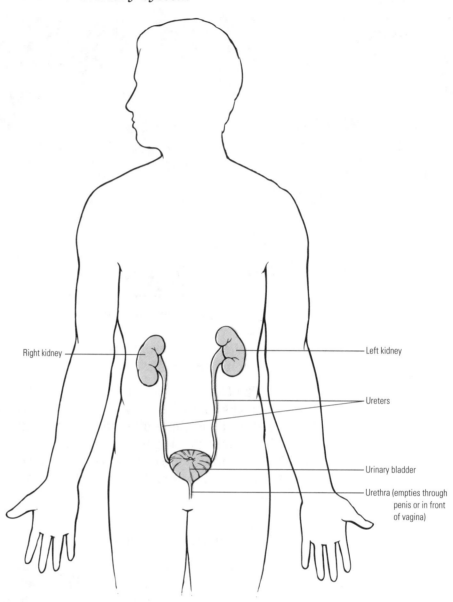

Right kidney

Left kidney

Ureters

Urinary bladder

Urethra (empties through penis or in front of vagina)

This capture approach uses a threadlike element at the end that forms a loop and is used to snare and extract the stent from the bladder. Code **50384** is reported only for removal of **ureteral stent** via percutaneous approach. Code **50387** is reported for removal and replacement of an externally accessible ureteral stent via the transnephric approach. As indicated in the parenthetical instructions following these three codes, for bilateral procedure, append the modifier **50**. Code **50389** is reported for those instances in which a ureteral stent has been placed with the loops in the renal pelvis and urinary bladder. Following clearance of blood after the stent placement, the nephrostomy catheter removal is performed under fluoroscopic guidance. When performing the introduction of a catheter into the renal pelvis (**50392**), the physician inserts

FIGURE 4-80 *Drainage of Renal Abscess*

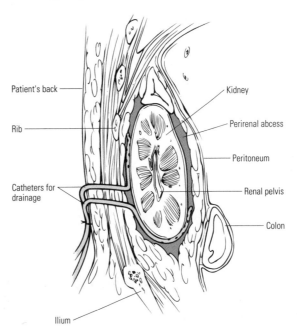

FIGURE 4-81 *Nephrolithotomy with Calculus Removal*

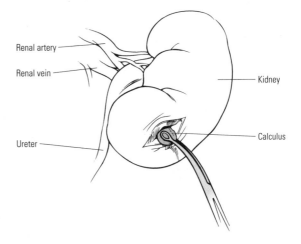

a catheter into the renal pelvis in order to drain urine and/or give an injection. See Figure 4-82. Code **50395** is reported for the introduction of a guide into the renal pelvis and/or ureter with dilation to establish a nephrostomy tract, percutaneously (see Figure 4-83).

Key Term

Ureteral stents: Thin catheters threaded into the ureter for diversion of the urine either internally into the bladder or externally into a collection system.

FIGURE 4-82 *Introduction of Catheter into Renal Pelvis*

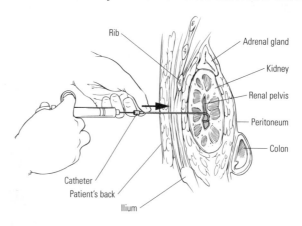

FIGURE 4-83 *Percutaneous Nephrostolitotomy or Pyelostolithotomy*

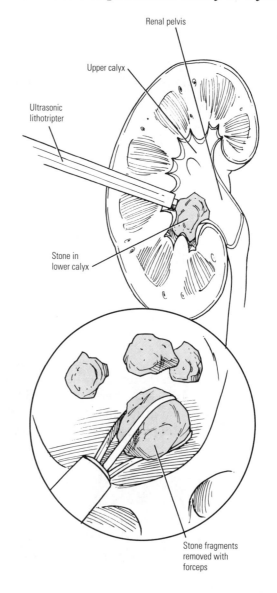

Coding Tip

The removal of a nephrostomy tube not requiring fluoroscopic guidance is considered inherent to the E/M service. Report the appropriate level of E/M service provided.

✓ Check Your Knowledge

1. Codes **50382**, **50384**, and **50387** are unilateral procedures. Is it appropriate to append modifier 50 if a bilateral procedure is performed?

When performing a laparoscopic radical nephrectomy (**50545**), the radical nephrectomy includes removal of Gerota's fascia and surrounding fatty tissue, removal of regional lymph nodes, and adrenalectomy. (See Figure 4-84.) When performing a laparoscopic nephrectomy (**50546**), a kidney is dissected and removed under laparoscopic guidance. (See Figure 4-85.)

When lithotripsy (**50590**) is performed, the physician breaks up a kidney stone (calculus) by directing shock waves through a liquid surrounding the patient. (See Figure 4-86.)

FIGURE 4-84 *Laparoscopic Radical Nephrectomy*

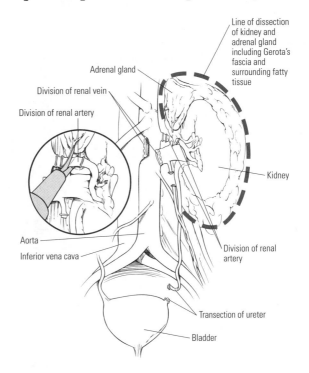

Ureter

With the indwelling of a ureteral stent procedure (**50605**), the physician makes an incision in the ureter (ureterotomy) and inserts a stent. (See Figure 4-87.) For placement using cystourethroscopic technique, use **52332**. When a ureteroileal conduit procedure (**50820**) is performed, the ureters are connected to a segment of intestine to divert urine flow through an opening in the skin. (See Figure 4-88.) The laparoscopic

FIGURE 4-85 *Laparoscopic Nephrectomy*

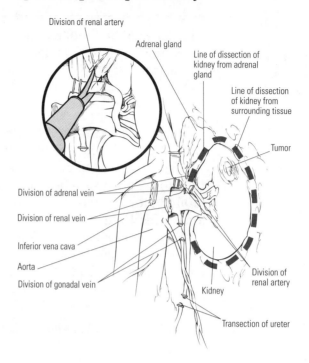

FIGURE 4-86 *Lithotripsy*

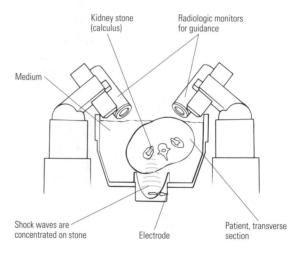

ureteroneocystostomy with cystoscopy and ureteral stent placement is reported with code **50947**. (See Figure 4-89.)

Bladder

The measurement of postvoiding is reported with code **51798**, *Measurement of post-voiding residual urine and/or bladder capacity by ultrasound, non-imaging.* (See Figure 4-90.)

When a laparoscopic sling suspension for urinary incontinence is performed (**51990**), nonabsorbable sutures are placed laparoscopically

FIGURE 4-87 *Indwelling Ureteral Stent*

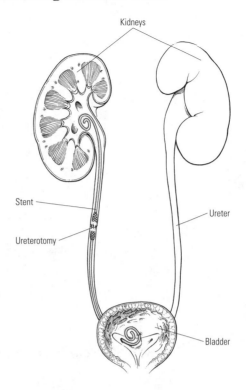

FIGURE 4-88 *Ureteroileal Conduit*

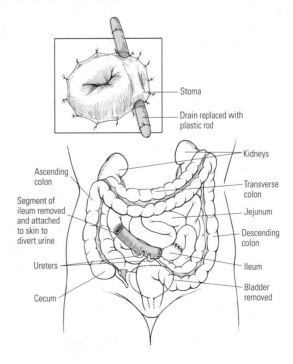

Chapter 4

FIGURE 4-89 *Laparoscopic Ureteroneocystostomy*

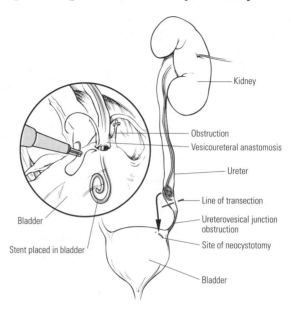

Kidney

Obstruction
Vesicoureteral anastomosis

Ureter

Line of transection

Ureterovesical junction
obstruction

Site of neocystotomy

Bladder

Bladder

Stent placed in bladder

FIGURE 4-90 *Measurement of Postvoiding*

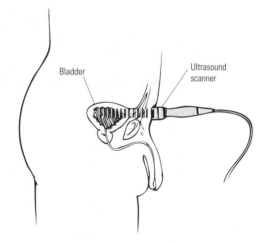

Bladder

Ultrasound
scanner

into the endopelvic fascia at the bladder neck region on each side and secured to the ipsilateral pectineal ligament. The sutures are tied using extra vaginal-urethral knots so as to create a hammock-type suspension of the bladder neck, without urethral occlusion. (See Figure 4-91.)

When a cystourethroscopy is performed with ureteral catheterization (**52005**), a cystourethroscope is passed through the urethra and bladder in order to view the urinary collecting system. (See Figure 4-92.)

Endoscopy Procedures

Some of the most frequently used procedures listed in the Urinary System subsection of the CPT codebook are endoscopic, including the use of:

FIGURE 4-91 *Laparoscopic Sling Suspension for Urinary Incontinence*

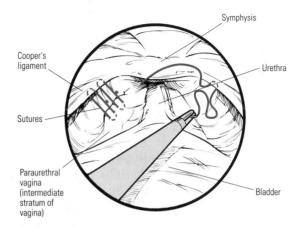

FIGURE 4-92 *Cystourethroscopy with Ureteral Catheterization*

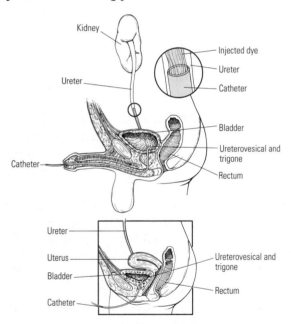

- Cystoscopy,
- Urethroscopy,
- Cystourethroscopy,
- Ureteroscopy,
- Pyeloscopy, and
- Renal endoscopy.

An endoscopy can be used as a diagnostic tool performed before proceeding with a more intensive surgical procedure or to check on the progress, completion, or a complication during the surgical procedure. CPT descriptors indicate whether an endoscopic procedure is included in the surgical procedure. An example of the use of cystourethroscopy

Coding Tip

Multiple endoscopic procedures performed at the same session by the same provider can be separately reported.

before, during, or after a urological procedure is a sling operation for stress incontinence (**57288**). There are times, however, when one endoscopic procedure must be performed before a more extensive endoscopic procedure because of anatomic locations. In this case, modifier **51** is appended to indicate that multiple procedures were performed at the same session by the same provider.

EXAMPLE

A patient presented for a cystourethroscopy and removal of a calculus located in the ureter. However, to remove the calculus, the urethral stricture must be dilated to provide access. Codes **52352**, *Cystourethroscopy, with ureteroscopy and/or pyeloscopy; with removal or manipulation of calculus (ureteral catheterization is included),* and **52281 51**,*Cystourethroscopy, with calibration and/or dilation of urethral stricture or stenosis, with or without meatotomy, with or without injection procedure for cystography, male or female,* are reported.

Laterality

Cystourethroscopy codes that are inherently unilateral are **52005**, **52007**, and **52320-52355**. When unilateral procedures are performed bilaterally, modifier **50** should be appended to the appropriate code(s). (For Medicare purposes only, code **52005** is inherently bilateral; therefore, modifier **50** is not appended to code **52005** for Medicare reporting. When code **52005** is reported for non-Medicare purposes, modifier **50** should be appended for bilateral procedures.)

Cystourethroscopy codes that should never be reported with modifier **50** are **52000**, **52010**, **52204-52285**, and **52305-52318**.

Code **52351** is not routinely reported with codes **52341-52346** and **52352-52355**, as it describes a diagnostic cystourethroscopy when performed on the same side. However, there are instances when a diagnostic cystourethroscopy and a procedure described by a code from the **52341-52346** or **52352-52355** series are performed on contralateral (opposite) sides of the body. When these are performed, code **52351** is reported separately with modifier **59**, *Distinct procedural service,* appended.

Prostate Procedures

Codes in the **52450-52700** series are used to report transurethral procedures of the vesical neck and prostate. Codes **53850-53853** are also used to report transurethral destruction of prostatic tissue. Code **52601** is used to report a procedure commonly referred to as *TURP* (transurethral resection of the prostate). This procedure uses electrical current to heat a wire loop on a resectoscope that slices through urethral or prostatic tissue like a knife. Two settings exist to regulate the current:

high-voltage current is used to cut the tissue and low-voltage current to coagulate the bleeding. As indicated in the code descriptor, when code **52601** is reported, vasectomy, meatotomy, cystourethroscopy, urethral calibration and/or dilation, and internal urethrotomy are included, when performed, and not reported separately. This code is intended to describe an initial resection of the prostate as well as a complete TURP. (See Figure 4-93.)

FIGURE 4-93 *Transurethral Resection of Prostate, Complete*

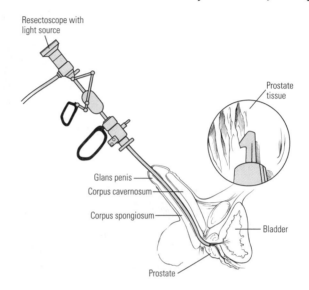

Prostate resection can be performed in two stages. Code **52612** is used to report the first stage of a two-stage resection. Code **52614** describes the second stage of a two-stage resection procedure and is reported when the resection is completed.

Other procedures involving the prostate include:

- Laser coagulation (**52647**),
- Laser vaporization (**52648**),
- Transurethral destruction of prostate tissue by microwave thermotherapy (**53850**),
- Transurethral destruction of prostate tissue by radiofrequency thermotherapy (**53852**), and
- Transurethral destruction of prostate tissue by water-induced thermotherapy (**53853**).

Code **52647** describes laser coagulation of the prostate. This code is intended to describe laser procedures that primarily heat the prostate and require sloughing for the treatment to be complete. This code is reported even if an incision or small amount of vaporization is done in combination with the coagulation. In this case, it is not appropriate to separately report code **52648** for the small amount of vaporization performed. Code **52648** describes laser vaporization with or without **transurethral resection of the prostate**. Vaporization is usually accomplished by moving a laser tip across the surface of the prostate, causing immediate vaporization of tissue and an end result that looks like a cavity (similar to the effect of a TURP). (See Figure 4-94.)

FIGURE 4-94 *Contact Laser Vaporization of Prostate*

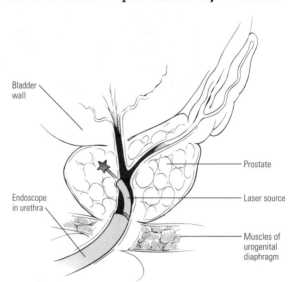

Bladder wall

Prostate

Endoscope in urethra

Laser source

Muscles of urogenital diaphragm

✓ Check Your Knowledge

2. When code **52601** is reported, would it be appropriate to report vasectomy, meatotomy, cystourethroscopy, urethral calibration and/or dilation, and internal urethrotomy separately?

Key Terms

- **Transurethral resection of the prostate (TURP)**
- **Transurethral microwave thermotherapy**

Code **53850** describes transurethral microwave thermotherapy, which is the selective destruction of prostate cells by therapeutic levels of heating. **Transurethral microwave thermotherapy** is a process of delivering sufficient microwave heating to destroy prostatic tissue without causing unnecessary damage to surrounding structures. The technique combines the principles of microwave radiative heating and conductive cooling to destroy tissue deep within the prostate while preserving surrounding structures such as the bladder neck, urethral mucosa, and distal sphincter.

Code **53852** describes transurethral destruction by radiofrequency thermotherapy, where low-power radiofrequency energy is used to cause tissue ablation and coagulation of prostate tissue. Insulated needles are pierced through the prostatic urethra to deliver radiofrequency energy directly into the prostate while the insulation on the needles protects the urethra. This procedure creates areas of necrosis within the prostate while preserving the urethral tissue.

Code **53853** describes transurethral destruction of prostate tissue by water-induced thermotherapy, where water is heated outside the body and circulated through the prostate in heat-shielded catheters; only the balloon emits heat. At 60°C, coagulative necrosis of the prostatic tissue occurs to an average depth of 1.0 cm from the urethra. Because water is heated and pumped from outside the body, there is no need to use internal temperature probes as is necessary with benign prostatic hypertrophy treatments such as microwave (**53850**) and radiofrequency-based

(**53852**) procedures. When a temporary prostatic urethral stent is inserted, it is reported with code **53855**. (See Figure 4-95.)

FIGURE 4-95 *Temporary Prostatic Urethral Stent Insertion*

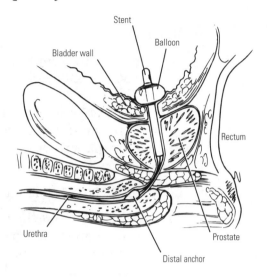

Key Terms

Transurethral resection of the prostate (TURP): A procedure that uses electrical current to heat a wire loop on a resectoscope that slices through urethral or prostatic tissue like a knife.

Transurethral microwave thermotherapy: The process of delivering sufficient microwave heating to destroy prostatic tissue without causing unnecessary damage to surrounding structures.

✓ Check Your Knowledge Answers

1. Yes. It would be appropriate to append modifier **50** to codes **50382**, **50384**, and **50387** if a bilateral procedure is performed.

2. No. Vasectomy, meatotomy, cystourethroscopy, urethral calibration and/or dilation, and internal urethrotomy are included, when performed, and not reported separately.

Urinary System Exercises

Match the following CPT codes to the correct procedures:

a. **52612**
b. **52614**
c. **52647**
d. **53850**

1. Describes laser coagulation of the prostate.
2. Is used to report the first stage of a two-stage prostate resection.
3. Describes the second stage of a two-stage resection procedure and is reported when the resection is completed.
4. Describes transurethral microwave thermotherapy.

True or False

5. Cystourethroscopy codes that should never be reported with modifier **50** are **52000**, **52010**, **52204-52285**, and **52305-52318**. **True or False**
6. Code **52647** describes laser coagulation of the prostate. This code is reported even if an incision or small amount of vaporization is done in combination with the coagulation. **True or False**

Choose the correct code for the following procedure report

7. A 70-year-old male had severe obstructive symptoms secondary to benign prostatic hyperplasia/hypertrophy. During cystoscopic examination under anesthesia, a 25-gram obstructive prostate was noted. A right-angle Nd:YAG laser fiber was passed into the prostatic fossa through a continuous-flow resectoscope, and 60 W of laser energy was delivered for 90 seconds in each of four quadrants and to the median lobe. The procedure was 45 minutes in duration. The patient had a catheter placed and was discharged the next day on drainage. He returned to the office on the fifth postoperative day, and his Foley catheter was removed. He was treated with intermittent catheterization until he began to void well, by the second postoperative week. How is this procedure reported?

Surgery: Female Genital System

Section Objectives

- Understand the codes for reporting procedures performed on the female genital system
- Understand the difference between open and hysteroscopic procedures
- Understand the global maternity care concept
- Undertand the different types of abortion

The Female Genital System subsection includes codes for reporting procedures on the vulva, perineum, and introitus (codes **56405-56821**); vagina (codes **57000-57426**); cervix uteri (codes **57452-57800**); corpus uteri (codes **58100-58579**); oviduct/ovary (codes **58600-58770**); and ovary (codes **58800-58960**) as well as in vitro fertilization (codes **58970-58976**). (See Figure 4-96.)

FIGURE 4-96 *Female Genital System*

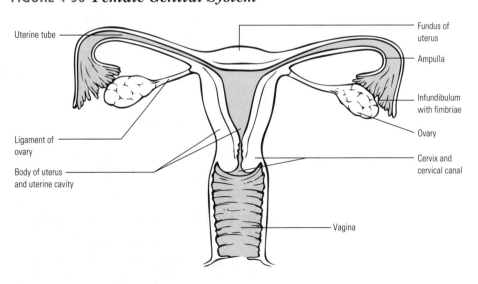

Uterine tube

Ligament of ovary

Body of uterus and uterine cavity

Fundus of uterus

Ampulla

Infundibulum with fimbriae

Ovary

Cervix and cervical canal

Vagina

Vulvectomy

Vulvectomy is performed on the external genitalia of the female. Definitions for simple, radical, partial, and complete vulvectomy are included under the Vulva, Perineum, and Introitus heading of the CPT codebook. They include the following:

- Simple vulvectomy: Removal of skin and superficial subcutaneous tissues
- Radical vulvectomy: Removal of skin and deep subcutaneous tissue
- Partial vulvectomy: Removal of less than 80% of the vulvar area
- Complete vulvectomy: Removal of more than 80% of the vulva

EXAMPLE

A patient has cancer of the vulva. Portions of the vulva are removed including the outer skinfolds of the vulva and the clitoris and terminal portions of the urethra, vagina, and other vulvar structures. CPT code **56630**, *Vulvectomy, radical, partial*, describes this surgery.

✓ Check Your Knowledge

1. Name the different vulvectomy procedures.

Key Term

- **Hysteroscopy**

Hysterectomy

Various hysterectomy procedures are described under the headings Corpus Uteri and Ovary. The extent of the procedure performed should be clearly documented in the operative report. Removal of the fallopian tube(s) and/or ovary(s) or ovaries when performed with an abdominal hysterectomy procedure is not reported separately because the code descriptors for abdominal hysterectomy procedures include the language "with or without removal of tube(s), with or without removal of ovary(s)." In addition, if an enterocele or urethrocystopexy repair is performed at the same session as a vaginal hysterectomy procedure, it should be determined whether the appropriate codes in the **58260-58294** series are available before referring to procedures from the **57200-57330** series of codes.

Hysterectomies can be abdominal (**58150-58210, 58951, 58953, 58956**), vaginal (**58260-58294**), or laparoscopic (**58541-58544, 58548-58554**). (See Figures 4-97 and 4-98.)

Laparoscopic/Hysteroscopic Surgery

The CPT code series **58541-58579** reports laparoscopic and hysteroscopic surgeries that occur on the uterus. Code series **58660-58679** reports laparoscopic surgeries on the oviduct or ovaries.

Chapter 4

FIGURE 4-97 *Total Abdominal Hysterectomy, With or Without Removal of Tube(s), With or Without Removal of Ovary(s)*

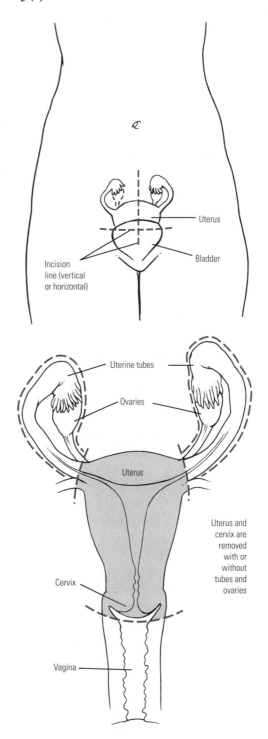

Uterus

Bladder

Incision line (vertical or horizontal)

Uterine tubes

Ovaries

Uterus

Uterus and cervix are removed with or without tubes and ovaries

Cervix

Vagina

When laparoscopic procedures are performed, a small surgical incision (cut) is made in the abdominal wall to permit the laparoscope to enter the abdomen or pelvis so that internal structures can be viewed. Tubes and probes are then introduced through the incision. This allows surgical procedures to be performed without the need for a large

Chapter 4

FIGURE 4-98 *Vaginal Hysterectomy, With Total or Partial Vaginectomy; With Repair of Enterocele*

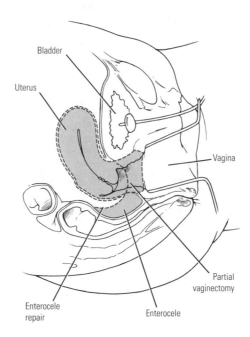

surgical incision. A surgical laparoscopy always includes a diagnostic laparoscopy.

The following steps will assist in selecting the appropriate CPT code to report when a laparoscopic procedure is performed:

- Look up *laparoscopy* in the index, and locate the organ and/or system being examined or treated using a scope.
- Look at the codes in that system/organ section to find a *laparoscopy* heading.
- If there is a laparoscopy heading in that section, look for a code with a descriptor that includes a suffix –*oscopy* and describes the procedure performed.
- If there is no heading of *laparoscopy* or there is no specific code describing the use of a scope in its descriptor, the codes described in that section are "open" surgical procedures and should not be used to report a procedure using a laparoscope approach.
- Clarify with the physician that the procedure was performed using a laparoscope.
- If it is determined that there is no specific code for the laparoscopic procedure one is attempting to code, the unlisted procedure laparoscopy code is used to report the procedure.
- If there is no specific unlisted laparoscopy code, use the general unlisted procedure code from the appropriate anatomic subsection of the CPT codebook. When reporting an unlisted code to describe a procedure/service, a copy of the operative report should be submitted to the insurance company with the claim.

Key Term

Hysteroscopy: Visual instrumental inspection of the uterine cavity. (See Figure 4-99.)

Coding Tip

It is not appropriate to report the "open" procedure code to describe a procedure performed laparoscopically.

EXAMPLE

The following is an example of a laparoscopic procedure performed on the ovary:

58661 Laparoscopy, surgical; with removal of adnexal structures (partial or total oophorectomy and/or salpingectomy)

The code series **58600-58770** (oviduct/ovary) is intended to report procedures involving ligation or transection of fallopian tube(s), tubal ligation, and occlusion of the fallopian tube(s) by device.

EXAMPLE

The following is an example of a procedure performed on the fallopian tube(s).

58600 Ligation or transection of fallopian tube(s), abdominal or vaginal approach, postpartum, unilateral or bilateral, during same hospitalization (separate procedure)

FIGURE 4-99 *Hysteroscopy*

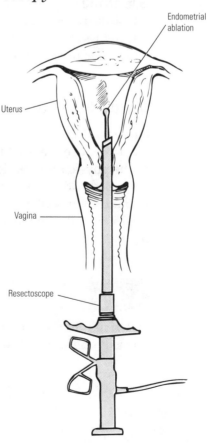

Endometrial ablation

Uterus

Vagina

Resectoscope

Coding Tip

Codes designated as separate procedures may be additionally reported when the procedure or service is performed as an integral component of another procedure or service.

The code series **58800-58960** is intended to report procedures performed on the ovary including biopsy, resection, cyst removal, and excisions in instances of tubal, ovarian, or peritoneal malignancy.

Some of the codes listed in this section include the phrase, "separate procedure" in the code descriptor. This designation indicates that the procedure may be considered an integral component of another procedure/service, performed independently, unrelated, or distinct from other procedure(s)/service(s) provided at that time.

EXAMPLE

Integral Component

58720 Salpingo-oophorectomy, complete or partial, unilateral or bilateral (separate procedure)

58150 Total abdominal hysterectomy (corpus and cervix), with or without removal of tube(s), with or without removal of ovary(s)

When reporting a total abdominal hysterectomy with removal of the tube(s) and ovary(s) or ovaries, it would **not** be appropriate to separately report code **58720** in conjunction with code **58150**. This would be considered unbundling. The procedure described by code **58720** is considered an integral component of the procedures described by code **58150**.

However, codes designated as separate procedures should be additionally reported when performed independently, unrelated, or distinct from other procedure(s) or service(s) provided.

In Vitro Fertilization

There is a separate series of CPT codes (**58970-58976**) used for reporting procedures related to in vitro fertilization, procedures performed by the physician in which egg cells are fertilized outside the woman's body. Code **58970** describes *follicle puncture for oocyte retrieval, any method*; code **58974** describes *embryo transfer, intrauterine*; and code **58976** describes *gamete, zygote, or embryo intrafallopian transfer, any method*.

Key Term

In vitro fertilization: Procedures in which egg cells are fertilized outside the woman's body.

Chapter 4

Maternity Care and Delivery

Coding Tip

If ultrasound guidance for aspiration of ova is used, CPT code **76948** is coded in addition to **58970**.

The services normally provided in uncomplicated maternity cases include routine **antepartum care**, delivery, and **postpartum care**. This is the global obstetric package for maternity care and delivery. The guidelines at the beginning of the Maternity Care and Delivery subsection in the CPT codebook define the services included when antepartum care, delivery services, and postpartum care are reported. (See Figure 4-100.)

Maternity patients are described by the number of pregnancies (including previous and current) and the number of births. **Gravida** refers to the number of pregnancies a women has had, a woman pregnant for the first time is referred to as a **primigravida** (or gravida I), during the second pregnancy gravida II or secundigravida, during the third pregnancy gravida III or tertigravida. The number of pregnancies that have resulted in the birth of viable offspring is referred to as **para**, followed by a Roman numeral to designate the number of pregnancies (eg, para 0 is no births yet; para I is one birth; para II is two births, etc). Since the number indicates how many pregnancies, a multiple birth counts as just one in the calculation. See the following example:

Key Terms

- **Antepartum care**
- **Postpartum care**
- **Primigravida**
- **Para**
- **Gravida**

EXAMPLES

Gravida 1, Para 0 (G_1P_0) means the first pregnancy, which has not resulted in the birth yet.

Gravida 3, Para 2 (G_3P_2) means the third pregnancy, two previous births.

FIGURE 4-100 *Vaginal Delivery*

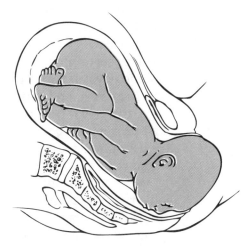

Key Terms

Antepartum care: Care during the first trimester.

Postpartum care: Care following delivery.

Primigravida: A woman pregnant for the first time; also written gravida I.

Para: A woman who has produced viable young regardless of whether the child was living at birth. Used with Roman numerals to designate the number of pregnancies that have resulted in the birth of viable offspring, as para 0 (none), para I (one), para II (two), para III (three), para IV (four), etc. Since the number indicates how many pregnancies, a multiple birth counts as just one in the calculation.

Gravida: A pregnant woman. Called gravida I or primigravida during the first pregnancy.

Global Services for Routine Obstetric Care

Antepartum care includes the following:

- The initial and subsequent history
- Physical examinations
- Recording of weight, blood pressures, and fetal heart tones
- Routine chemical urinalysis
- Monthly visits up to 28 weeks' gestation, biweekly visits to 36 weeks' gestation, and weekly visits until delivery

The E/M services (visits) provided with those services included in the provision of antepartum care are not separately reported. However, any other visits or services provided within the antepartum period, other than those listed above, should be coded and reported separately. When the same physician (solo practice) or same physician group (group practice) provides the global routine obstetric care (including antepartum care, delivery, and postpartum care), the appropriate global code is reported to describe the services rendered. Codes **59400**, **59510**, **59610**, and **59618** describe the global services for routine obstetric care.

Under certain circumstances, the same physician (solo practice) or same physician group (group practice) does not provide the global maternity care and delivery services. Under these circumstances the use of the global codes is not appropriate. Codes in the CPT codebook exist for reporting the specific services provided when the global codes are not appropriate. Codes **59425** and **59426** are available for reporting antepartum care only. Codes **59409**, **59514**, **59612**, and **59620** describe delivery services only. Codes **59410**, **59515**, **59614**, and **59622** describe delivery services including postpartum care. The provision of postpartum care only is reported with code **59430**.

The following services are not included in the global obstetric package:

- Management of inpatient or outpatient medical complications not related to pregnancy, such as cardiac problems, neurologic problems, pneumonia, chronic hypertension, diabetes, etc.
- Management of inpatient or outpatient medical complications related to pregnancy, such as bleeding, preterm labor, pregnancy-induced hypertension, toxemia, hyperemesis, premature rupture of membranes, etc.
- If there are more than 13 outpatient visits or inpatient visits.
- The laboratory tests performed during pregnancy, excluding dipstick urinalysis.
- Routine venipuncture (code **36415**).
- Management of surgical complications and problems of pregnancy, such as incompetent cervix, hernia repair, ovarian cyst, Bartholin cyst, ruptured uterus, appendicitis (reported separately with the appropriate codes from the Surgery section of the CPT codebook [eg, codes **44950**, **59320**, **59325**, **59350**])
- Amniocentesis, chronic villous sampling, and cordocentesis (reported separately when performed [codes **59000**, **59001**, **59015**, **59012**])
- Fetal contraction stress test and fetal nonstress test (reported separately when performed [codes **59020**, **59025**])
- Insertion of cervical dilator by physician (eg, laminaria, prostaglandin [code **59200**])
- External cephalic version with or without tocolysis (code **59412**)
- The obstetric limited or complete ultrasound (reported separately with codes **76805**, **76810**, **76815**, **76816**, **76830**)
- Fetal biophysical profile (code **76818**, **76819**)
- Fetal echocardiography (codes **76825**, **76826**, **76827**, **76828**)
- Administration of RH immune globulin (code **90772**)

Coding Tip

Hospital visits within 24 hours of delivery are generally considered part of the global service.

✓ Check Your Knowledge

2. What's included in the global obstetric care?

Cesarean Delivery

Separate codes exist for reporting routine obstetric care associated with cesarean delivery. CPT code **59510**, *Routine obstetric care including antepartum care, cesarean delivery, and postpartum care,* reports the global care provided to obstetric patients including those who have had a previous cesarean section delivery and return for elective repeat cesarean section delivery. Code **59514** describes cesarean delivery only. If postpartum care is also provided by the same physician or physician group, code **59515**, *Cesarean delivery only; including postpartum care,* is reported. If a subtotal or total hysterectomy is performed after cesarean delivery, code **59525** is reported in addition to the code for primary procedure. Codes **59618**, **59620**, and **59622** can be reported for cesarean deliveries. (See Figure 4-101.)

Chapter 4

FIGURE 4-101 *Cesarean Delivery*

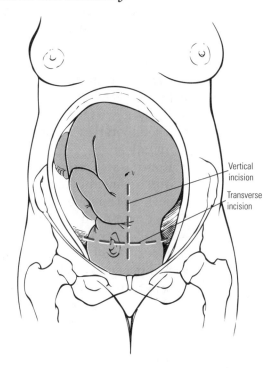

Vertical incision

Transverse incision

Abortion

The definition of **abortion** is the premature expulsion from the uterus of the products of conception, the embryo, or a nonviable fetus. Abortions may be categorized as either *spontaneous,* the natural (with no active interference) termination of pregnancy prior to the 20th week of gestation, or *induced*, in which a deliberate attempt has been made to terminate the pregnancy.

Key Term

Abortion: The premature expulsion from the uterus of the products of conception, the embryo, or a nonviable fetus.

The different types of abortions that are reportable with CPT codes as follows.

Threatened Abortion

A threatened abortion is diagnosed when vaginal bleeding occurs in the first 20 weeks of pregnancy. The differential diagnosis of this bleeding that occurs in early pregnancy in approximately 20% of all patients is usually included in the antepartum care component of routine obstetric care of the patient who successfully delivers. In the event that the patient being treated for a threatened abortion requires additional visits, these should be coded separately using E/M services codes, according to the services the physician provides.

Spontaneous Abortion (Miscarriage)

Spontaneous abortions are also known as *miscarriages*. The types of spontaneous abortion include:

- Complete abortion
- Incomplete abortion
- Missed abortion
- Septic abortion
- Blighted ovum

Complete Abortion. When a spontaneous abortion that is *complete* (any trimester) occurs and the physician manages the patient medically with no surgical intervention, the physician should report the appropriate level of E/M code, dependent on the place where the patient is seen (**99201-99233**).

Incomplete Abortion. An *incomplete* abortion occurs when the uterus is not entirely emptied of its contents. Fragments of the products of conception may remain within the uterus, may protrude from the external os of the cervix, or can be found in the vagina. Some fragments of the products of conception may have spontaneously passed out of the vagina. Code **59812**, *Treatment of incomplete abortion, any trimester, completed surgically,* is used to report the dilation and curettage (either sharp or suction curettage) for the surgical management of an incomplete abortion. However, if the patient is septic and is diagnosed as experiencing an incomplete abortion, do not use code **59812**. (See septic abortion.)

Missed Abortion. A missed abortion refers to the prolonged retention of a fetus that died in the first half of pregnancy. The evacuation of the uterus in these cases is coded according to the trimester in which the procedure is performed, ie, **59820**, *Treatment of missed abortion, completed surgically; first trimester,* and **59821** for the second trimester.

Septic Abortion. Septic abortions are those in which intrauterine infection is present. Most often this infection is confined to the uterus, but peritonitis and septicemia are not rare. Treatment of the infection involves, in addition to treatment with antibiotics, the prompt evacuation of the products of conception. Code **59830**, *Treatment of septic abortion, completed surgically,* is used to report these services.

Blighted Ovum. The advent of diagnostic tools that aid in the very early detection of pregnancy, such as beta subunit human chorionic gonadotropin (HCG) and ultrasound, has had an impact in defining when early "abortion" occurs. The instance of a positive pregnancy test with a blighted ovum identified on ultrasound (a pathologic ovum in which the embryo was degenerated or absent) raises the question of whether a code for treatment of abortion should be selected or a code for dilation and curettage, since there was no (viable) product of conception present. In many of these cases, women who did not seek medical attention for early diagnosis of pregnancy would not have previously identified a delayed menstrual cycle as the loss of a pregnancy nor have been aware that any conception had occurred. However, if a pregnancy is diagnosed and terminates, either by spontaneous or induced means, the abortion codes should be used to report the physician services related to the abortion.

Induced Abortion

Both therapeutic and elective abortions may be classified as induced abortions. Therapeutic abortion is the termination of pregnancy before the time of fetal viability for medical indications. Elective abortion is the interruption of pregnancy before viability at the request of the woman.

Coding for an induced abortion is done based on the technique used. This may be done surgically, by dilating the cervix and performing curettage or using vacuum aspiration. Medical induction may be performed by the administration of oxytocin or the administration of prostaglandins. Intra-amniotic injections of saline or urea are also used to induce abortions.

When an induced abortion is performed by dilating the cervix and performing sharp and/or suction curettage, code **59840**, *Induced abortion, by dilation and curettage,* is reported.

If the cervix is dilated and the uterus mechanically evacuated, code **59841**,*Induced abortion, by dilation and evacuation,* is reported. In the event that a small amount of sharp curettage is needed to complete the dilation and evacuation, this is included when reporting **59841**.

Abortions performed during the second trimester are sometimes performed using intra-amniotic hyperosmotic solutions (saline or urea). These solutions are injected to stimulate uterine contractions and cervical dilation to deliver the products of conception. This is coded using **59850** and includes admission to a facility, necessary hospital visits, and follow-up care.

59850 Induced abortion, by one 1 or more intra-amniotic injections (amniocentesis-injections), including hospital admission and visits, delivery of fetus and secundines);

59851 with dilation and curettage and/or evacuation

59852 with hysterotomy (failed intra-amniotic injection)

In the event that the intra-amniotic injections facilitate the evacuation of the uterus but curettage and/or dilation is necessary to complete the procedure, code **59851** is reported.

If other methods are not successful or if there are additional indications, an abdominal hysterotomy may be necessary to terminate pregnancy. This technique is similar to the technique of cesarean delivery except that the abdomen and uterus are generally smaller. In this case, code **59852** is reported and encompasses both the attempted intra-amniotic injections as well as the surgical hysterotomy.

If a laminaria is inserted prior to any of the procedures discussed in this chapter, code **59200**, *Insertion of cervical dilator (eg, laminaria,* *prostaglandin) (separate procedure),* may also be reported because it is not included as a part of any of the other procedures.

✓ Check Your Knowledge

3. List the different types of spontaneous abortion.

4. What is the difference between spontaneous abortion and induced abortion?

✓ Check Your Knowledge Answers

1. Simple, partial, radical, and complete

2. Antepartum care, delivery, and postpartum care

3. Incomplete, missed septic, blighted ovum, complete

4. Spontaneous abortion is non-elective vs induced abortion, which is elective.

Female Genital System Exercises

Check your answers in Appendix B.

1. A 28-year-old patient was seen by her family physician for a well-woman examination. The Papanicolaou smear report indicated an abnormality. The family physician requested that the patient be seen in consultation by a gynecologist. The family physician wrote the gynecologist that, in addition to the abnormal Papanicolaou smear, the patient had a one-year history of vulvar irritation and itching that had been unresponsive to antifungal and antibiotic cream preparations. The gynecologist subsequently saw the patient, reviewed the intake history, and discussed the year-long complaint and treatment of the vulvar irritation. The patient reported that the itching had persisted for more than a year. It was not related to her menstrual cycle. The creams were of little help, as the patient experienced a sensation of mild burning irritation all the time. Her vital signs included blood pressure of 124/82 mm Hg, height of 5 ft 7 in, and weight of 156 lb. Her orientation, mental status, and appearance were normal.

   After discussing the Papanicolaou smear report and receiving informed consent, the gynecologist performed vulvar and cervical colposcopies. Suspicious lesions were noted on the vulva and just inside the endocervical canal. A biopsy specimen of the vulvar lesion was obtained, and an endocervical curettage was performed. The gynecologist sent a letter back to the family physician describing the findings and the proposed treatment plan. How is this procedure reported?

2. **History:** A 32-year-old female was diagnosed with infertility caused by adhesions of both fallopian tubes. After a discussion of the risks, the physician scheduled a fimbrioplasty.

Preoperative diagnosis: Infertility caused by adhesions

Postoperative diagnosis: Same

Operation: Bilateral fimbrioplasty

Procedure: Through an incision just above the pubic hairline, the existing fimbriae were reconstructed in the obstructed oviducts. The fimbrial adhesions on the left and right were lysed, and material was applied to prevent future adhesions. After the procedure, a chromotubation was performed to ensure that the tubes were patent.

How is this procedure reported?

3. **Preoperative diagnosis:** Endometriosis of uterus; vaginal enterocele

   Postoperative diagnosis: Same

   Operations: Supracervical abdominal hysterectomy; repair of enterocele

   Procedure: A horizontal incision within the pubic hairline was made. The uterus and left ovary and fallopian tube were removed. The supporting pedicles containing the tubes, ligaments, and arteries were clamped and cut free. The uterus was cut free from the cervix, leaving the cervix still attached to the vagina. The abdominal incision was closed with sutures. Through the vagina, the enterocele sac was incised and ligated and the uterosacral ligaments and endopelvic fascia were approximated anterior to the rectum. The vaginal epithelium was closed. How is this procedure reported?

4. A diagnostic laparoscopy was performed on a patient with genuine stress urinary incontinence. During the diagnostic laparoscopy, multiple small subserosal or intramural fibroids were noted. A laparoscopic vaginal hysterectomy and a laparoscopic Burch procedure were performed during the same surgical session on the patient. The pathology report indicated that the uterus weighed 230 g and that there were seven fibroid tumors ranging in size from 0.8 cm to 3.5 cm. How is this procedure reported?

5. **Preoperative diagnosis:** Endometriosis of fallopian tube; uterine polyp

   Postoperative diagnosis: Same

   Operation: Laparoscopic removal of endometrial implants; polypectomy

   A 28-year-old patient underwent a laparoscopy for pelvic pain and a hysteroscopy for abnormal uterine bleeding. The preoperative diagnoses were endometriosis of the fallopian tube and uterine polyp. During the laparoscopy, multiple endometriotic implants were identified, and cautery was used to destroy them. During the hysteroscopy, a polyp was identified, and a dilation and curettage and polypectomy were performed. How is this procedure reported?

6. A patient presented with enlarged bilateral labia majora, 9 in in length, that interfered with daily activities, coitus, and self-esteem. The physician removed part of the labia. The underlying superficial subcutaneous fatty tissue was removed along with the large portion of excised skin. How is this procedure reported?

7. An established patient, 58 years old, presented with stress incontinence, and stated she felt a bulge in her vagina. After an examination, the physician diagnosed both a cystocele and a rectocele. After a 15-minute discussion of treatment options, the patient decided on surgical repair. The total encounter time was 25 minutes. The surgery was scheduled for two weeks. The day before the surgery, she came into the office again to review the surgery risks and benefits and sign consent forms.

In the operating room, the physician began with repair of the cystocele. She made an incision from the apex of the vagina to within 1 cm of the urethral meatus. Plication sutures were placed along the urethral course from the meatus to the bladder neck. A suture was placed through the pubourethral ligament to the posterior symphysis pubis on each side of the urethra. The sutures were tied and the posterior urethra was pulled upward to a retropubic position. The cystocele was repaired using mattress sutures placed in the paravesical tissue.

Next, the physician turned to the posterior repair. The rectovaginal fascia were plicated and closed with layered suture. A perineorrhaphy was also performed, including midline approximation of the levator and perineal muscles. Excess fascia in the posterior vaginal wall was excised and the incisions were closed with sutures.

In order to prevent formation of an enterocele, a McCall culdoplasty was performed. The vaginal mucosa was then closed. How is this procedure reported?

8. A 48-year-old new patient presented for evaluation of an abnormal cervical cytology result that showed "atypical glandular cells." An expanded problem-focused history and physical examination, including a pelvic exam, were performed with straightforward medical decision making. Colposcopy of the cervix was performed, and the exocervix appeared normal. Both an endocervical curettage and an endometrial biopsy were performed to determine the source of the atypical glandular cells in the lower genital tract.

At the completion of the colposcopy, biopsy, and endocervical curettage, the speculum was removed. A sterile Graves speculum was inserted, and the cervix was prepared with an antiseptic solution. The anterior lip of the cervix was grasped with a tenaculum, and the uterus was sounded with a uterine sound to gauge the depth of the endometrial cavity. The endometrial curette was passed through the cervix to the fundus of the uterus. The endometrial biopsy was performed. The curette was withdrawn, and the tissue was placed in formalin. The tenaculum was removed. Pressure was applied to the cervix to control any postoperative bleeding. The speculum was removed, and the patient was taken down from the lithotomy position. How is this procedure reported?

9. A 28-year-old patient presented with complaint of very heavy and long menstrual periods and pelvic pain. After an examination, she was diagnosed with myomas. The physician discussed her options for treatment. The discussion took 20 minutes of the total

Chapter 4

30 minutes for the encounter. The patient said she wanted to discuss the options with her family. Two weeks later, she called to say she would like to have the surgery. An abdominal hysterectomy was scheduled for two weeks.

The physician removed three intramural myomas along with the uterus. The total weight of the specimen (myomas and uterus) was 265 g. The patient's fallopian tubes and ovaries were left intact. How is this procedure reported?

10. A 48-year-old established patient who had undergone a prior vaginal hysterectomy for abnormal bleeding was found to have bilateral pelvic masses. She was seen in consultation and was advised to undergo an exploratory laparotomy. She was counseled for 40 minutes about the possibility that an ovarian cancer might be present. She was taken to surgery the next day. An exploratory laparotomy was performed, confirming the presence of bilateral ovarian masses. A bilateral salpingo-oophorectomy was performed, and a frozen section obtained intraoperatively confirmed the presence of a well-differentiated mucinous carcinoma. In addition, an omentectomy was also performed. How is this procedure reported?

Maternity Care and Delivery Exercises

Check your answers in Appendix B.

1. A 27-year-old, gravida 1, para 0, patient had been managed in the antepartum period by her family physician, who saw her for 12 visits. At 40 weeks, three days, she was admitted to the hospital in active labor at 10 a.m. She progressed well with artificial rupture of the membranes, and an epidural catheter was placed when her cervix was 5 cm dilated. Fetal heart tones remained normal. The cervix was completely dilated and 0 station at 5 p.m. However, after one and one-half hours of pushing, the vertex was firmly wedged in the pelvis at 0 station. The family physician requested a consultation from an obstetrician. The obstetrician reviewed the patient's prenatal history, assessed her mental status, performed an abdominal examination, listened to her heart and lungs, palpated the fetus abdominally, and performed a pelvic examination to assess the bony pelvis, cervix, and presenting vertex of the fetus. The obstetrician discussed the situation with the patient and her husband and recommended a cesarean delivery. This discussion took 20 minutes, during which informed consent was obtained. The patient was taken to the operating room for a cesarean delivery by the obstetrician at 7:15 p.m. The obstetrician provided her hospital care and six-week postpartum office care. How is this procedure reported?

2. A 22-year-old female presented with heavy vaginal bleeding of one day's duration. She was 14 weeks pregnant. She denied passing tissue but had had large clots. On exam, she had a dilated cervical os with tissue at the os. Following the administration of local anesthesia, the patient underwent surgical treatment of incomplete abortion. The uterine cavity was emptied of the products of conception using a suction apparatus. Instrumentation was removed and hemostasis

was maintained. Discharge instructions were given to the patient, and routine follow-up care during the 90-day global period was scheduled. How is this procedure reported?

3. A 32-year-old primigravida with no prenatal care presented to the emergency department at 39 weeks gestation in active labor. Following examination by the emergency department physician, the patient was transferred to labor and delivery. Labor progressed normally, and she delivered a healthy infant. Hospital course was uneventful. The patient was instructed to follow up with Dr Jansen in the obstetrics/gynecology clinic in six weeks. How is this procedure reported?

4. A 34-year-old gravida 3, para 2 female was admitted with ruptured bags of water at 38 weeks gestation. Patient received prenatal care with no complications. Previous deliveries had been vaginal. She had a twin pregnancy.

The first stage of labor was uneventful, with fetal heart tones looking good on both babies. She did not develop spontaneous labor after the water was ruptured, so she was placed on a Pitocin drip. The second stage of labor showed some dips in the heart tones on Twin A, so a forceps delivery was done from the occiput anterior position with a low outlet presentation. The baby did fine.

The obstetrician broke the water of Twin B; it was meconium stained. The head did not come down and the baby showed deep decelerations of heart tones with each contraction, so a cesarean section was performed under general anesthesia. The incision was made one minute after the anesthesia was started, and the baby was delivered one minute after the incision. This baby also did fine.

The postoperative course was uneventful. The patient was discharged with instructions to follow up in six weeks. How is this procedure reported?

5. A 29-year-old G_1P_0 new patient presented because her period was late. A pregnancy test was positive. The physician saw her briefly to discuss the results of the pregnancy test, give her a prescription for prenatal vitamins, and schedule her first prenatal visit in one month.

At six-weeks gestation, she was seen because of a complaint of vomiting for the last three days. This was a problem-focused visit.

At eight weeks, she was seen for her first prenatal visit. She indicated that she still had nausea, but the vomiting was less frequent. This was an expanded problem-focused visit.

She was seen monthly up to 28-weeks gestation and biweekly to 36-weeks gestation. Five days after her visit at 38 weeks, she delivered vaginally a healthy 8-lb female. She was seen for 13 antepartum visits. The postpartum course was uneventful. How is this procedure reported?

6. The patient was 24 years old and presented to her obstetrician for her first pregnancy. At 17 weeks, an ultrasound was performed for increased uterine growth. It was determined that she was carrying twins.

Starting at 32-weeks gestation, the physician performed fetal nonstress tests in his office during her routine antepartum visits. A report was prepared describing the findings for each fetus. She had a total of 13 antepartum visits.

At 35 weeks she went into active labor, and her physician admitted her to the hospital. She progressed well with spontaneous rupture of membranes, and an epidural was placed. The fetal heart tones remained normal.

She was complete and 0 station at 5 p.m. After 1.5 hours of good pushing, a girl was delivered vaginally. However, the other fetus (a boy) was breech and was delivered by cesarean. How is this procedure reported?

7. The physician had seen the patient for all of her obstetric care. The physician was called out of town for the weekend and asked another physician to cover his patients. On Saturday afternoon, the patient presented to labor and delivery in active labor. The covering physician was called and went to the hospital. The covering physician delivered vaginally a healthy female. The first physician returned and provided the postpartum visit at six weeks. How is this procedure reported?

8. An obstetric patient, 31 years old, was seen for five antepartum visits. At 12-weeks gestation she called her obstetrician stating that she had started bleeding and cramping a few hours before and had passed some clots. Her obstetrician advised her to go to the emergency room and he would meet her there. Once in the emergency room, he examined her, diagnosed an incomplete abortion, and admitted her to the maternity ward. The obstetrician took her to the operating room and removed the remaining products of conception with a dilation and curettage. He released her from the hospital the next day and saw her in a follow-up visit after four weeks. How is this procedure reported?

Surgery: Nervous System

Section Objectives

Recognize the differences in the Nervous System subsections

- Understand the Nervous System guidelines
- Distinguish between the various types of diagnostic and therapeutic procedures
- Know the difference between Stereotactic Radiosurgery (Intracranial vs Spinal) and Neurostimulators (Intracranial vs Spinal vs Peripheral Nerve)
- Understand the differentiation of intracranial vs extracranial anatomy

The Nervous System subsection describes diagnostic and therapeutic procedures on the following:

- The central nervous system (CNS), comprising the brain and spinal cord
- The peripheral nervous system, controlling nerves that relay and receive messages connecting the CNS and other body parts
- The autonomic nervous system, controlling involuntary functions of internal organs

The Nervous System subsection attempts to list procedures in an anatomical brain to peripheral nerves format. However, from a procedural perspective, a strict anatomic separation is not entirely possible, as certain procedures inherently affect communication and coordination of information to and from the **central nervous system** and the **peripheral nervous system**. It is important to become familiar with the differentiation of intracranial vs extracranial anatomy in order to appropriately use these codes. (See Figures 4-102 and 4-103.)

Coding Tip

Injection, Drainage, or Aspiration codes **61000-61070** do not include imaging guidance. When performed, the appropriate imaging guidance code from the Radiology section should be additionally reported.

Key Terms

Central nervous system: The brain and spinal cord.

Peripheral nervous system: The voluntary and autonomic systems.

Chapter 4

FIGURE 4-102 *The Nervous System*

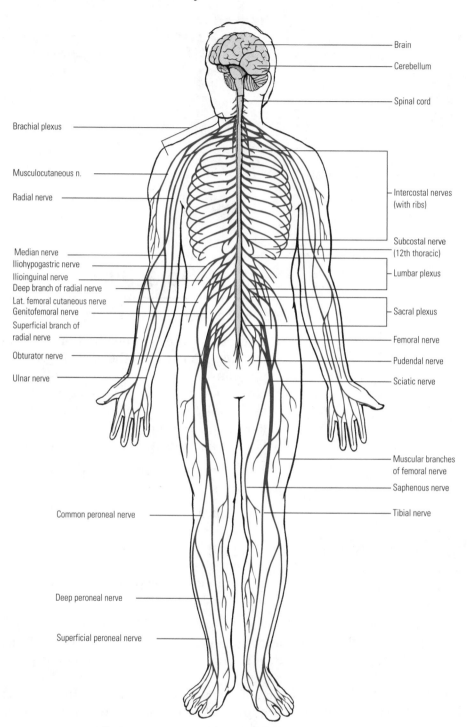

Craniectomy or Craniotomy (61304-61576)

This series of codes describes craniotomy and craniectomy procedures involving various surgical approaches through the skull to reach a specific area of the brain because of disease or trauma (eg, **61546**) or for reconstructive procedures related to congenital or acquired defect (eg, **61556**). To select the correct code, make sure the approach and method are known (eg, hematoma or lesion or abcess). For example, the excision

FIGURE 4-103 *The Brain*

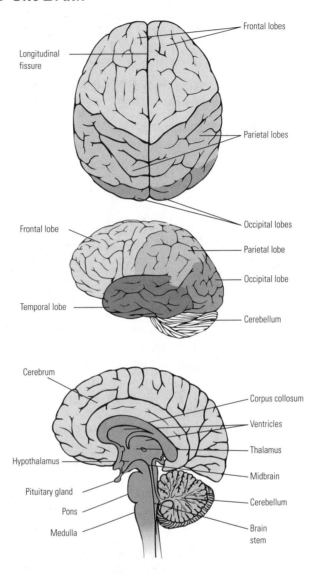

of a cerebellopontine angle tumor of the infratentorial or posterior fossa is reported with code **61520**, as opposed to the excision of a cerebello-pontine angle tumor (ie, acoustic neuroma) involving a transtemporal craniectomy/bone flap craniotomy, which is reported by code **61526**. If harvest of graft material requiring separate incision is performed, this should be additionally reported by means of the appropriate graft code.

Some of the craniotomy procedures (codes **61340**, **61490**) may be performed unilaterally or bilaterally, depending on the involved anatomy. If a bilateral procedure is performed, modifier **50** should be appended to the appropriate code.

Surgery of Skull Base

Skull base surgery can be performed as the initial treatment for lesions of the base of the skull or to excise a lesion after the initial surgery to excise a lesion has failed because of a recurrence of the initial tumor. Coding for skull base procedures requires a thorough understanding of anatomy of the brain and adjoining structures, a good anatomy and physiology text, and a medical dictionary. (See Appendix E, Other Resources.)

Surgery of Skull Base Codes Guidelines

The format of the skull base procedures is based on the division of the cranium into three parts:

1. Anterior,
2. Middle,
3. Posterior fossae.

For each of these anatomic regions, codes were developed that describe the surgical approach, the definitive procedure, and the defect reconstruction. Within this format, any number of surgeons can use the appropriate codes for their specific role in the overall treatment of a patient with a cranial base lesion. Surgical management of lesions involving the skull base often requires the skills of several surgeons of varying specialties working together during the operative session. These operations are single-staged and require primary closure of the surgical defect to avoid life-threatening infectious complications such as meningitis and/or osteomyelitis. The procedures are categorized into the following three groups:

1. **Approach procedure(s)** necessary to obtain adequate exposure to the lesion
2. **Definitive procedure(s)** necessary to biopsy, excise, or otherwise treat the lesion
3. **Reconstruction/repair** of the defect present after the definitive procedure(s)

Key Terms

Approach procedure(s): Described according to anatomical area involved, ie, anterior cranial fossa, middle cranial fossa, posterior cranial fossa, and brain stem or upper spinal cord.

Definitive procedure(s): Describes the repair, biopsy, resection, or excision of various lesions of the skull base and, when appropriate, primary closure of the dura, mucous membranes, and skin.

Reconstruction/repair: Reported separately if extensive dural grafting, cranioplasty, local or regional myocutaneous pedicle flaps, or extensive skin grafts are required.

For Approach procedures, identify if the approach is:

1. Anterior cranial fossa,
2. Middle cranial fossa, or
3. Posterior cranial fossa, and
4. If it is performed by one or more physicians.

When a single surgeon performs the approach procedure, another surgeon performs the definitive procedure, and a third surgeon performs the reconstruction/repair procedure, each surgeon reports only the CPT code for the specific procedure performed. If one surgeon performs more than one procedure (eg, approach and definitive procedure), then both CPT codes are reported, with modifier **51**, *Multiple procedures,* appended to the secondary additional procedure(s). However, it should be noted that add-on procedures cannot be performed if the basic procedure was not performed. Parenthetical notes following add-on codes will instruct which basic procedure the code must be reported with. It is not appropriate to append the modifier **51** to any add-on codes.

When performing both definitive procedures and approach procedures, the definitive procedure has to match the anatomy of the approach procedure. For example, it would not be correct for a coder to select **61582** (base of *anterior* cranial fossa) and **61616** (base of *posterior* cranial fossa). Code **61616** is a definitive procedure for the base of posterior, and the surgery was an anterior cranial fossa.

✓ Check Your Knowledge

1. Explain why the following codes cannot be reported together: approach procedure code **61590** (middle cranial fossa) and definitive procedure code **61600** (anterior cranial fossa)?

Endovascular Therapy

Endovascular Therapy codes represent balloon and catheter codes performed for occlusion on the vessels in the brain. Endovascular intracranial or extracranial vessel *temporary* balloon occlusion uses radiological imaging to facilitate the placement of an intravascular occlusion device in the vasculature of the head or neck to reversibly occlude blood flow to the brain.

The descriptor of codes **61623** and **61624** is differentiated by the terms *temporary* and *permanent* endovascular balloon occlusion procedures. These codes represent different device(s), procedural techniques, and intended outcomes. For code **61623**, the selective catheter placement, positioning, and inflation of the balloon occlusion and the radiological supervision and interpretation (RS&I) of the vessel to be occluded are included in the procedural code **61623**, and therefore are not separately reportable. However, when catheterization is performed for angiography **outside** of the cerebral artery to be occluded, additional nonselective codes (eg, **36005**, **36010**) or selective codes (eg, **36215**, **36216**) may be reported as well. Code **61623** includes fluoroscopic monitoring used to guide placement of a catheter into the target vessel (eg, internal carotid artery, vertebral artery, etc). After vessel selection and angiographic confirmation, fluoroscopic guidance is used for placement of a neuroexchange wire that is then used to monitor placement of the temporary balloon occlusion catheter. Code **61624** represents endovascular therapy that specifically describes *permanent*

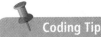
Coding Tip

Certain third-party payers may require modifier **59** be appended to diagnostic angiography codes when reported in conjunction with a therapeutic RS&I code on the same date of service.

occlusion of target vessel. With permanent endovascular vessel occlusion of the central nervous system, selective catheterization and all appropriate RS&I are separately reportable.

Balloon Dilatation of Intracranial Vasospasm

Codes **61640-61642** include all selective vascular catheterization of the target vessel, contrast injection(s), vessel measurement, roadmapping, postdilatation angiography, and fluoroscopic guidance for the balloon dilatation. Complete cerebral angiography (even if performed on the same day) may be reported separately.

For the intracranial aneurysm by intracranial approach (code **61700**), the placement of the ligating clip goes across the neck of an intracranial aneurysm. See Figure 4-104.

Stereotactic Radiosurgery (Cranial) (61796-61800)

Stereotactic radiosurgery/therapy (SRS/SRT) is a method of treating brain disorders with a precise delivery of a single high dose of radiation in a one-day session. Through the use of three-dimensional computer-aided planning and a degree of immobilization, the system can

FIGURE 4-104 *Intracranial Aneurysm, Intracranial Approach*

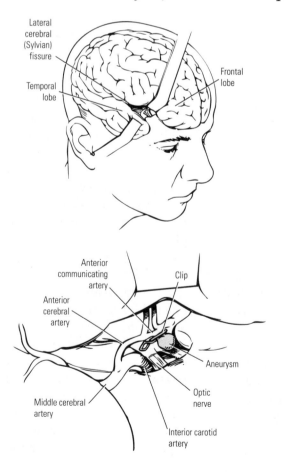

minimize the amount of radiation to healthy brain tissue. Treatment involves the use of focused radiation beams delivered to a specific area of the brain to treat cerebral arteriovenous malformations, benign or malignant primary brain tumors, other metastatic brain tumors, or functional disorders. Although stereotactic radiosurgery can be performed with more than one planning session and in a limited number of treatment sessions (up to a maximum of five sessions), do not report stereotactic radiosurgery more than once *per lesion per course* of treatment when the treatment requires more than one session.

Neurostimulators (Intracranial)

Codes **61850-61888** apply to both simple and complex neurostimulators. Implantation of neurostimulator arrays in subcortical sites is used for control of moderate to severe functional disorders occurring from diseases such as Parkinson is intractable resting tremors, multiple sclerosis, or severe pain from noncancer and cancer causes. (See Figure 4-105.) The Neurostimulator codes do **not** include programming or analysis of neurostimulators. For the initial or subsequent electronic analysis and programming of neurostimulator pulse generators, report codes from the Medicine section (eg, **95970-95982**).

FIGURE 4-105 *Placement of Cranial Neurostimulator*

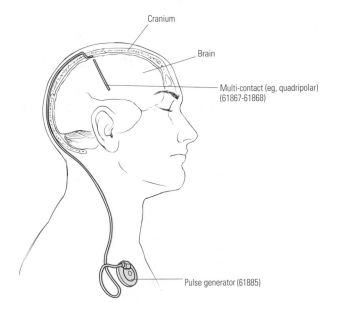

Injection, Drainage, or Aspiration

The spine injection series of codes (**62263-62319**) differentiate by:

- Specific spinal anatomy (subarachnoid, epidural)
- Levels (cervical, thoracic, lumbar, sacral)
- Types of substances injected (neurolytic, opioid, anesthetic, steroid, antispasmodic) to treat intractable pain.

Coding Tip

Code **62263** is not reported for each adhesiolysis treatment, but should be reported once to describe the entire series of injections/infusions spanning two or more treatment days.

Coding Tip

Codes **62310-62319** do not differentiate the type of agent(s) (eg, narcotic, anesthetic, steroid, antispasmodic) injected but focus upon the route of injection (subarachnoid). They do exclude injection of a neurolytic substance, since that procedure is represented by codes **62280-62282**.

Fluoroscopic assistance may or may not be required to visualize and identify specific spinal anatomy in the performance of either epidural or subarachnoid injection procedures. The injection of contrast material during fluoroscopic guidance and localization is **included** in this code series, and therefore is not a separately reportable service. However, if fluoroscopic guidance is performed to assist in accurately localizing specific spinal anatomy for placement of a needle or catheter tip for spinal therapeutic or diagnostic injections, then fluoroscopic guidance code **77003** may be reported. It is important to note that code **77003** does not represent a formal contrast study such as myelography, epidurography, or sacroiliac joint arthrography. If any of these formal contrast studies are performed, fluoroscopy code **77003** is considered to be an inclusive component and should not be separately reported. For example, if doing an injection procedure under fluoroscopic guidance, the injection of *contrast* **is** included, but the *fluoroscopic guidance* can be reported with **77003** if a formal study is done.

Code **62263** includes percutaneous insertion and removal of an epidural catheter that remains in place over a several-day period, for the administration of multiple injections of a neurolytic agent or agents performed during consecutive treatment sessions (ie, spanning two or more treatment days). Code **62264** represents a procedure essentially the same as described for **62263** but differs in that the technique is performed on a one-day basis where the catheter is removed after injecting the drugs or performing mechanical lysis (using a percutaneously deployed catheter), rather than leaving the catheter in the patient over two or more days.

Stereotactic Radiosurgery (Spinal)

Spinal stereotactic radiosurgery is a distinct procedure that utilizes externally generated ionizing radiation to inactivate or eradicate defined target(s) in the spine without the need to make an incision. The target is defined by and the treatment is delivered using high-resolution stereotactic imaging. These codes are reported by the surgeon. Spinal stereotactic radiosurgery is typically performed in a single planning and treatment session using a stereotactic image-guidance system, but can be performed with a planning session and in a limited number of treatment sessions, up to a maximum of five sessions. Do not report stereotactic radiosurgery more than once per lesion per course of treatment when the treatment requires more than one session.

Neurostimulators (Spinal) (63650-63688)

Spinal neurostimulators have been used to treat chronic pain of spinal origin since the 1970s. This treatment involves implanting **electrodes** into the spinal canal to pulse energy across the cord or nerve roots that are involved in transmitting pain sensation. They have been useful for patients with Failed Back Syndrome (pain after multiple surgical interventions), Complex Regional Pain Syndrome (a very difficult syndrome

Key Terms

- Array
- Catheter
- Contact
- Electrode
- Plate/Paddle

in which patients have pain, skin and muscle changes, alteration in blood flow, and loss of function in a limb or other body part), and even in pain due to peripheral ischemia or angina pectoris. The electrode **arrays** are first tested in a patient, placed via an epidural needle, or, if there is a great deal of scar tissue, through an incision with some cutting away of the vertebral lamina to facilitate placement. (See Figures 4-106 and 4-107.)

FIGURE 4-106 *Percutaneous Implantation of Neurostimulator Electrodes*

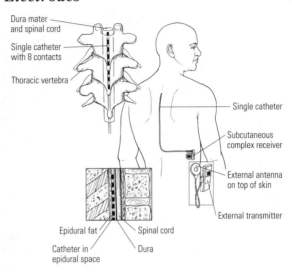

FIGURE 4-107 *Placement of Neurostimulator Electrodes through Laminectomy*

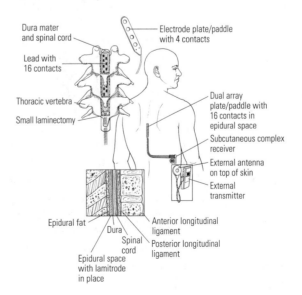

Key Terms

Array: The collection of electrodes or contacts that are on one catheter.

Catheter: A very small plastic tube often implanted in a patient to allow continuous movement of fluid in (local anesthetic) or out (urine).

Contact: The portion of a stimulator array that allows the flow of electrical current between the electrodes and the adjacent patient tissue.

Electrode: The conductor that allows transmission of electrical impulses (created by the generator and carried by the lead) to be translated into energy in the tissue of the patient.

Plate/Paddle: Four or more contacts or electrodes providing electrical stimulation in the epidural space; this design allows a large and complex stimulation design to be used to try to "cover" the patient's pain distribution.

Coding Tip

All neurostimulator electrode arrays have leads with multiple contact electrodes. Reporting is based per electrode catheter or electrode plate or electrode paddle array inserted. A catheter has four to eight bands, each a few millimeters apart around the end of the lead; these bands are the actual contact electrodes. Paddle electrodes can also be used for either peripheral or spinal cord stimulation; named, because they look more like a little paddle at the end of a lead and have four to eight contacts all on one side. It is not appropriate to report based on the number of contact electrodes on a single catheter, plate, or paddle surface.

During this temporary lead placement, the patient is awake in order to determine if the electrical impulses are "covering" the area of pain. If that placement is successful, then the patient is typically sent home with the electrodes exiting the skin and connected to a trial stimulator about the size of a pager, and with which the patient can alter the electrical signal (and sensations) on his or her own over the next few days to determine the likely benefit. If the patient has more than 50% improvement in pain over those days, then he or she will return to have those electrodes buried under the skin and connected to a device similar to a pacemaker, which is also placed under the skin. The patient is also given a wand to program the device to customize the sensations.

It should be noted that the descriptions in codes **63661**, **63662**, **63663**, and **63664** specifically state "array(s)" and "**plate/paddle(s)**" in the plural form, whereas existing code **63650**, *Percutaneous implantation of neurostimulator electrode array, epidural*, and code **63655**, *Laminectomy for implantation of neurostimulator electrodes, plate/paddle, epidural*, reference a single electrode array and single plate/paddle. The rationale is that CPT makes no distinctions in the number of sites required for the placement of electrode catheters. For example, CPT code **63650** is reported for the placement of the initial neurostimulator electrode catheter.

As stated in the parenthetical instructions, removal codes **63661** and **63662**, *Removal of spinal neurostimulator electrode plate/paddle(s) placed via laminotomy or laminectomy, including fluoroscopy, when performed*, are not reported in addition to codes **63663** or **63664**. The work of removing the existing permanent lead array is valued within the code for replacement (**63663**, **63664**), and is therefore not separately reportable.

Because of the spinal cord stimulation's broad indications, it is used for numerous neuropathic pain disorders that require either simple or complex treatment (eg, management of postamputation neuralgia [stump pain], postherpetic neuralgia). Codes **63650-63688** apply to both simple and complex neurostimulators.

For more complex pain patterns:

- two catheter electrode arrays can be percutaneously placed,
- one plate/paddle with two arrays (two lines of multiple electrode contacts), or
- two plates/paddles can be placed.

These types of systems allow the delivery of complex stimulation patterns for conditions not amenable to stimulation by single catheter electrode array. If the physician implants one neurostimulator paddle containing four electrodes, code **63655** should be reported once. Each reporting of this code describes placement of only one such plate/paddle containing multiple **contacts**. For percutaneously placed systems, the contacts are on a catheter (**63650**); for systems placed via an open surgical exposure, the contacts are on a plate- or paddle-shaped surface (**63655**). The contacts are permanently attached to the catheter or the plate-paddle surface. After placement of the stimulation system, the catheter or plate-paddle is left permanently implanted. Fluoroscopy to position the catheter or plate-paddle containing the electrode array is considered an inclusive component of code **63655** and therefore is not separately reportable (eg, **76000, 77002, 77003**).

Paravertebral Facet Joint Injections

The facet joints are a complex system of joint space, meniscal covering, nerves, and ligaments that allow each spinal vertebra to interact with its neighbors, and is the site of interaction between the vertebral bone above and below, and can be a source of pain. These joints and ligaments are subject to impressive stress, and may develop arthritis and other joint diseases. Injections or lesions can be made either:

- into the joint, or
- at each of the nerves that supply the joint (these are the medial nerve branches).

Codes **64490-64495** are differentiated from each other based on the anatomic location and the number of levels where the procedures are performed (ie, single, second, and any additional level[(s]). The lumbar facet injection codes (**64490-64495**) and cervical/thoracic facet joint injection codes (**64479** and **64480**) are reported **once** when the injection procedure is performed, irrespective of whether a single or multiple puncture is required to anesthetize the target joint at a given level and side. Commonly, physicians use a technique that involves insertion of the needle once, with attachment of a short piece of extension tubing through which the first drug is injected. The syringe is then changed, and the next drug is injected through the same tubing/needle. Should the physician choose to perform separate needle punctures, this multiple needle technique does not alter reporting.

Coding Tip

Because a lead array contains at least four to eight electrodes, the plural use of the term electrodes occurs in the descriptors of the peripheral nerve neurostimulator codes (**64553-64565**). There are multiple electrode contacts on the catheter, plate, or paddle type of electrode array used in brain, spinal cord, sacral, and peripheral nerve stimulation. However, reporting is per insertion of either a single electrode array or a single plate or paddle. Again, it is not appropriate to report based on the number of contact electrodes on a single catheter, plate, or paddle surface.

Coding Tip

The fluoroscopic guidance (eg, **76000, 77003**) is considered inherent in the performance of the percutaneous implantation of the neurostimulator electrode array in the epidural space as represented by code **63650**, *Percutaneous implantation of neurostimulator electrode array, epidural.* Therefore, it would not be appropriate to additionally report the fluoroscopic guidance used.

Add-on codes **64492** and **64495** are reported once as a line item irrespective of the number of spinal levels treated. Therefore, codes **64492** and **64495** are not reported more than once.

Only one facet injection code should be reported at a specified level and side injected (eg, right L4-5 facet joint), regardless of the number of needle(s) inserted or number of drug(s) injected at that specific level.

Neurostimulators (Peripheral Nerve) (64550-64595)

Codes **64553-64595** apply to both simple and complex neurostimulators. For initial or subsequent electronic analysis and programming of neurostimulator pulse generators, see codes **95970-95975**. (See Figure 4-108.)

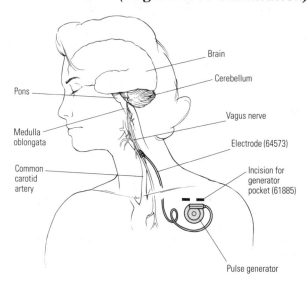

FIGURE 4-108 *Implantation of Neurostimulator Electrodes, Cranial Nerve (Vagal Nerve Stimulation)*

Destruction by Neurolytic Agent (eg, Chemical, Thermal, Electrical, Radiofrequency, or Chemodenervation)

Although this heading includes codes for reporting destruction by neurolytic agent to somatic and sympathetic nerves, the term *destruction* does not apply to all of the **64600-64681** series of codes. Destruction does not apply to codes **64611-64614** and **64650-64653** because the nerve is technically not destroyed but is chemodenervated, meaning that the effect of the drug injection (eg, type A botulinum toxin) is largely or completely reversible. To innervate muscles of the limb or trunk muscles, botulinum toxin is injected directly into the muscle through an electrode to treat dystonia, spasticity, cerebral palsy, multiple sclerosis, muscle spasms, spinal cord injuries, and multiple sclerosis. Codes **64611-64614** and **64650-64653** are reported **once**, even though multiple injections are performed in sites along a particular muscle (several muscles are typically injected). (See Figure 4-109.) If the Botox injection is performed on muscle(s) not specified in these codes, then the unlisted code **64999**, *Unlisted procedure, nervous system,* is reported.

When performing both approach and definitive procedures, the definitive procedure has to match the anatomy of the approach procedure.

FIGURE 4-109 *Chemodenervation of Extremity*

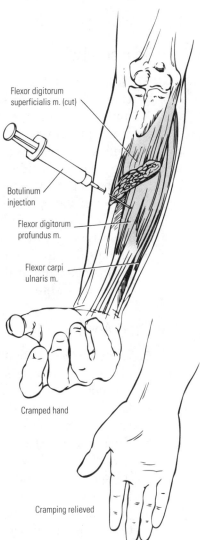

Flexor digitorum
superficialis m. (cut)

Botulinum
injection

Flexor digitorum
profundus m.

Flexor carpi
ulnaris m.

Cramped hand

Cramping relieved

Therefore, it would not be correct to select code **61590** (*middle* cranial fossa) and **61600** (*anterior* cranial fossa).

✓ Check Your Knowledge Answer

1. When performing both approach and definitive procedures, the definitive procedure has to match the anatomy of the approach procedure. Therefore, it would not be correct to select code **61590** (*middle* cranial fossa) and **61600** (*anterior* cranial fossa).

Nervous System Exercises

Check your answers in Appendix B.

True or False

1. Both codes **62263** and **62264** should be reported only one time for the entire series of injections/infusions or mechanical lysis procedures performed, not per adhesiolysis treatment. **True or False**
2. It is **not** appropriate to report based on the number of contact electrodes on a single catheter, plate, or paddle surface. **True or False**
3. Fluoroscopic guidance is considered not inherent in the performance of the percutaneous implantation of the neurostimulator electrode array in the epidural space (code **63650**) and may be reported separately. **True or False**
4. If destruction by a neurolytic agent of the paravertebral facet joint on both left and right sides at the L5 level of the lumbar spine is performed, then code **64622** is reported only once for the L5 level. **True or False**

Short Answer

5. If the surgeon, Dr A, performs the Approach and Definitive procedures and another surgeon, Dr B, performs the reconstruction/repair procedure, which procedures can Dr A report?
6. List the three parts the cranium is divided into.
7. List the three groups the skull base procedures are categorized in.
8. Choose the correct code for the following procedure report.

   A 27-year-old woman was receiving the dopamine-receptor blocking agent, pimozide, for treatment of Tourette syndrome. She developed tardive dystonia with severe arching of her back. The patient was unresponsive to and had side effects from oral medications. Using clinical examination and available electrodiagnostic information, the erector spinae muscles were identified. The sites were prepped and localized. Injections of botulinum toxin were administered to the multiple sites along the muscle. Several muscles were injected. A report was dictated. How is this reported?
9. Choose the correct code for the following procedure report.

   A 45-year-old male with extensive rectal carcinoma involving the left lumbosacral plexus had intractable left perirectal pain but had lost much of his control of both bladder and bowel function. Various systemic medications (oral narcotic and nonnarcotic), physical therapy, radiation therapy, and chemotherapy all failed to provide significant long-term pain relief. There were no further operative resections possible for the tumor.

   This patient was a good candidate for a neurolytic injection because of the severity of the pain and the diminished control of bladder and bowel function. A neurolytic injection to ablate the left S2-4 nerve roots was recommended. The injection could be performed subarachnoid or epidural, depending upon the extent of tumor and any scarring from previous therapy in either the subarachnoid or epidural space. How is this reported?

Surgery: Eye and Ocular Adnexa

Section Objectives

- Recognize the differences in the Eye and Ocular Adnexa subsections
- Understand the Eye and Ocular Adnexa guidelines

Coding of surgical procedures on the eye and its surrounding tissues can be complex because of the numerous anatomic structures in the ocular system. It is essential to review the eye anatomy (see Figure 4-110), as these terms are critical to understanding the operative procedures performed on the eye and the CPT codes that describe them. Therefore, it is important to pay close attention to eye anatomy, each code descriptor, and its location in the Eye and Ocular Adnexa subsection, as well as the appropriate guidelines. A key concept used throughout this subsection is that of *separate procedure,* which serves to identify those procedures that may be considered a part of a surgical procedure on certain visual system anatomy. For example, code **65860**, *Severing adhesions of anterior segment, laser technique (separate procedure),* may be an integral part of another procedure on the anterior segment; however, it is not a part of surgical procedures on the sclera.

FIGURE 4-110 *Eye Anatomy*

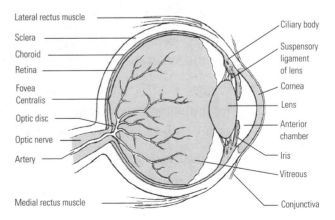

Lateral rectus muscle
Sclera
Choroid
Retina
Fovea Centralis
Optic disc
Optic nerve
Artery
Medial rectus muscle

Ciliary body
Suspensory ligament of lens
Cornea
Lens
Anterior chamber
Iris
Vitreous
Conjunctiva

Coding Tip

The diagnostic and noninvasive tests of the eye are not reported from the Eye and Ocular Adnexa subsection. These are listed in the Medicine section of the CPT codebook, under the Ophthalmology subheading or in the appropriate section, such as Diagnostic Ultrasound.

Chapter 4

Coding Tip

For orbital implant insertion (implant outside the muscle cone), use code **67550** for the implant and code **67560** for removal.

The codes in the Eye and Ocular Adnexa subsection of the CPT codebook represent procedures of the eyeball (the globe) and the ocular adnexa. The codes describing procedures performed on the eyeball are divided anatomically into:

- Divisions among the globe in its entirety
- The anterior segment
- The posterior segment

The codes describing procedures performed on the ocular adnexa are divided anatomically into:

- The extraocular muscles
- The eyelids
- The conjunctiva
- The orbit

The further subheadings are anatomically based and then broken into procedure categories. The orbital bones are ordinarily considered part of the musculoskeletal system, but incision and excision of bone(s) of the orbit are described in the Eye and Ocular Adnexa subsection for convenience of the user of the CPT codebook. However, treatments of fractures of the orbital bones are described and coded in the Musculoskeletal System subsection.

Eyeball

Codes **65091-65114** describe removal of the eye, contents of the eye, or the eye and surrounding adnexa (associated anatomic sites). This series of codes is differentiated by the types of procedures performed; evisceration, enucleation, and exenteration.

When implants are placed in the orbit at a time **after** the initial surgery to enucleate or eviscerate the eye, they are called *secondary implant procedures*. Codes **65125-65175** describe secondary implant(s) procedures. Ocular and orbital implants are used to replace the volume loss created by removing the eye and/or orbital contents.

EXAMPLE

Evisceration with implant and placement of a regional orbital block catheter.

Code **65093**, *Evisceration of ocular contents; with implant*. The placement of the pain pump or catheter during other surgery in the operative site is *not* separately reported. When the pump or catheter is placed during a surgical procedure in the same site for pain management, only the surgical code identifying the definitive/main procedure for that surgical site should be used (no additional codes should be used to identify the placement of the catheter or pump device when other surgery is performed for that site).

To select the correct code for the removal of a foreign body, it is important to note the anatomical area and the approach. For example, code the removal of a foreign body from:

- The eyelid (embedded), use **67938**
- The lacrimal system, use **68530**
- The orbit
  - frontal approach, use **67413**
  - lateral approach, use **67430**
  - transcranial approach, use **61334**

- **Secondary implant procedures**
- **Lamellar**
- **Penetrating**
- **Endothelial**

Codes **65205-65265** apply to the removal of foreign bodies of the globe, conjunctiva, cornea, and inside the eye (anterior chamber, posterior chamber, posterior segment, or lens). When coding for removal of an intraocular foreign body from the eye, check the patient's medical record to see if any imaging procedures were performed. If so, remember to code the echography procedure (eg, code **76510**) when appropriate.

Laceration repairs of the conjunctiva, cornea, and sclera are reported using codes from the **65270-65290** series. Repair of a laceration includes use of a conjunctival flap and restoration of the anterior chamber by air or saline injection, when indicated. Repair of wounds of the eyelid and the skin of the face surrounding the orbit are coded in the integumentary system (eg, simple repair codes **12011-12018**; intermediate, layered closure codes **12051-12057**; and linear, complex repair codes **13150-13153**.) For repair of a wound of the lacrimal system, use code **68700**. For repair of an operative wound, use code **66250**.

✓ Check Your Knowledge

1. Is the following statement true or false, and why?
   When removing a foreign body from the orbit using the frontal approach, code **67430** may be reported.

Anterior Segment

The Anterior Segment subsection of the CPT codebook includes the codes describing procedures of the cornea, anterior chamber, limbus, iris, ciliary body, and lens. The structure follows a template of excision (**65400-65426**) and removal or destruction (**65430-65600**) procedures. With code **65450**, a freezing probe is applied directly to the corneal defect to destroy it. (See Figure 4-111.)

For codes **65710-65757**, the term *keratoplasty* specifically refers to corneal transplants differentiated by three terms (ie, lamellar, penetrating, and endothelial). **Lamellar** refers to a transplant method

FIGURE 4-111 *Cryotherapy of Lesion on Cornea*

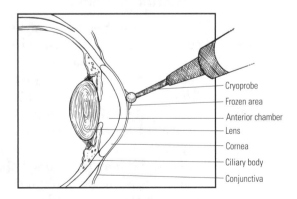

Key Terms

Secondary implant procedures: When implants are placed in the orbit at a time **after** the initial surgery to enucleate or eviscerate the eye.

Lamellar: Transplant method that removes the anterior layers of the diseased cornea and replaces them with a piece of donor cornea cut to the same size and shape.

Penetrating: Full-thickness replacement of the cornea following removal of the diseased corneal tissue.

Endothelial: Replacement of only the innermost layer of the cornea containing the corneal endothelium.

that removes the anterior layers of the diseased cornea and replaces them with a piece of donor cornea cut to the same size and shape. **Penetrating** refers to the full-thickness replacement of the cornea following removal of the diseased corneal tissue. **Endothelial** refers to the replacement of only the innermost layer of the cornea containing the corneal endothelium. The work associated with preparation or sizing of the donor graft corneal tissue performed by the physician is included in this series of codes, and therefore, not separately reported.

In addition to the corneal transplant codes, the CPT codebook contains codes describing other corrective procedures performed on the cornea. Codes **65760-65775** identify distinct procedural techniques that may be used to improve visual acuity. Codes **65772** and **65775** describe procedures used to correct astigmatism resulting from a prior surgical procedure. Astigmatism may occur following, for example, corneal transplant surgery, lens implant surgery, or glaucoma or cataract surgery. The goal of these procedures is to alter the corneal surface to correct the astigmatism. Codes for procedures on the lens, **66820-66986**, can be described as incisions, removal of lens, and placements of intraocular lens prostheses.

Posterior Segment

The Posterior Segment subsection, codes **67005-67299**, includes procedures performed on the vitreous, the retina or choroid, and the posterior sclera. The parenthetical notes are key for referral to other codes that are closely related to these procedures. The Retina or Choroid subsection, codes **67101-67229**, delineates those procedures performed for repair, prophylaxis, and destruction. **Repair** refers to treatment of retinal detachments. When repair of retinal detachments is coded, the codes refer to the series of treatments needed. This treatment series may be accomplished at one or more treatment sessions on the same day or different days. (Refer to the discussion in this chapter regarding reporting codes with the phrase "one or more sessions.")

Coding Tip

If more than one method is used to treat the holes, tears, or detachment, such as diathermy, cryotherapy, and/or photocoagulation, select the code that corresponds to the principal modality that the physician uses. For example, when the repair of retinal tears is treated by both cryotherapy, but predominantly photocoagulation, code **67105** should be selected in this instance.

Prophylaxis in these codes refers to the goal to seal a retinal tear and prevent a retinal detachment from extending. With code **67027**, a drug delivery system that releases medication into the vitreous is implanted into the vitreous by pars plana incision. (See Figure 4-112.)

With code **67107**, the retinal tear is treated externally by placing a hot or cold probe over the sclera and then depressing it. The burn seals the choroid to the retina at the site of the tear. The healing scar is supported by the encircling band, which buckles the eye. (See Figure 4-113.)

FIGURE 4-112 *Intravitreal Drug Delivery System*

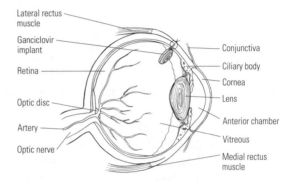

EXAMPLE

Procedure: Ocular photodynamic therapy is a noninvasive treatment for age-related macular degeneration.

Rationale on how to report: Laser photocoagulation (**67220**, *Destruction of localized lesion of choroid (eg, choroidal neovascularization); photocoagulation (eg, laser), 1 or more sessions)* relies on the laser to ablate the abnormal tissue by heating, which involves greater work intensity and usually more than one treatment session. Ocular Photodynamic therapy (**67221**, *Destruction of localized lesion of choroid (eg, choroidal neovascularization); photodynamic therapy (includes intravenous infusion),* usually requires a single session. However, this procedure may also be performed on both eyes at a single session. In that instance, report the bilateral add-on code (**✚67225**, *Destruction of localized lesion of choroid [eg, choroidal neovascularization]; photodynamic therapy, second eye, at single session (List separately in addition to code for primary eye treatment])* in addition to **67221**. Do not append modifier **50** to code **67221**.

One or More Sessions

A number of codes in the Eye and Ocular Adnexa section contain the phrase "one or more sessions" in their descriptor. When this phrase appears in a code descriptor, the code should be reported only once for the entire defined treatment period, regardless of the number of sessions necessary to complete the treatment. In other words, the code

FIGURE 4-113 *Repair of Retinal Detachment*

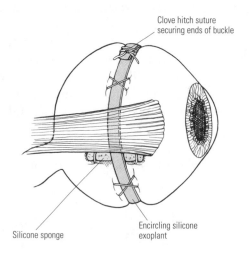

Clove hitch suture securing ends of buckle

Silicone sponge

Encircling silicone exoplant

would not be reported for each session in which the patient was seen if it was a visit included in a defined treatment period. The defined treatment period is determined by the physician and varies depending on the patient, diagnosis, and, often, the area to be treated. However, if the patient experiences a recurrence of the condition and retreatment is necessary, then these subsequent retreatment sessions would not be considered included in the first treatment series. This retreatment would be reported with the appropriate code, since it represents a new defined treatment period of one or more sessions performed to treat the problem.

Ocular Adnexa

The Ocular Adnexa subsection includes codes **67311-67999** describing strabismus surgery (operation on the extraocular muscles). This surgery is performed to realign the eyes so that they are both aimed in the same direction. The correction of extraocular muscle misalignment may allow restoration of depth perception, single binocular vision, and expansion of the visual field. The coding of modern strabismus surgery often requires the use of multiple procedural codes. (See Figure 4-114.)

FIGURE 4-114 *Extraocular Muscles of the Right Eye*

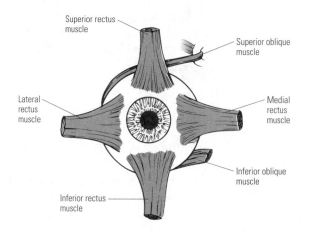

Superior rectus muscle

Superior oblique muscle

Lateral rectus muscle

Medial rectus muscle

Inferior oblique muscle

Inferior rectus muscle

See Figure 4-115 for the strabismus surgery horizontal muscles codes **67311-67312**. In Figure 4-115A, the medial or lateral rectus muscle is made weaker by recession (retroplacement of the muscle attachment). Use **67311** for one horizontal muscle and **67312** for two muscles of the same eye. In Figure 4-115B, it is made stronger by resection (removal of a segment).

FIGURE 4-115A *Strabismus Surgery—Horizontal Muscles*

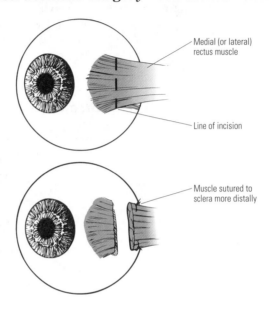

Medial (or lateral) rectus muscle

Line of incision

Muscle sutured to sclera more distally

FIGURE 4-115B *Strabismus Surgery—Horizontal Muscles*

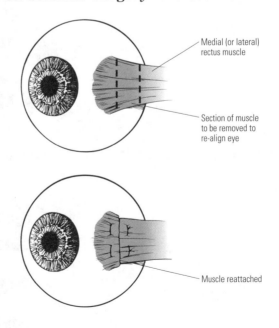

Medial (or lateral) rectus muscle

Section of muscle to be removed to re-align eye

Muscle reattached

Chapter 4

> **EXAMPLE**
>
> One horizontal muscle in each eye is operated on for the first time. In this case, code **67311 50** is reported to indicate that one horizontal muscle in each eye was operated on.
>
> With the strabismus surgery vertical muscles codes **67314-67316**, either the superior or inferior rectus muscle is strengthened or weakened. Use **67316** for two muscles of the same eye. For the transposition procedure code **67320**, the extraocular muscles are transposed. With strabismus surgery adjustable sutures code **67335**, sutures are tied in such a way as to allow the tension on the muscle to be adjusted after the anesthetic is not affecting the position of the globe. (See Figures 4-116 through 4-118.)

FIGURE 4-116 *Strabismus Surgery—Vertical Muscles*

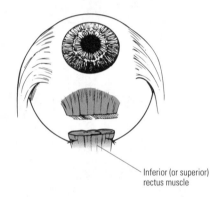

Inferior (or superior) rectus muscle

FIGURE 4-117 *Transposition Procedure*

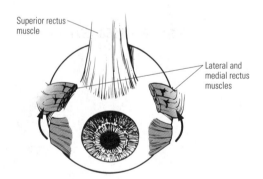

Superior rectus muscle

Lateral and medial rectus muscles

FIGURE 4-118 *Strabismus Surgery—Adjustable Sutures*

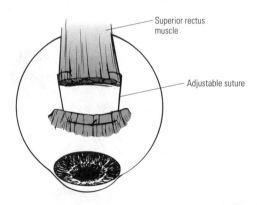

Superior rectus muscle

Adjustable suture

Conjunctiva

Surgical procedures performed on the conjunctiva include:

- Incision and drainage
- Excision and/or destruction
- Injection
- Conjunctivoplasty
- Other procedures

These conjunctiva procedures are described by codes **68020-68399**. Excluded from this series are the removal of foreign body procedures from the conjunctiva, which are coded using **65205-65222**.

Coding Tip

When the eyelashes are ingrown or misdirected (trichiasis), the physician uses a biomicroscope and forceps to remove the offending eyelashes. Report **67825** when cryosurgery or electrosurgery is used to destroy the follicles. (See Figure 4-119.)

FIGURE 4-119 *Trichiasis*

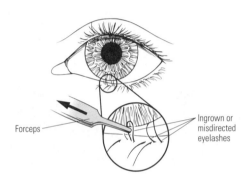

Forceps

Ingrown or misdirected eyelashes

Coding Tip

Because there is one punctum in **each** eyelid, if **both** puncta of one side are occluded, then code **68761** would be reported twice. If **both** eyes are treated *(all four puncta),* then code **68761** is reported four times.

EXAMPLE

One horizontal muscle of the right eye is operated on for the first time, and the superior oblique muscle of the left eye is also operated on. In this case, modifier **50**, *Bilateral procedure,* is not used. The individual codes for these specific services are reported (**67311** and **67318**). Modifier **51**, *Multiple procedures,* is appended to code **67311**.

Lacrimal System

Codes **68400-68899** describe procedures on the lacrimal system and include:

- Incision
- Excision repairs
- Probing and/or related procedures

Coding Tip

Nasolacrimal duct probing is included in the descriptor for code **68815**. It would not be appropriate to separately report codes **68810** and **68811** for probing the nasolacrimal duct and insertion of a tube or stent.

The incisional procedures typically involve drainage-type procedures. The excisional procedures include biopsies of the lacrimal gland and lacrimal sac. Closure of the lacrimal puncta (the entrance to the tear drainage system from the eye surface to the nose) is one of the most common procedures performed. Code **68760** describes closure of the lacrimal punctum by thermocauterization, ligation, or laser surgery. Code **68761** is reported if the closure is performed with a punctal plug.

With code **68761**, the physician inserts a lacrimal duct implant into a lacrimal punctum. (See Figure 4-120.)

When performing code **68816**, *Probing of nasolacrimal duct, with or without irrigation; with transluminal balloon catheter dilation*, a balloon catheter is passed through the superior puncture, canalicular system, and into the nasolacrimal duct. (See Figure 4-121.)

FIGURE 4-120 *Closure of Lacrimal Punctum by Plug*

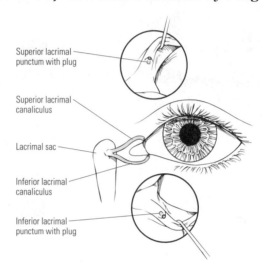

FIGURE 4-121 *Probing of Nasolacrimal Duct*

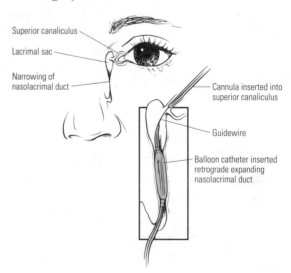

Operating Microscope

A surgical operating microscope is used to obtain good visualization of the fine structures in the operating field. The lens system may be operated by hand or foot controls to adjust to working distance, with interchangeable oculars providing magnification as needed. The surgical microscope is used when the surgical services are performed using the techniques of microsurgery. (See Figure 4-122.) Code **69990** should be reported in addition to the code for the primary procedure performed. Do not use **69990** for visualization with magnifying loupes or corrected vision. Do not report code **69990** in addition to procedures in which use of the operating microscope is an inclusive component (codes **15756-15758, 15842, 19364, 19368, 20955-20962, 20969-20973, 22551, 22552, 22856-22861, 26551-26554, 26556, 31526, 31531, 31536, 31541, 31545, 31546, 31561, 31571, 43116, 43496, 49906, 61548, 63075-63078, 64727, 64820-64823, 65091-68850, 0184T, 0226T, 0227T**). As with all add-on codes, **69990** should be reported with modifier **51** appended.

EXAMPLE

For what types of procedures would one additionally report use of the operating microscope for microsurgical technique?

- Some types of procedures for which the operating microscope may be reported include **61700**, *Surgery of intracranial aneurysm, intracranial approach; carotid circulation.* When procedure **61700** is performed with the use of an operating microscope, it is appropriate to also report the use of the operating microscope code **69990**, *Use of operating microscope (List separately in addition to code for primary procedure).*
- If an operating microscope was used to perform microsurgery techniques in conjunction with **55400**, *Vasovasostomy, vasovasorrhaphy,* the use of the operating microscope may be reported separately using **69990**.
- Code **35206** describes the repair of each blood vessel (thoracodorsal artery to inferior epigastric artery and thoracodorsal vein to inferior epigastric vein). Code **35206** does not describe a microvascular technique, so the add-on code **69990** should be reported for each anastomosis performed by microvascular technique.

✓ Check Your Knowledge Answers

1. False. When selecting the correct code for the removal of a foreign body, it is important to note the anatomical area and the approach. This removal is taken from the orbit using the frontal approach, which would be reported with code **67413**. The code **67430** is for the lateral approach.

FIGURE 4-122 *Operating Microscope*

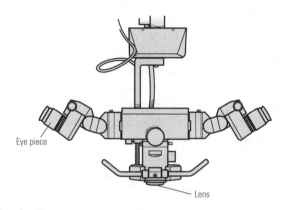

Eye piece

Lens

Eye and Ocular Adnexa Excercises

Check your answers in Appendix B.

True or False

1. The treatments of fractures of the orbital bones are described and coded in the Eye and Ocular Adnexa subsection. **True or False**
2. If performing a *photodynamic therapy destruction of a lesion of choroid* (code **67221**), modifier **50** is appended. **True or False**
3. When the phrase "one or more sessions" appears in a code descriptor, the code may be reported only for each session in which the patient was seen if it was a visit included in a defined treatment period. **True or False**

Short Answer

4. Exploration, excision, and decompression procedures as well as injections and orbital implants are described by codes _____.
5. Does the ciliary body destruction described by code **66710**, *Ciliary body destruction; cyclophotocoagulation, transscleral*, include an endoscopic approach as in code **66711**, *Ciliary body destruction; cyclophotocoagulation, endoscopic*? Explain.

Multiple Choice

6. A patient visited his ophthalmologist because of tears in the retina in his left eye. The ophthalmologist recommended laser photocoagulation treatment(s) for prophylaxis of retinal detachment and documented this in the record. In the outpatient setting, the patient underwent laser photocoagulation on April 1, April 15, and May 15. How are these treatments coded?
   a. **67145, 67145 51, 67145 51**; reported three times for each date and modifier **51** appended to indicate multiple procedures
   b. **67145**; reported once for all dates
   c. **67145, 67145 59, 67145 59**; reported three times for each date and modifier **59** appended to indicate separate procedures

Match the following terms to the correct definitions:

7. keratoplasty
8. blepharoplasty
9. enucleation
10. exenteration
11. cataract
12. punctum
13. lacrimal gland
14. pterygium
15. iris
16. evisceration
17. strabismus
18. lamellar
19. lacrimal sac
20. sclera
21. tarsal plate
22. uvea
23. conjunctiva
24. choroid
25. lens
26. retina

    a. opaque covering on or in the lens
    b. extensive removal of entire contents of orbit
    c. removing intraocular contents of the eyeball
    d. removing the entire eyeball
    e. degenerative hyperplastic process of ocular surface
    f. responsible for the form/shape of each eyelid
    g. "the whites of your eyes," the white outer coat of the eyeball that surrounds the cornea all the way back to the optic nerve
    h. produce tears to lubricate the eye
    i. middle layer of tissue of the eyeball (includes iris and ciliary body)
    j. repair of the eyelid
    k. colored portion of the eye, an anterior extension of the uvea
    l. a corneal transplant method
    m. surgical repair of the cornea
    n. entrance to the tear drainage system from the eye to the nose
    o. defect due to excess contraction or to excess relaxation of one or more extraocular muscles
    p. vascular network in the posterior portion of the uvea
    q. multilayered, inner portion of the eye through which light is focused on the retina
    r. the part of the eye (containing rods and cones) that converts light into nervous signals
    s. site in lacrimal bone where tears fill
    t. a mucous membrane that lines the inner surfaces of the eyelids and folds back to cover the front surface of the eyeball, except for the central clear portion of the outer eye cornea

Surgery: Auditory System

Section Objectives

- Recognize the differences in the Auditory subsection
- Understand the guidelines that apply to the Auditory System

The auditory system subsection of the CPT codebook is further divided into code ranges for reporting procedures of the following:

- External ear: **69000-69399**
- Middle ear: **69400-69799**
- Inner ear: **69801-69949**
- Temporal bone, middle fossa approach: **69950-69979**

Read the parenthetical note at the beginning of this subsection that provides direction for reporting diagnostic services of the auditory system. Those services are not described here but rather are reported with codes from the Special Otorhinolaryngologic Services subsection in the Medicine section of the CPT codebook (**92502-92700**).

External Ear

In the section for procedures of the external ear (**69000-69399**), separate headings indicate:

- Incision
- Excision
- Removal
- Repair
- Other procedures

The external ear (see Figure 4-123) consists of the portion on the side of the head called the auricle or pinna and the tube that connects the auricle to the temporal bone, called the external auditory meatus or ear canal. The tympanic membrane stretches across the inside end of the canal to separate it from the middle ear. Code **69399** is used to report unlisted procedures of the external ear. Use of this code is appropriate

FIGURE 4-123 *Ear*

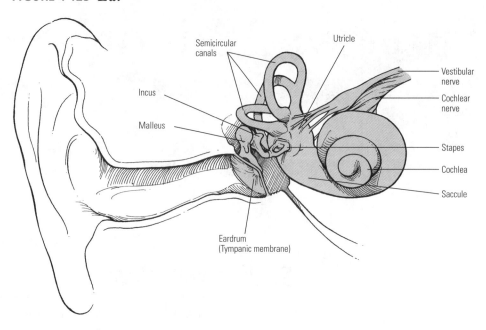

when a procedure is performed on the external ear that is not described with a more specific code from the external ear section. Code **69210** is used to report removal of impacted cerumen from one or both ears. This procedure involves direct visualization generally with magnification for removal of impacted cerumen by means of suction, a cerumen spoon, or delicate forceps. If the use of an operating microscope is necessary during this procedure, separately code **69990**.

Middle Ear

In the section of procedures of the middle ear (**69400-69799**), separate headings indicate:

- Introduction
- Incision
- Excision
- Repair
- Other procedures

The middle ear consists of several parts:

- Malleus
- Incus
- Stapes
- Ossicles with the tympanic cavity

The ossicles cavity has several openings including the oval window, the round window, and the eustachian tube. One will notice these terms throughout the middle ear section. This section of codes also contains unlisted code **69799** that is used to report unlisted procedures of the middle ear. When performing codes **69433-69436**, a ventilating tube is inserted into the opening of the tympanum.

Removal of Tubes

The subsequent removal of ventilating tubes, when performed by the same or another physician who performed the original placement procedure, is a separately reportable service. When ventilating tubes are removed by a physician with the patient under general anesthesia, code **69424** is used to report this procedure. Ventilating tube removal may be performed in those instances where the tympanostomy tube has failed or is causing problems (ie, local infection, granulation, cholesteatoma formation). Code **69424** is considered a unilateral procedure. Therefore, if tubes are removed from both ears, then modifier **50** should be appended to procedure code **69424**. The code should not be reported if performed along with a more complex procedure involving the tympanic membrane (eg, myringoplasty or tympanoplasty).

✓ Check Your Knowledge

1. When a physician performs the removal of ventilating tubes under general anesthesia, subsequent to the original placement of the tubes, how is this reported? Explain.

Tympanoplasty

Tympanoplasty is a microsurgical technique that repairs or removes disease involving the tympanic membrane or the middle ear. This type of surgery is performed either transcanal (through the external auditory canal) or postauricularly (behind the ear). The tympanoplasty family of codes **(69631-69646)** describes tympanic membrane and middle ear repair procedures to treat disease and restore hearing. Occasionally, when disease processes or previous surgery has caused damage to the middle ear bones (ossicles) and resultant conductive hearing loss, a surgeon will reconstruct middle ear structure(s) with the patient's own ossicles or a synthetic prosthesis. Tympanoplasty must be distinguished from myringoplasty, a procedure limited solely to the drumhead or eardrum. Code **69620** describes an operation to repair the tympanic membrane only and includes the harvesting of a donor graft when performed. The middle ear is not entered. However, a tympanoplasty as described by codes **69631-69646** requires entry and inspection of the middle ear. When performing tympanoplasty procedure codes **69635-69646**, a graft is used to repair the tympanic membrane perforation. (See Figure 4-124.)

There are three families of tympanoplasty codes **(69631-69633, 69635-69637, 69641-69646)**, each representing unique techniques, approach, anatomy, and prosthetic or graft placement procedures. Therefore, the tympanoplasty code descriptors have distinct structure differentiating the procedural services:

- The descriptors reference canalplasty, atticotomy, and/or middle ear surgery as inclusive procedures, when performed.
- Mastoidectomy may or may not be performed.

Chapter 4

FIGURE 4-124 *Tympanostomy*

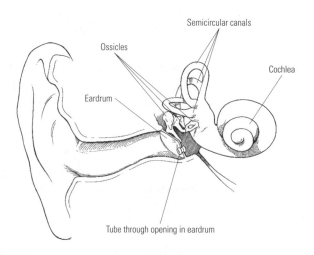

Coding Tip

Although not specifically stated in the descriptor nomenclature, code **69610** is considered a unilateral procedure code. If it is done bilaterally, modifier **50**, *Bilateral procedure*, should be appended to code **69610**. CPT codes **69631-69646** are unilateral procedures. Therefore, if the surgeon performs one of these procedures in both ears (although clinically infrequently performed), then it would be appropriate to append modifier **50**, *Bilateral procedure*, to the code describing the definitive surgical procedure.

- Reconstruction may or may not be performed on the middle ear's three tiny bones (ossicles—malleus, incus, and stapes) that form a chain attached to the inner side of the eardrum in the middle ear.
- Synthetic ossicular replacement prosthesis (partial or total) may be used.
- Tympanoplasties can be either an "initial" or "revision" procedure.

Inner Ear

In the section of procedures of the inner ear (**69801-69949**), separate headings indicate:

- Incision and/or destruction (**69801-69840**)
- Excision (**69905-69915**)
- Introduction (**69930**)
- Other procedures (**69949**)

Procedure code **69930** involves an internal coil being attached to the temporal bone with its ground wire attached to the temporalis muscle. The electrode array is implanted into the cochlea. This procedure is intended to stimulate cochlear nerve fibers and to aid sound perception. (See Figures 4-125 and 4-126.)

✓ Check Your Knowledge Answer

1. The subsequent removal of ventilating tubes, when performed by the same or another physician who performed the original placement procedure, is a separately reportable service. When ventilating tubes are removed by a physician with the patient under general anesthesia, code **69424** is used to report this procedure.

FIGURE 4-125 *Cochlear Device Implantation*

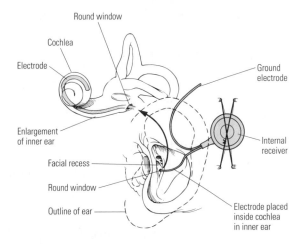

FIGURE 4-126 *Vestibular Nerve Section, Transcranial Approach*

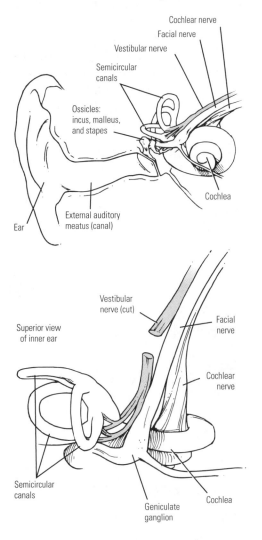

Auditory System Exercises

Check your answers in Appendix B.

True or False

1. Tympanoplasty can be either an "initial" or "revision" procedure. **True or False**

Short Answer

2. List the anatomy comprising the external ear, middle ear, and inner ear.

Assign the appropriate code(s) for the following procedures

3. Bilateral tympanostomy with insertion of ventilating tubes under general anesthesia.
4. Removal and replacement of an osseointegrated implant to the temporal bone (with mastoidectomy) with percutaneous attachment to external speech processor or cochlear stimulator.
5. What code is used to report removal of impacted cerumen from one or both ears?
6. List the three codes representing unlisted procedures of the external, middle, and inner ear.

Radiology

Chapter Objectives

- Understand the organization and features of the Radiology section of the CPT® codebook
- Understand definitions pertaining to radiology services
- Understand guidelines for various subsections listed in the Radiology section
- Learn coding tips for reporting radiology services

Introduction

This chapter reviews the Radiology section of the CPT® codebook. A fundamental understanding of the organization and instructional features of the Radiology section is key to coding radiological services. The CPT code set lists both diagnostic and therapeutic procedures according to the various types of imaging modalities. The structure and features of the Radiology section extend reporting functionality as these codes may do the following:

- Describe the total service
- Describe a portion of a procedure performed
- Require reporting of procedure codes outside the 70000 series (eg, surgical procedure code)
- Allow reporting of the same radiology code for different procedures outside the 70000 series
- Require reporting of multiple radiology codes
- Require use of modifiers
- Disallow reporting of additional radiology codes

The Radiology section includes anatomical subsections listed according to organ or anatomic site (ie, head and neck, chest, spine and pelvis, heart, vascular, etc). See Figures 5-1A–5-1C. Typically, the imaging technique is either delineated by the subheading title or specified in

- **Computed tomography (CT)**
- **Ultrasound**
- **Fluoroscopy**

the code descriptor. Careful review of each descriptor is recommended, as the imaging modality (eg, conventional X-ray imaging, **computed tomography [CT]**, magnetic resonance [MR], **ultrasound**, stereotaxis, mammography, **fluoroscopy**) may or may not be specified. For example, codes **70030-70330** are listed in the Diagnostic Radiology (Diagnostic Imaging) subsection under the Head and Neck anatomic heading. Although not specifically stated in the descriptor nomenclature, this series of codes (**70030-70330**) represents radiological examinations using conventional X-ray imaging. Codes **70450-70498** are also listed in this subsection and anatomic heading, but the descriptor nomenclature specifies CT as the imaging modality used.

To further clarify, the type of imaging supervision and interpretation provided may change while the procedure remains the same. For example, a physician may perform a percutaneous needle biopsy of the liver (**47000**). However, this procedure may be performed under fluoroscopic, ultrasound, magnetic resonance imaging (MRI), or CT guidance. Therefore, depending on the imaging service performed, code **76942**, **77002**, **77012**, or **77021** would be reported in addition to the liver biopsy (code **47000**).

FIGURE 5-1A *Body Planes—3/4 View*

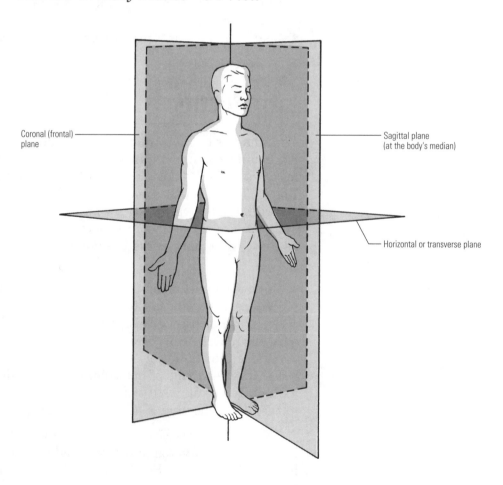

Coronal (frontal) plane

Sagittal plane (at the body's median)

Horizontal or transverse plane

FIGURE 5-1B *Body Aspects—Side View*

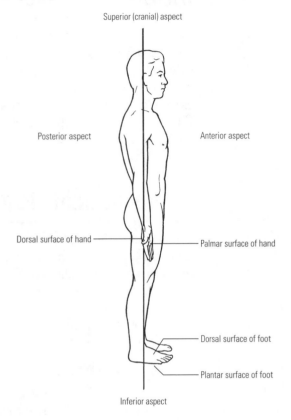

Superior (cranial) aspect

Posterior aspect

Anterior aspect

Dorsal surface of hand —

— Palmar surface of hand

— Dorsal surface of foot

— Plantar surface of foot

Inferior aspect

FIGURE 5-1C *Body Planes—Front View*

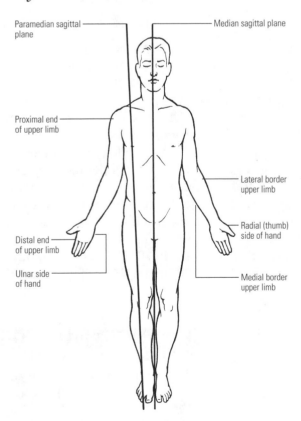

Paramedian sagittal plane

Median sagittal plane

Proximal end of upper limb

Lateral border upper limb

Radial (thumb) side of hand

Distal end of upper limb

Ulnar side of hand

Medial border upper limb

Chapter 5

Introductory Notes

To better understand certain types of imaging modalities, introductory or instructional notes provide information such as definitions of procedural elements, specific reporting instruction, and requirements related to image documentation and the final written report. An example of introductory notes can be found in the Diagnostic Radiology (Diagnostic Imaging) subsection following the Vascular Procedures/Aorta and Arteries subheadings.

Parenthetical Notes and Cross-References

Throughout the Radiology section, parenthetical notes also provide instructional reporting information when combinations of imaging modalities are performed. The following is an example of the instructional notes pertaining to the use of fluoroscopy following code **77002**:

77002 Fluoroscopic guidance for needle placement (eg, biopsy, aspiration, injection, localization device)

(See appropriate surgical code for procedure and anatomic location)

(77002 includes all radiographic arthrography with the exception of supervision and interpretation for CT and MR arthrography)

▶(Do not report 77002 in addition to 70332, 73040, 73085, 73115, 73525, 73580, 73615, 0232T)◀

▶(For injection(s) of platelet rich plasma, use 0232T)◀

(77002 is included in the organ/anatomic specific radiological supervision and interpretation procedures 49440, 74320, 74355, 74445, 74470, 74475, 75809, 75810, 75885, 75887, 75980, 75982, 75989)

Cross-references provide quick reference to related procedures and services inside and outside the **70000** series. For example, the cross-reference following radiological supervision and interpretation code **74190** directs the user to code **49400** for the actual procedure. The parenthetical instruction following code **70332** indicates that it would not be appropriate to additionally report code **77002**. Instructions may appear following multiple codes. For example, the same parenthetical instruction appears following codes **70470**, **70482**, **70488**, **70492**, **71270**, **72133**, **72194**, **73202**, **73702**, and **74170** directing users to codes **76376** and **76377** for three-dimensional rendering.

Coding Tip

It is the radiologist who ultimately should decide the number of views performed to answer the clinical question at hand.

✓ Check Your Knowledge

1. Why is it important to read the cross-references in parenthetical material in the CPT codebook?

Diagnostic Radiology (Diagnostic Imaging)

This Radiology subsection is organized according to organ or anatomic site (ie, head and neck, chest, spine and pelvis, heart, vascular, etc) with each code representing the imaging modality (eg, conventional X-ray imaging, CT, MR) and imaging-guided procedures (eg, cisternography, myelography, arthrography). There are no individual subheadings for CT, **computerized tomographic angiography (CTA)**, MRI, MRA, angiography, venography, mammography, or fluoroscopy. Specific codes for the various diagnostic imaging techniques are distributed throughout the anatomic series of codes.

Conventional X-Ray Imaging

The term **radiologic examination** is used in the CPT code set for conventional X rays.

A conventional X-ray imaging system consists of a high-voltage generator, an X-ray tube, an Al filter, a collimator, a grid, an intensifying screen, and a film; ultimately, an image that is a "shadow" of the anatomy of the body is generated. Conventional and digital systems provide the capability for a wide range of applications from examinations of the skull, spinal column, or abdomen to the extremities. These procedures can be performed on patients in a lying, sitting, or standing position. For example, code **73565**, *Radiologic examination, knee; both knees, standing, anteroposterior,* describes the anatomy, position, and type of views performed. Some of the codes representing diagnostic imaging using conventional X-ray imaging include **70030-70160, 70190-70328, 70360-70370, 70380, 71010-71035, 71100-71130, 72010-72120, 72170-72190, 72220, 73000-73030, 73050-73140, 73500-73520.**

> ### Key Terms
>
> **Radiologic examination:** conventional X rays.
>
> **Computed tomography (CT) imaging:** combines the use of a digital computer together with a rotating X-ray device to obtain image data from different angles around the body. Computer processing of the image data is then performed to show a cross-section of body tissue, bone, and organs.
>
> **Computed tomographic angiography (CTA):** noninvasive technique for imaging vessels.
>
> **Magnetic resonance angiography (MRA):** noninvasive diagnostic study used to evaluate disorders of the arterial and venous structures.
>
> **Fluoroscopy:** imaging technique commonly used by physicians to obtain real-time images of the internal structures of a patient through the use of a fluoroscope.
>
> **Ultrasound:** noninvasive imaging technique that uses high-frequency sound waves and their echoes.

Chapter 5

- **Computed tomography imaging (CTI)**

Number and Types of Views

Besides specifying the involved anatomy, the descriptor nomenclature of the Radiology codes includes references to the number (eg, **73140**, *Radiologic examination, finger(s), minimum of 2 views*) and/or type of views (eg, **74010**, *Radiologic examination, abdomen; anteroposterior and additional oblique and cone views)* performed. In order to assign and report appropriate CPT codes, the documentation should reflect the number and type of views taken and the method of examination performed and interpreted.

If the number of views is not mentioned in the report, the coder should **not** assume the procedure performed. Instead, the coder should work closely with the interpreting physician to clarify and obtain the appropriate information. This will help ensure that all pertinent information has been captured, allowing for submission of the correct procedural CPT code that reflects the level of work performed.

Computed Tomography

Computed tomography (CT) imaging, also known as *CAT scanning* (computed axial tomography scanning), combines the use of a digital computer together with a rotating X-ray device to obtain image data from different angles around the body. Computer processing of the image data is then performed to show a cross-section of body tissue, bone, and organs. CT imaging is particularly useful because it can show several types of tissue with great clarity, including organs like the liver, spleen, pancreas, and kidneys. In addition, CT is a very useful diagnostic method because it can display and distinguish many different types of tissue in the same region, including bone, muscle, soft tissue, and blood vessels.

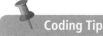
Coding Tip

The term *axial* does not appear in many of the CT code descriptors because direct acquisition imaging may be performed in any plane (eg, axial, coronal, sagittal, or multiplanar).

✓ Check Your Knowledge

2. How does the CPT code set list both diagnostic and therapeutic procedures?

EXAMPLE

The patient is a 52-year-old female with suspected intracranial bleeding. In this study, CTA (**70496**) allows visualization of intracranial vessels and provides valuable information regarding an aneurysm if identified, illustrating the value of the modality for this particular disorder (aneurysm).

Magnetic Resonance Imaging

This radiology technique produces images of internal structures of the body using magnetism, radio waves, and a computer to produce the

Key Term

- **Magnetic resonance angiography (MRA)**

Coding Tip

Functional MRI involves identification and mapping of stimulation of brain function. When neurofunctional tests are administered by a technologist or other nonphysician or nonpsychologist, see **70554**. When neurofunctional tests are entirely administered by a physician or psychologist, use **70555**.

images of body structures, particularly in the soft tissue, brain and spinal cord, abdomen, and joints. The existing CPT codes for MRI are silent with regard to patient positioning. Some MRI studies require more images and positioning and some require less. It may be appropriate to append **modifier 22** to these studies to indicate more work, but only if one routinely appends **modifier 52** to easier studies. For example, the coding of MRI with flexion and extension views is appropriately coded based on the anatomy studied (eg, MRI of the spine), not the type of views acquired or the type of equipment used. If a few additional pulsing sequences are acquired or dynamic positional changes are made in a given anatomic region, they are included in the base procedure code and not coded separately. If the work for these additional dynamic position changes is greater than that usually provided, this may be a case to use **modifier 22**.

EXAMPLE

An MRI of the hand is performed with concentration on only two of the metacarpals (eg, second and third metacarpophalangeal joints). An MRI of the foot is performed with concentration on only two of the metatarsophalangeals (eg, fourth and fifth metatarsophalangeal joints).

The appropriate number of units to report is one, either for the entire hand or the entire foot. All hand and finger joints are included in an MRI of the hand. Therefore, a provider would not report a unit greater than one. This same logic carries forward for the corresponding small joints of the foot.

Magnetic Resonance Angiography

Magnetic resonance angiography (MRA) is a noninvasive diagnostic study used to evaluate disorders of the arterial and venous structures. Currently, the MRA procedure entails two- or three-dimensional time-of-flight or phase contrast gradient echo sequences sensitive to blood flow covering the anatomic region of interest.

EXAMPLE

The patient is a 45-year-old male with severe headache and altered mental status. Noncontrast CT exam shows intracranial bleeding. The patient is allergic to iodinated contrast media. Magnetic resonance angiography is requested to look for a source of bleeding such as aneurysm.

This example illustrates an MRA (**70544**) used to evaluate the anterior and posterior circulation vessels within the cranial vault for aneurysms. Cranial MRA is also used for the evaluation of

Chapter 5

Coding Tip

Scout films generated prior to and during MRI or MRA sequences are considered inclusive of the study and not separately reportable.

atherosclerotic occlusive disease, acute thrombosis, dissection, vascular malformations, vascular loop syndromes, arterial causes of pulsatile tinnitus, and arteriovenous malformations as well as to assess the vascularity of tumors. The examination can also be tailored to assess the intracranial venous structures to exclude sinovenous thrombosis or to evaluate venous malformations or fistulae.

EXAMPLE

Views included in a spine survey study (72010) of an adult.

CPT code **72010**, *Radiologic examination, spine, entire, survey study, anteroposterior and lateral,* is intended to be used to report a survey study of the entire spine. A survey study is commonly performed to obtain scoliosis measurements or evaluate for spine metastasis. This radiological examination involves obtaining anteroposterior (AP) and lateral views of the entire spine. The number of films required will vary depending on the size of the film available and the size of the patient examined. For an adult patient, the study may require six films (the AP and lateral views of the cervical, thoracic, and lumbar spine). For smaller patients (eg, a pediatric patient), it may be possible to obtain the AP and lateral views of the entire spine with fewer films. These films are then interpreted as a single study (ie, one study is reported regardless of the number of films taken).

Besides specifying the involved anatomy, the descriptor nomenclature of the radiology codes include references to the number (eg, **73140**, *Radiologic examination, finger(s), minimum of two views*) and/or type of views (eg, **74010**, *Radiologic examination, abdomen; anteroposterior, additional oblique and cone views*) performed. In order to assign and report appropriate CPT codes, the documentation should reflect the number and type of views taken and the method of examination performed and interpreted.

Coding Tip

In order to assign and report appropriate CPT codes, the documentation should reflect the number and type of views taken and the method of examination performed and interpreted.

Report code **72275**, *Epidurography, radiological supervision and interpretation,* only when an epidurogram is performed, images documented, and a formal radiologic report is issued. See Figure 5-2.

The terms *complete* (eg, **76700**) and *limited* (eg, **76705**) are found in certain Radiology code descriptors and refer to the elements comprising the examination for that anatomic region. The written report should contain a description of these elements or the reason that an element could not be visualized. If fewer than required elements for a complete exam are reported (eg, limited number of organs or limited portion of region evaluated), the limited code for that anatomic region should be used once per patient exam session. A limited exam of an anatomic region should not be reported for the same exam session as a complete exam of that same region.

Chapter 5

FIGURE 5-2 *Epidurography*

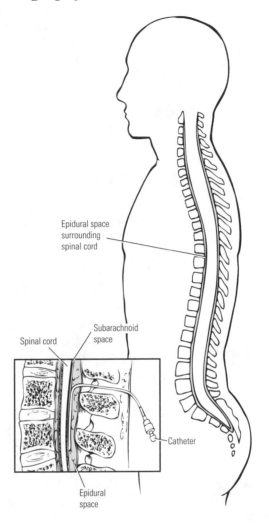

Epidural space
surrounding
spinal cord

Subarachnoid
space

Spinal cord

Catheter

Epidural
space

EXAMPLE

A three-view X ray of the hand with a three-view X ray of the wrist when obtained on three films vs. six films.

When three views of the hand and three views of the wrist are performed, it is appropriate to code **73130**, *Radiologic examination, hand; minimum of 3 views,* and **73110**, *Radiologic examination, wrist; complete, minimum of 3 views,* for the professional component, irrespective of whether these studies are performed together on three films or separately on six films. Both procedures should be coded if the physician performed a full and complete interpretation of both anatomic sites.

Certain code descriptors delineate a unilateral or bilateral study. For example, code **73500** describes a unilateral examination of the hip, with code **73520** describing a bilateral examination. Also, be aware that the descriptor nomenclature may not specifically include the terms *unilateral* or *bilateral* (for anatomy where the study may be performed on one or both sides of the body). An example is code **70336**, *Magnetic resonance (eg, proton) imaging, temporomandibular joint(s)*. This single code is intended to report unilateral *or* bilateral imaging of the temporomandibular joint(s). Hence, the option of either the singular or plural word *joint(s)*. If bilateral imaging of the temporomandibular joints is performed, then code **70336** is reported only one time. Therefore, report the code that most accurately describes the anatomy, number and type of views taken, and the method of examination performed and interpreted.

> ## EXAMPLE
>
> A bilateral hip X ray with two views on each side without an AP view of the pelvis.
>
> An AP view of the pelvis as well as additional views of both hips is the appropriate method of examination when a bilateral hip study is ordered. In addition to the AP view of the pelvis, at least one more view of each hip, typically a coned-down frog-leg lateral view is obtained, amounting to three views: one AP view of the pelvis that includes both hips, one frog-leg lateral of the right hip, and one frog-leg lateral of the left hip.
>
> If a bilateral study is performed without an AP view of the pelvis, code **73520**, *Radiologic examination, hips, bilateral, minimum of 2 views of each hip, including anteroposterior view of pelvis*, may be reported with modifier 52, *Reduced services*, appended to indicate that the study was not performed in its entirety. CPT code **73510**, *Radiologic examination, hip, unilateral; complete, minimum of 2 views*, is not intended to describe a bilateral hip study but a complete radiologic examination with a minimum of two views performed on a single hip.
>
> If right and left hip studies are separately ordered and performed and there are separate interpretations and written reports signed by the interpreting physician, it would be appropriate to report the code **73510** two times. In this case, modifier(s) to designate a bilateral study (eg, ***RT, LT, 50***) should be appended to the code(s) to indicate that bilateral procedures were performed. (**Modifier 59** is used only when a more appropriate modifier is not reported.)

For combinations of CT of the abdomen with CT of the pelvis performed at the same session, use Table 5-1. Do not report more than one CT of the abdomen or CT of the pelvis for any session.

Interventional Radiology

Interventional radiology is the branch of medicine that diagnoses and/or treats a wide range of diseases by using percutaneous or minimally invasive techniques with imaging guidance. Understanding how to code for interventional radiology services requires a thorough knowledge of

Key Terms

- Professional (physician) component
- Technical component

TABLE 5-1 *Combination of CT of Abdomen and CT of Pelvis*

▶ Stand Alone Code	74150 CT Abdomen WO Contrast	74160 CT Abdomen W Contrast	74170 CT Abdomen WO/W Contrast
72192 CT Pelvis WO Contrast	74176	74178	74178
72193 CT Pelvis W Contrast	74178	74177	74178
72194 CT Pelvis WO/W Contrast ◀	74178	74178	74178

anatomy and physiology as well as an in-depth knowledge of the use of CPT codes unique to this specialty. Often, diagnostic and therapeutic services are delivered in a variety of combinations determined by the underlying disease process, the clinical evaluation of the patient, and the intraprocedural interpretation of the diagnostic portion of the service (including physiologic data and images obtained).

Supervision and Interpretation

When a procedure that is a combination of an interventional radiology procedure and imaging study is performed, the *imaging portion* of the procedure is designated as "radiological supervision and interpretation." When a physician both performs the procedure and provides the radiological imaging supervision and interpretation, a combination of procedure codes (outside the **70000** series) and imaging supervision and interpretation codes (**70000** series) are necessary to completely and accurately report the procedure(s) performed. When a radiological supervision and interpretation procedure is performed and the radiologist does not perform the supervision, **modifier 52**, *Reduced services*, should be appended to the procedure code to designate a reduced level of service.

Professional vs Technical Procedural Components

Certain procedures described by the CPT code set are a combination of a **professional (physician) component** and a **technical component** (ie, diagnostic tests that involve a physician's interpretation, such as cardiac stress tests and electroencephalograms and physician pathology services). For diagnostic or therapeutic radiological services, the professional component includes the physician work and associated overhead and professional liability insurance costs involved in the diagnostic or therapeutic radiological service. The technical component of a service includes the cost of equipment, supplies, technician salaries, etc. The global charge refers to both components when billed together.

Coding Tip

For radiological services, the term *component* may refer to:
a. Specific (integral) part of a total service or procedure,
b. Type of endovascular graft extension/module, or
c. Coding concept wherein multiple code combinations are used to describe complex services.

Chapter 5

Because CPT codes are intended to represent physician and other health care practitioner services, the CPT nomenclature does not contain a coding convention to designate the technical component for a procedure or service. CPT coding does provide **modifier 26**, *Professional component for separately reporting the professional (or physician) component of a procedure or service.* This is because a hospital or other facility may be reporting the technical component of the procedure. Unmodified CPT codes are intended to describe both the technical and professional components of a service. When reporting the technical component of a procedure or service, become familiar with the various reporting requirements of individual insurance companies. For example, the Healthcare Common Procedure Coding System (HCPCS) Level II modifier TC is not one of the CPT modifiers, but rather it is required for Medicare reporting purposes to differentiate the professional vs technical components of the service (radiological in this instance) provided.

Key Terms

Professional (physician) component: Includes the physician work and associated overhead and professional liability insurance costs involved in the diagnostic or therapeutic radiological service.

Technical component: Includes the cost of equipment, supplies, technician salaries, etc. The global charge refers to both components when billed together.

Coding Tip

If the technical and professional components of the service are performed by the same provider, it is not appropriate or necessary to report the components of the service separately.

Administration of Contrast Material(s)

Contrast material is commonly used for imaging enhancement. It improves visualization and evaluation of the body structure or organ studied. Some of the procedures listed in the Radiology section of the CPT codebook may be performed with or without the use of contrast material for imaging enhancement. The phrase "with contrast" used in the codes for procedures using contrast for imaging enhancement represents contrast material administered intravascularly, intra-articularly, or intrathecally. For example, a brain CT may be done with intravenous contrast (**70460**), without contrast (**70450**), or without contrast followed by injection of intravenous contrast (**70470**). In procedures in which contrast material is always used, the CPT descriptor will not indicate that contrast material is used. For instance, intravenous pyelogram and abdominal aortogram do not list "with contrast" because contrast is an intrinsic part of the procedure. When contrast materials are administered only orally and/or rectally, the study does not qualify as "with contrast" and should be coded "without contrast." See the following examples:

- A CT scan of the abdomen with oral contrast should be coded as a CT of the abdomen without contrast (**74150**).
- For intra-articular injection, the appropriate joint injection code is used. If radiographic arthrography is also performed, the

arthrography supervision and interpretation code for the appropriate joint (which includes fluoroscopy) is also used.

- If CT or MR arthrography is performed without radiographic arthrography, the appropriate joint injection code, the appropriate CT or MR code ("with contrast" or "without followed by contrast"), and the appropriate imaging guidance code for needle placement for contrast injection would be used. Spine examinations using CT, MRI, or magnetic resonance angiography (MRA) with contrast may be performed with intrathecal (within either the subarachnoid or the subdural space) or intravascular contrast injection. However, for intrathecal injection of contrast material, the injection procedure is separately reported with either code **61055** or **62284**, as appropriate. Injection of intravascular contrast material is part of the "with contrast" CT, CT angiography, MRI, or MRA procedure.

Coding Tip

The physician should document in the report the administration of intravenous contrast when used. Coders should take care to determine from the report which studies were performed and evaluated with or without contrast.

✓ Check Your Knowledge

3. When contrast materials are administered, whether intravenously orally, or rectally, is the study reported as "with contrast"? Why or why not?

Coding Tip

Mercer views of both patellae are reported using **73564**, *Radiologic examination, knee; complete, 4 or more views.*

Medicare's National Level II HCPCS codes should be used to report the use of diagnostic and therapeutic radiopharmaceutical supplies. The A, C, and Q sections of the HCPCS codebook refer to medical and surgical supplies. (For example, see codes A4641, A4642, and A9500-A9699 for a listing of diagnostic and therapeutic radiopharmaceutical imaging agents used for radiological procedures.) It is important to separately report and charge for these items in the hospital outpatient setting, even though they may not trigger additional payment for the procedure (based on payer), because this charge data are used in the Medicare hospital outpatient prospective payment system and by other payers to set or determine current and future payments.

Computed Tomographic Angiography

Coding Tip

The key distinction between CTA and CT is that CTA includes reconstruction postprocessing of angiographic images and interpretation. If reconstruction postprocessing is not done, it is not a CTA study.

Computed tomographic angiography (CTA) is a noninvasive technique for imaging vessels. The information obtained from the CTA is used in the evaluation of vascular anatomy (eg, renal or liver transplant donors, congenital anomalies), vascular disorders (eg, aortic or intracranial aneurysms, renal artery or carotid stenosis), vascular trauma (eg, aortic laceration), and in the follow-up of organ transplantation. A radiogoraphic contrast study performed on the carotid artery vascular family is reported with codes **75660-75680**. See Figure 5-3.

Injection of contrast material is part of the "with contrast" CTA procedure; therefore, it is not appropriate to separately report the code for the administration of contrast. The supply of contrast, however, may be reported separately with CPT code **99070**, *Supplies and materials*

FIGURE 5-3 *Angiography, Carotid Artery*

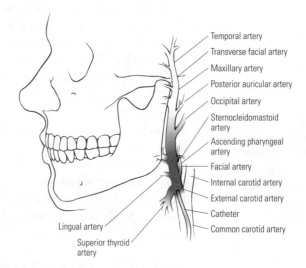

Temporal artery
Transverse facial artery
Maxillary artery
Posterior auricular artery
Occipital artery
Sternocleidomastoid artery
Ascending pharyngeal artery
Facial artery
Internal carotid artery
External carotid artery
Catheter
Common carotid artery
Lingual artery
Superior thyroid artery

(except spectacles) provided by the physician over and above those usually included with the office visit or other services rendered (list drugs, trays, supplies, or materials provided), or with the appropriate HCPCS Level II code for the contrast material used.

Typically, noncontrast sequences are performed for localization of the anatomic region to be evaluated during the contrast scan. This is indicated in the "without" component of the CTA code and is not separately reported. Evaluation of the source images is an ***inclusive*** component of the CTA interpretation.

✓ Check Your Knowledge

4. How is the radiologic subsection structured in the CPT codebook?

Vascular Procedures

The introductory notes of the Aorta and Arteries, Veins and Lymphatics, and Transcatheter Procedures subsections provide comprehensive coding instructions for the use of these codes. The stated instruction correlates with the Cardiovascular System chapter discussion of the vascular and nonvascular interventions using component coding. For procedures reported using component codes, the surgical components of the service are described by the codes preceding the **70000** series, whereas the radiological or imaging services are described by these **70000** codes. When a radiographic contrast study is performed on the abdominal or thoracic aorta, it is reported with codes **75600-75630**. See Figure 5-4. When a radiographic contrast study is performed on the veins of the lower extremities, it is reported with codes **75820-75822**. See Figure 5-5.

- **Ultrasound**

FIGURE 5-4 *Aortography*

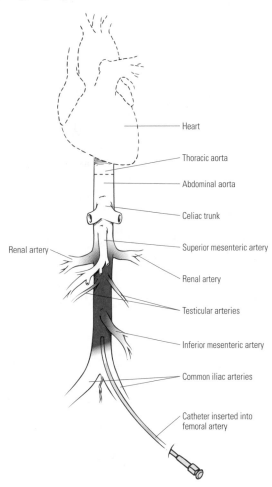

- Heart
- Thoracic aorta
- Abdominal aorta
- Celiac trunk
- Superior mesenteric artery
- Renal artery
- Testicular arteries
- Inferior mesenteric artery
- Common iliac arteries
- Catheter inserted into femoral artery

Renal artery

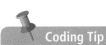

Coding Tip

There are ultrasound procedures located in sections other than Radiology. For instance, located in the Medicine section of the CPT codebook there are ultrasounds involving Cerebrovascular Arterial Studies of the extremities (**93875-93893**), Extremity Arterial Studies (**93922-93931**), Extremity Venous Studies (**93965-93971**), Visceral and Penile Vascular Studies (**93975-93982**), Extremity Arterial-Venous Studies (**93990**), and ultrasounds of the heart (Echocardiography) (**93303-93352**).

Diagnostic Ultrasound

Ultrasound is a noninvasive imaging technique that uses high-frequency sound waves and their echoes. Simplistically, using a transducer probe, sound waves are generated and received to the computer. Ultrasound displays real-time images, so it is helpful for guiding invasive procedures (eg, biopsy) and also can display movement and function of organs and blood vessels.

There are four types of diagnostic ultrasounds recognized:

1. *A-mode ultrasound* implies a one-dimensional ultrasonic measurement procedure.
2. *M-mode ultrasound* implies a one-dimensional ultrasonic measurement procedure with movement of the trace to record amplitude and velocity of moving echo-producing structures.
3. *B-scan ultrasound* implies a two-dimensional ultrasonic scanning procedure with a two-dimensional display.
4. *Real-time scan* implies a two-dimensional ultrasonic scanning procedure with display of both two-dimensional structure and motion with time.

Chapter 5

FIGURE 5-5 *Venography*

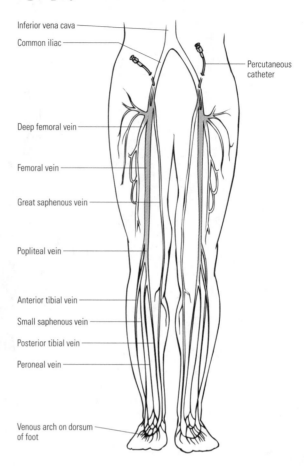

Inferior vena cava

Common iliac

Percutaneous catheter

Deep femoral vein

Femoral vein

Great saphenous vein

Popliteal vein

Anterior tibial vein

Small saphenous vein

Posterior tibial vein

Peroneal vein

Venous arch on dorsum of foot

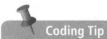

Coding Tip

All diagnostic ultra-sound examinations require permanently recorded images with measurements.

Use of ultrasound without thorough evaluation of organ(s) or anatomic region, image documentation, and final written report is not separately reportable. If fewer than the required elements for a *complete* exam are reported (eg, limited number of organs examined or limited portion of region evaluated), the *limited* code for that anatomic region should be used once per patient exam session. If a complete exam is performed as defined in the CPT introductory language but certain organs are not visible, the reason (eg, bowel gas) should be documented in the report to justify submission of a complete exam code. The introductory language in the Diagnostic Ultrasound subsection of the CPT codebook provides additional guidance on the use of these codes.

✓ Check Your Knowledge

5. What are the four types of recognized diagnostic ultrasounds?

————————, ————————, ————————, ————————.

Coding Tip

Intraoperative ultrasonic guidance (**76998**) should be reported *once* per operative field. Do not report **76998** in conjunction with **36475-36479**, **37760**, **37761**, **47370-47382**, **0249T**. For ultrasound guidance for open and laparscopic radiofrequency tissue ablation, report **76940**.

EXAMPLE

Ultrasound of two quadrants of the abdomen.

An ultrasound of two quadrants of the abdomen should be reported once using code **76705**, which is reported for a limited ultrasound examination of either a single organ or a limited area of the abdomen. If one study is performed involving two quadrants of the abdomen, this study is considered to be a *limited* area of the abdomen.

Ultrasonic Guidance Procedures

Certain imaging modalities are used during many diagnostic and therapeutic radiological procedures to observe the action of instruments being used. Among these are ultrasound (**76930**, **76932**, **76936**, **76937**, **76940**, **76941**, **76942**, **76945**, **76946**, **76948**, **76950**, **76965**, **76998**), fluoroscopy (**77001**, **77002**, **77003**), CT (**77011**, **77012**, **77013**, **77014**), MR (**77021**, **77022**), stereotaxis (**77031**), and mammography (**77032**).

EXAMPLE

Placement of peripherally inserted central venous catheter (PICC) under ultrasound and fluoroscopic guidance.

In this instance, two types of imaging guidance may be required to complete the procedure. For example, the documentation reflects that the ultrasound guidance was used for assessment of the potential venous access site with the selected vessel patency documented in the report, actual real-time guidance of needle passage into the supracondylar segment of the right basilic vein was provided, and permanent images were created; it is, therefore, appropriate to code for the ultrasound guidance (**+76937**). The use of ultrasound to locate a vein or mark a skin entry point for a nonguided puncture is not considered an ultrasound-guided procedure and, therefore, does not meet the requirements to report **+76937**. Should the documentation reflect that fluoroscopic guidance was provided to advance the PICC line to the level of the junction of the superior vena cava and right atrium, fluoroscopy (**+77001**) is coded in addition to the ultrasound guidance used for access.

Fluoroscopic guidance can be used independently or in combination with other imaging methods; therefore, it is important to refer to the code descriptors, parenthetical instructions, and introductory notes for specific reporting instructions. For example, fluoroscopic guidance (**77002**) is inclusive of all radiographic arthrography with the exception of supervision and interpretation for CT and MR arthrography.

Chapter 5

- **Fluoroscopy**

Therefore, it is not appropriate to report **77002** in addition to **70332**, **73040**, **73085**, **73115**, **73525**, **73580**, and **73615**. Because fluoroscopic imaging requires personal supervision, if the physician is not present in the operating room during a procedure that uses fluoroscopy or fluoroscopic guidance, that physician should not submit a code for fluoroscopy. However, the appropriate radiographic code to report the anatomy evaluated should be submitted in the event that:

a. the radiologist's contract with the hospital requires that a radiologist issue a formal interpretation, or

b. the physician performing the study requests that a radiologist produce a formal report of the procedure from permanent images recorded.

For computer-aided detection applied to a screening mammogram, code **77057**, *Screening mammography, bilateral (2-view film study of each breast)*, is reported in conjunction with add-on code **77052**, *Computer-aided detection (computer algorithm analysis of digital image data for lesion detection) with further physician review for interpretation, with or without digitization of film radiographic images; screening mammography (List separately in addition to code for primary procedure)*. For a bilateral screening mammography code **77057**, *Screening mammography, bilateral (2-view film study of each breast)*, is reported. See Figure 5-6.

CT is used as guidance for surgical and therapeutic procedures. Some examples in which CT imaging guidance is used for invasive procedures include code **77012** for CT-guided needle placement (eg, biopsy, aspiration, injection, localization device). Code **77011** describes CT-guided stereotactic localization. Code **77014** describes CT guidance used for placement of radiation therapy fields. The listed radiology codes represent the radiological portion of the procedure. Should the same physician perform both the procedure and the radiological portion of the procedure, refer to the cross references following each CT code to additionally report the appropriate organ or site-specific procedure code. For example, the parenthetical following code **77013** instructs the coder that for percutaneous radiofrequency ablation, use codes **32998**, **47382**, **50592**, and **50593**.

Fluoroscopy

Fluoroscopy is an imaging technique commonly used by physicians to obtain real-time images of the internal structures of a patient through the use of a fluoroscope. A fluoroscope consists of an X-ray source and fluorescent screen between which the patient is positioned. The fluorescent screen is electronically and optically coupled to an image intensification system and television camera, allowing the images to be seen on a monitor, recorded, and stored.

Fluoroscopy (**76000**) may be considered inclusive of the imaging portion of the procedure (**50590**) or radiographic service (**74300**) performed. See the appropriate surgical code for procedure and anatomic location for instruction regarding the additional reporting of

FIGURE 5-6 *Screening Mammography*

Mammogram

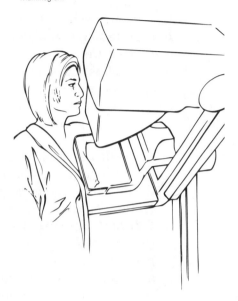

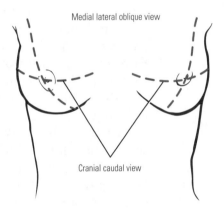

Medial lateral oblique view

Cranial caudal view

Coding Tip

Fluoroscopic guidance is inclusive of organ/anatomic-specific radiological supervision and interpretation procedures **74320, 74355, 74445, 74470, 74475, 75809, 75810, 75885, 75887, 75980, 75982,** and **75989**.

fluoroscopy. (Refer to the Radiologic Guidance subsection of the CPT codebook for further discussion of the fluoroscopic guidance codes [eg, **77001-77003**]).

Radiation Oncology

CPT Radiation Oncology codes (**77261-77263**) describe the therapeutic radiology used for planning radiation to treat diseases, especially neoplastic tumors. To treat certain types of malignancies, such as early stages of Hodgkin's disease, radiation therapy may be used as the primary therapy.

A course of radiation therapy is composed of six steps that involve distinct activities of varying complexity. A clinical team led by the radiation oncologist provides the medical services associated with the steps in the process of care. Other team members in the patient's planning and treatment regimen include the medical physicist, dosimetrist,

Chapter 5

Key Terms

- **Port**
- **Stereotactic radiation therapy**
- **Block**
- **Fraction**

radiation therapist, and nursing staff. Many of the procedures within each step will be carried to completion before the patient's care is taken to the next step. Others will occur and reoccur during the course of treatment. Each of these distinct steps involves medical evaluation, interpretation, management, and decision making by the radiation oncologist. Certain steps, of necessity, are repeated during treatment because of patient tolerance, changes in tumor size, necessity for boost field or port size changes, protection of normal tissue, or as other clinical circumstances may require.

Steps in the course of radiation therapy are as follows:

1. **Consultation: clinical management.** The radiation oncologist often provides consultative services before a treatment plan is developed for the patient. This initial consultation is reported with Evaluation and Management (E/M) codes from the CPT codebook.
2. **Clinical treatment planning.** If the determination is made that the patient should receive radiation treatment, clinical treatment planning occurs. The planning that occurs before treatment involves a complex decision-making process that includes interpretation of testing, choice of treatment modality, selection of treatment devices, etc. The planning process becomes the foundation upon which subsequent decisions are made. CPT codes corresponding to clinical treatment planning are **77261-77263**.
3. **Simulation.** After the completion of clinical treatment planning including tumor mapping, it is necessary to establish the treatment portals to deliver the radiation to the volume selected. Therapeutic radiology simulation is the process of establishing radiation treatment portals that most efficiently and precisely encompass the treatment volume. Simulation is usually performed on a dedicated simulator, but it can be performed on other pieces of equipment such as virtual reality-based, three-dimensional simulation systems or other dedicated diagnostic X-ray, MR, ultrasound, or nuclear medicine equipment that is modified to localize treatment volume to define the area that requires treatment. (Simulation is also used for determination of radioactive implant location within the body.) Simulation may be performed more than once during a course of therapy, but only once per day. CPT codes corresponding to simulation are **77280**, **77285**, **77290**, and **77295**.
4. **Medical radiation physics, dosimetry, treatment devices, and special services.** This phase of the process of care involves the radiation oncologist in collaboration with the medical physicist, dosimetrist, and radiation therapist staff. This team develops dosimetry, builds treatment devices to modify and refine treatment delivery, and performs other special services required for the measurement of precision dose delivery (including quality assurance and the identification and review of complicated situations requiring special medical physics consultation). The CPT codes used are in the **77300-77399** series.
5. **Radiation treatment delivery and radiation treatment management.** Radiation treatment delivery described by CPT codes

77401-77416, **77418**, **77422**, **77423**, and **77520-77525** are technical codes only and describe the delivery of external beam radiation therapy. Brachytherapy CPT codes (interstitial implants) are described in the **77750-77799** series and include both professional work and technical reimbursement. While the patient is undergoing radiation therapy, the radiation oncologist is responsible for the care of the patient and the overall management of the course of treatment. External beam services, reported by codes **77427**, **77431**, **77432**, and **77470**, are used depending on the complexity and modality of treatment. For external beam radiation therapy, radiation therapy management is reported in units of five fractions (or treatment sessions) for CPT code **77427**.

6. **Patient follow-up.** This final step in the course of radiation therapy is covered by CPT E/M codes for follow-up evaluation of an established patient. This phase involves periodic patient visits and examinations. These services are performed after a course of radiation therapy is completed. Follow-up exams within 90 days of completion of therapy (the global period) are considered part of treatment management and are not reported separately. However, diagnostic tests such as endoscopy furnished within the 90-day global period are reported separately. If a patient returns within the 90-day global period with a new or different clinical problem, a new and separate E/M code may be reported. After the completion of the 90-day global period, usual and customary use of the CPT E/M codes for follow-up evaluation of an established patient is appropriate.

Frequently Asked Questions on Reporting Radiation Oncology

1. On what occasion can therapeutic radiology treatment planning codes (**77261-77263**) be used?

Therapeutic radiology treatment planning, as described by codes **77261**, **77262**, and **77263**, is a process of developing a course of action for treating a patient's disease and involves numerous issues that the radiation oncologist must take into account, including planning for devices, simulation, choice of modality, dose, fractionation, and specific anatomic constraints.

2. How many times per course of treatment should treatment planning codes be used?

Treatment planning is typically performed once for each course of therapy and generally takes place before the treatment or simulation.

3. Should these codes be reported at the beginning of treatment?

There may be occasions when a patient under therapy develops a new and unexpected problem that requires another course of therapy to

Coding Tip

A *port* (often referred to as a *field*) is the area encompassed by a single radiation beam. It may be defined either on a patient's surface or inside the body. Multiple intersecting ports combine to produce the three-dimensional treatment volume. A *block* is a radiation-shielding device placed into the beam that allows for a change in the shape or projected configuration of the port. It may be a simple multiuse device that is placed by hand, a custom-designed block that is inserted on the linear accelerator, or a physician-designed multileaf collimator pattern generated by the physician using a computer.

a different site and for a different problem. Therefore, a change in clinical circumstances or diagnosis may require a new treatment plan. However, it would not be appropriate to use multiple codes in the **77261-77263** series for a change in treatment plan or treatment of multiple sites for the same diagnosis and circumstance.

Complexity Levels of Treatments

The level of complexity of a treatment device may be related to the clinical reason for the device or the method of construction. Not all devices are **blocks**. The following provides clarifying language for the terms *simple, intermediate,* and *complex* blocks as listed in CPT codes **77332**, **77333**, and **77334**.

77332 Treatment devices, design, and construction; simple (simple block, simple bolus)

77333 intermediate (multiple blocks, stents, bite blocks, special bolus)

77334 complex (irregular blocks, special shields, compensators, wedges, molds or casts)

An example of a *simple* treatment device (code **77332**) might be a prefabricated reusable block selected by the physician for a particular indication. An *intermediate* treatment device (code **77333**) is appropriate when multiple such reusable blocks are used. The code for *complex* devices (**77334**) is reserved for those cases in which a highly complex field is required and a unique device is constructed for treatment or protection of sensitive vital tissues. A complex device is unique to a particular patient and port. Examples of complex devices would be a mantle field block, head and neck treatment blocks, and a custom fabricated immobilization device.

Key Terms

Port: Area encompassed by a single radiation beam.

Stereotactic radiation therapy: General term for stereotactic-based radiation treatment. This treatment usually consists of one to five high-dose radiation treatments delivered by either a linear accelerator or a Cobalt 60 unit.

Block: Radiation-shielding device placed into the radiation beam that allows for a change in the shape or projected configuration of the port.

Fraction: Term for treatment sessions for radiation therapy management.

Stereotactic Radiation Treatment Delivery

Stereotactic radiation therapy is the general term for stereotactic-based radiation treatment. This treatment usually consists of one to five high-dose radiation treatments delivered by either a linear accelerator (**77372**) (sometimes called *linac radiosurgery* or *robotic-based radiosurgery*) or a Cobalt 60 unit (**77371**) (sometimes referred to as the *GammaKnife* or *radiosurgery*). Stereotactic radiotherapy is often used to treat tumors in the brain as well as other parts of the body. With the advent of new technologies for stereotactic treatments to non-cranial areas, the term *stereotactic body radiation therapy* (SBRT) is used for designation of the extracranial targets (**77373**).

✓ Check Your Knowledge Answers

1. Cross-references in parentheticals provide quick references to related procedures and services inside and outside the **70000** series, indicate which codes it would not be appropriate to additionally report, and direct the user to additional appropriate codes to report.

2. The CPT code set lists both diagnostic and therapeutic procedures according to the various types of imaging modalities.

3. When contrast materials are administered only orally and/or rectally, the study does not qualify as "with contrast" and should be coded "without contrast."

4. The Radiology subsection is organized according to organ or anatomic site (ie, head and neck, chest, spine and pelvis, heart, vascular, etc) with each code representing the imaging modality (eg, conventional X-ray imaging, CT, MR) and imaging-guided procedures (eg, cisternography, myelography, arthrography).

5. The four types of diagnostic ultrasounds recognized are A-mode ultrasound, M-mode ultrasound, B-scan ultrasound, and real-time scan.

Chapter Exercises

Check your answers in Appendix B.

True or False

1. The professional component includes the physician work and associated overhead and professional liability insurance costs involved in the diagnostic or therapeutic radiological service. **True or False**
2. The technical component of a service includes the cost of equipment, supplies, technician salaries, etc. **True or False**

Matching

3. Component _____.

4. Stereotactic Radiation Therapy _____.

    a. is the general term for stereotactic-based radiation treatment.

    b. may refer to a specific (integral) part of a total service or procedure, a type of endovascular graft extension/module, or a coding concept wherein multiple code combinations are used to describe complex services.

Fill in the Blank

5. _____ is commonly used for imaging enhancement. It improves visualization and evaluation of the body structure or organ studied.

6. A course of radiation therapy is composed of _____ steps that involve distinct activities of varying complexity.

Code the Following Procedures

7. X-ray of the foot with three views. How is this procedure reported?

8. MRI of the lumbar spine without contrast. How is this procedure reported?

9. MRA of the lower extremity with contrast. How is this procedure reported?

Pathology and Laboratory

Chapter Objectives

- Understand the Pathology and Laboratory guidelines
- Understand the difference between drug testing and organ or disease-oriented panels
- Recognize the differences in the Pathology and Laboratory sections

Introduction

This chapter reviews the Pathology and Laboratory section of the CPT® codebook. The **80000** series of codes is for reporting the performance of the specific laboratory test only and does not include the collection of the specimen itself via venipuncture, arterial puncture, lumbar puncture, or other collection methodology. The collection of the specimen by venipuncture or by arterial puncture is not considered an integral part of the laboratory procedure(s) performed and therefore may be reported separately.

Just as throughout the CPT codebook, there are parenthetical notes following some of the codes, instructing which codes may not be reported in conjunction with that code, as well as instructing on which other codes should be reported for certain procedures.

Pathology and Laboratory Guidelines

Just as with all the sections in the CPT codebook, the Pathology and Laboratory Guidelines are located in the beginning of the Pathology and Laboratory section. When performing separate procedures or multiple procedures, it is appropriate to select the multiple procedure codes that are performed on the same date of service and list the codes as separate entries on the claim form. In order to show that a laboratory procedure was repeated or that different laboratory procedures were done on the same date of service for the same patient, you may need to append the appropriate modifiers (see Chapter 10, Modifiers).

Just as with the Surgery, Radiology, and Medicine sections of the CPT codebook, the Pathology and Laboratory section has codes for unlisted services or procedures. Due to advances in the field of medicine, there may be services or procedures performed by physicians that have not yet been designated by a specific CPT code. Please note, as listed in the "Instructions for Use of the CPT Codebook" in the Introduction of the CPT codebook, it is very important that a code similar to the actual procedure performed not be selected in lieu of an unlisted procedure code. If no such specific code exists, then report the service using the appropriate unlisted procedure or service code. Any service or procedure should be adequately documented in the medical record. When reporting an unlisted code to describe a procedure or service, it may be necessary to submit supporting documentation (eg, procedure report) along with the claim to third-party payers in order to provide an adequate description of the nature and extent of the procedure; the need for the procedure; and the time, effort, and equipment necessary to provide the service.

Drug Testing vs Organ or Disease-Oriented Panels

Organ or Disease-Oriented Panels

Organ or Disease-Oriented Panel codes consist of multiple tests that the physician performs to determine if there are any abnormalities with the patient. These Organ or Disease-Oriented Panel tests include both the technical component (which is the actual running of the test, HCPCS modifier TC) and the professional component (the physician is only reading and interpreting the test results, CPT modifier 26).

When reporting the panel codes, *all* the components listed under the code descriptor *must* be performed, with no substitutions. If fewer tests are performed than those listed in the panel code, the individual code number(s) for each test should be listed rather than the panel code. Even if only 1 of the components listed in the code descriptor is missing, the panel code cannot be reported. Instead, report each of the other codes separately. For example, see code **80047**, *Basic metabolic panel (Calcium, ionized)*. Under the code descriptor it lists the components that must be included in order to report that panel code along with the code for each individual component: Calcium, ionized (**82330**), Carbon dioxide (**82374**), Chloride (**82435**), Creatinine (**82565**), Glucose (**82947**), Potassium (**84132**), Sodium (**84295**), Urea Nitrogen (BUN) (**84520**). If, for example, the Glucose test was not performed and all the others listed in the code descriptor were performed, then it would not be appropriate to report code **80047**. Instead all of the other components would be reported individually by the codes provided in the parenthesis.

These panel components are not intended to limit the performance of other tests. If a physician performs tests in addition to those specifically indicated for a particular panel, those tests should be reported separately in addition to the panel code. The presence or absence of a specific code for a panel of tests in no way limits the physician's ability to order or perform a specific battery of tests. Whether a specific panel code exists or not affects only the method of reporting the tests performed. Some clinical laboratories may define their own panels for the ordering provider's convenience. When a panel of tests is not described by a specific CPT panel code, the tests contained within the laboratory-defined panels are reported with the individual component CPT codes. Consider the following coding example:

EXAMPLE

Dr E performs a lipid panel on automated equipment in his office. The battery of tests he provides includes high-density lipoprotein cholesterol, total serum cholesterol, triglycerides, and quantitative glucose. Although the test for quantitative glucose is not included in the code descriptor for the lipid panel, the test is reported in addition.

Dr E reports the following two codes for the panel performed:

80061 Lipid panel

This panel must include the following:

Cholesterol, serum, total (82465)

Lipoprotein, direct measurement, high density cholesterol (HDL cholesterol) (83718)

Triglycerides (84478)

82947 Glucose; quantitative, blood (except reagent strip)

On another note, if the same component is listed in more than one panel code, do not report those codes together. Said a different way, if the components of two groups of tests overlap in any respect, report the panel that incorporates the greater number of tests to fulfill the code definition and then report the remaining tests using individual test codes. For example, do not report **80047** in conjunction with **80053**, as the code descriptors list some of the same components in both panel codes. All of the components listed in code **80047** are also listed in code **88053**. If all of the components list in **80053** were performed, then only code **80053** would be reported.

✓ Check Your Knowledge

1. Can codes **80048** and **80051** be reported together? Why or why not?

Drug Testing

The CPT codes used to report drug testing are located in three sections of the Pathology and Laboratory chapter of the CPT codebook: Drug Testing (**80100-80104**), Therapeutic Drug Assays (**80150-80299**), and Chemistry (**82000-84999**). Qualitative assays are tests that detect whether a particular analyte, constituent, or condition is present and reported with the drug testing codes. The term **analyte** is the actual drug being tested for, such as amphetamines and barbiturates. Quantitative assays are tests that give results expressing the specific numerical amount of an analyte in a specimen and are reported with the therapeutic drug assay or chemistry codes. The term **assay** is the determination of the amount of a particular part of a mixture or the determination of the biological or pharmacological potency of a drug.

The codes used to report qualitative drug testing distinguish between screening tests and confirmation tests. When drugs or classes of drugs are assayed by qualitative screen and followed by confirmation with a second method, the confirmation is included and is not reported separately. These tests are looking to see if traces of the drug are present in the specimen.

Code **80100**, *Drug screen, qualitative; multiple drug classes chromatographic method, each procedure*, means that this one procedure detects multiple drug classes and is counted as one procedure, regardless of the number of drugs tested. Code **80101**, *Drug screen, qualitative; single drug class method (eg, immunoassay, enzyme assay), each drug class*, means that this method detects a single class of drugs and is to be reported as one drug class.

Therapeutic Drug Assays

The material for these examinations may be from any source, such as blood, tissue, feces, or urine. Therapeutic Drug Assay examinations are quantitative, meaning the physician is looking for the number or quantity of the drug present, or how much of the drug is there. When performing nonquantitative testing, the Drug Testing codes are used. The drugs in these sections are listed in alphabetical order.

Pathology Consultations

There are three different sets of codes in the Pathology and Laboratory section of the CPT codebook for reporting various types of pathology consultative services. The three different types of consultative services include the following:

- Clinical pathology consultations;
- Consultation on referred material; and
- Pathology consultation during surgery.

The various pathology consultation services codes are similar to the other CPT consultation codes found in the Evaluation and Management (E/M) section in that they describe physician pathology services provided at the *request* of another physician of the same facility or another facility or institution. In contrast to the E/M consultation services, pathology consultations do not require a face-to-face encounter with the patient. If there is a face-to-face encounter, then the pathologist may report the appropriate E/M consultation code(s) with the appropriate modifier(s), if needed. The pathology consultation codes are reported if the following services are performed:

- At the request of the attending physician of the same or another institution relevant to test result(s) requiring further medical interpretation;
- For consultation and report on material referred from another pathologist or facility;
- For consultation provided to another pathologist in a different practice site or facility;
- For consultation provided to another physician in the same facility or site on material from another institution (eg, review of slides before surgery or therapy at the consulting physician's facility); and
- During surgery or other invasive procedures.

Consultations (Clinical Pathology)

A clinical pathology consultation is a service that includes a written report and is rendered by the pathologist in response to a request from an attending physician regarding test result(s) that require additional medical interpretive judgment. Reporting of a test result without medical interpretive judgment is not considered a clinical pathology consultation.

Pathology Consultation During Surgery

To appropriately report these codes, it is necessary to understand the definitions of **tissue blocks** and **tissue sections**. A tissue block is a portion of tissue from a specimen that is frozen or encased in a support medium such as paraffin or plastic, from which sections are prepared. A tissue section is a thin slice of tissue from that tissue block prepared for microscopic examination.

Chapter 6

When a single frozen section (ie, the first and only tissue block) from a specimen is examined, the service is coded as **88331**, *Pathology consultation during surgery; first tissue block, with frozen section(s), single specimen*. When frozen sections from more than one tissue block from the same specimen are examined, the appropriate coding is one unit of service of code **88331** for the first tissue block and an additional unit of service with add-on code **88332**, *Pathology consultation during surgery; each additional tissue block with frozen section(s)*, for each block subsequent to the first.

Code **88332** is reported only when a single specimen requires multiple frozen section tissue blocks. CPT code **88332** cannot be reported for a specimen that has not already been examined initially, as indicated by code **88331**. If more than one specimen is submitted for consultation, the services for each specimen would be separately coded, as appropriate.

✓ Check Your Knowledge

2. If three frozen section tissue blocks from one specimen are examined, how is this reported?

Urinalysis

Codes in the Urinalysis section (**81000-81099**) are used to report various types of urinalysis. The note at the beginning of this section indicates that many specific quantitative analyses are not reported with codes from this section; rather, the user is directed to see the appropriate section where the specific test is described. For example, quantitative testing for urinary chloride is not in the Urinalysis section and would be reported with code **82436**, *Chloride; urine*, from the Chemistry section.

Appropriate code selection from the Urinalysis section depends on the type of test performed. In order to select the appropriate code, one must know whether the testing was automated or not and whether the testing was performed with or without microscopy. It is important to note that when urinalysis is reported, multiple tests described within a single code descriptor should not be ***unbundled*** to produce and report multiple codes.

EXAMPLE

Code **81000**, *Urinalysis, by dip stick or tablet reagent for bilirubin, glucose, hemoglobin, ketones, leukocytes, nitrite, pH, protein, specific gravity, urobilinogen, any number of these constituents; non-automated, with microscopy*, which describes urinalysis with microscopy, should not be coded as **81005**, *Urinalysis; qualitative or semiquantitative, except immunoassays*, for the urinalysis plus **81015**, *Urinalysis; microscopic only*, for the microscopic examination, as this would be considered unbundling.

Chemistry

The material for examination may be from ***any source*** unless otherwise specified in the code descriptor. When an analyte (or drug) is measured in multiple specimens from different sources (eg, urine, blood), the analyte is reported separately for each source and for each specimen. For instance, when the analyte Catecholamines is being tested from both the urine and the blood, both sources for the specimen are reported with code **82382**, *Catecholamines; total urine*, and code **82383**, *Catecholamines; blood*. Likewise, when an analyte (or drug) is measured in specimens that are obtained at different times, the analyte is reported separately for each source and for each specimen.

The Chemistry examinations are quantitative unless specified (eg, code **82127**, *Amino acids; single, qualitative, each specimen*).

The Chemistry section is in alphabetical order, which is helpful in locating the correct code. With the chemistry codes, it is appropriate to report for each test done (eg, if testing for calcium and aluminum, it is appropriate to report the code for each). The basic rule for coding these Chemistry codes is as follows:

1. Code for the analyte; and
2. Check for the source (eg, serum, urine, blood).

Cytopathology

The Bethesda system of reporting is a format for reporting cervical-vaginal cytologic diagnoses. The Cytopathology section has specific codes used for the manual screening of conventional Pap smears that are reported by means of the ***non-Bethesda system*** of reporting, as well as specific codes used for the manual screening of conventional Pap smears that are reported by means of the ***Bethesda system*** of reporting.

The Bethesda system has the following four basic elements:

1. Specimen type (conventional smear vs. liquid-based preparation vs. other);
2. Statement of specimen adequacy (an integral part of the report);
3. General categorization (aids clinicians in prioritizing cases for review or to assist laboratories in compiling statistical information); and
4. Interpretation or result (descriptive diagnoses grouped into categories).

Coding Tip

For the Chemistry codes, if you cannot find the analyte, code by general methodology using codes **83516-83520**. Molecular diagnostic codes **83890-83913** are coded by procedure rather than by analyte. Each technique used in the analyses is to be reported separately.

Coding Tip

To report Immunology codes (**86000-86849**):
1. Look for the analyte; and
2. Look for the general methodology if the specific analyte is not in the CPT codebook. If the general methodology code is not there, use the unlisted code (**86849**).

Coding Tip

In the event an automated screening procedure fails, it provides no information and testing is essentially not performed. Therefore, it is not appropriate to report a laboratory test that was not performed, regardless of whether the sample was unacceptable or if the analyzer failed.

Chapter 6

Note: although the general CPT guidelines state that when a code is not available for a particular procedure or service, a code similar to the actual procedure performed should **not** be selected in lieu of an unlisted procedure code. Instead the unlisted code should be reported. However, the one exception to this rule is for the Surgical Pathology codes, in which any unlisted specimen should be assigned the code that most closely reflects the physician work involved in securing it.

Surgical Pathology

Services **88300** through **88309** include accession, examination, and reporting. The unit of service for codes **88300** through **88309** is the specimen. A specimen is defined as tissue(s) that is submitted for individual and separate attention, requiring individual examination and pathologic diagnosis. Two or more such specimens from the same patient (eg, separately identified endoscopic biopsies, skin lesions) are each appropriately assigned an individual code reflective of its proper level of service.

Key Terms

Specimen: Tissue(s) that is submitted for individual and separate attention, requiring individual examination and pathologic diagnosis.

✓ Check Your Knowledge Answers

1. No, codes **80048** and **80051** cannot be reported together, because both codes contain the same component in the code descriptors (carbon dioxide, chloride, potassium, and sodium).

2. This is reported with 1 unit of **88331** and 2 units of **88332**. Code **88331** is reported for the first frozen section tissue block, and since there were two additional frozen tissue blocks examined, the add-on code **88332** would be reported twice—once for each additional tissue block.

Chapter Exercise

Check your answers in Appendix B.

True or False

1. If most of the components within an organ or disease-oriented panel are performed, the panel code may be reported. **True or False**
2. If one performs tests in addition to those specifically indicated for a particular organ or disease-oriented panel, those tests may be reported separately in addition to the panel code. **True or False**
3. CPT code **88332**, *Pathology consultation during surgery; each additional tissue block with frozen section(s)*, cannot be reported for a specimen that has not already been examined initially. **True or False**
4. When reporting a non-automated urinalysis dip stick test performed without microscopy, code **81000** is appropriate. **True or False**
5. The unit of service for Surgical Pathology codes **88300** through **88309** is the specimen. **True or False**

Matching

6. Qualitative assays are _____.
7. Quantitative assays are _____.

   a. tests that detect whether a particular analyte, constituent, or condition is present or absent.
   b. tests that give results expressing the specific numerical amount of an analyte in a specimen.

Fill in the Blank

8. For the Surgical Pathology codes, a _____ is defined as tissue(s) that is submitted for individual and separate attention, requiring individual examination and pathologic diagnosis.
9. Any _____ specimen should be assigned to the code which most closely reflects the physician work involved when compared to other specimens assigned to that code.
10. When urinalysis is reported, multiple tests described within a single code descriptor should not be _____ to produce and report multiple codes.
11. Although the general CPT guidelines state that when a code is not available for a particular procedure or service, a code similar to the actual procedure performed should **not** be selected in lieu of an unlisted procedure code. However, the one exception to this rule is for the _____ codes, in which any unlisted specimen should be assigned to the code that most closely reflects the physician work involved.

Medicine*

Objectives

- Identify services and procedures provided by nonphysician health care providers
- Recognize procedure-oriented subsections and medical specialty subsections
- Understand different categories of injection procedures

Introduction

The Medicine section of the CPT codebook is a single section, similar to the Surgery section, that includes a variety of codes for reporting procedures and services provided by many different types of health care providers. In addition, many services and procedures provided by nonphysician health care providers are also located in the Medicine section. For example, codes in the Physical Medicine and Rehabilitation subsection may be used to report the services and procedures provided by physical and occupational therapists. Audiologists and speech therapists can find codes in the Special Otorhinolaryngologic Services subsection to describe the procedures and services they provide.

There are two basic types of subsections: those that are procedure oriented and those that refer to particular medical specialties. It is very important to remember that the codes in a specialty subsection, such as Gastroenterology, are not limited to use by gastroenterologists. Any qualified physician or, as appropriate, any other qualified health care professional may use any code in the CPT codebook to designate the services rendered. As indicated in the CPT codebook, the listing of a service or procedure and its code number in a specific section of this book does not restrict its use to a specific specialty group.

Coding Tip

Codes in a specialty subsection, such as Gastroenterology, are not limited to use by gastroenterologists.

---

* Please refer to *CPT 2012* codebook for updates on codes and/or code descriptors.

Immune Globulins, Serum, or Recombinant Products; Immunization Administration for Vaccines/Toxoids; and Vaccines, Toxoids

Immune globulin, serum, or recombinant products, which include broad-spectrum and anti-infective immune globulins, antitoxins, and various isoantibodies, are reported with codes **90281-90399**. To report the administration of an immune globulin, serum, or recombinant product, the immune globulin product codes **90281-90399** are reported in addition to the administration code(s) **96365-96368**, **96372**, **96374**, and **96375**, as appropriate. Vaccines and toxoids are reported with codes **90476-90749**. To report the administration of a vaccine/toxoid, the vaccine/toxoid product codes **90476-90749** are reported in addition to the immunization administration code(s) **90460** and **90461**. For immunization administration of any vaccine that is not accompanied by counseling to the patient or family, or for administration of vaccines to patients over 18 years of age, report codes **90471-90474**.

In order to adequately identify and facilitate correct coding, the convention of using upper- and lower-case letters to distinguish between varying amounts of antigen components in related vaccine products is used. For example, in code **90702**, *Diphtheria and tetanus toxoids (DT) adsorbed when administered to individuals younger than 7 years, for intramuscular use,* the initials "DT" are used to reflect the increased diphtheria component for children younger than age seven, and in code **90718**, *Tetanus and diphtheria toxoids (Td) adsorbed when administered to individuals 7 years or older, for intramuscular use,* the initials "Td" are used to indicate the reduced antigen concentration of diphtheria for children ages seven and older.

New and Revised Vaccine Codes

To assist users in reporting the most recent new or revised vaccine product codes, the American Medical Association (AMA) currently uses the CPT Web site, which features updates of CPT Editorial Panel actions regarding these products. Vaccines pending US Food and Drug Administration (FDA) approval are indicated by the ⫫ symbol. CPT users should refer to the AMA Web site for updated information regarding FDA status of a specific vaccine (www.ama-assn.org/ama/pub/category/10902.html). As noted in the *CPT 2011* codebook, once approved by the CPT Editorial Panel, these codes will be made available for release on a semiannual basis (January 1 and July 1). As part of the electronic distribution, there is a six-month implementation period from the initial release date (eg, codes released on January 1 are eligible for use on July 1, and codes released on July 1 are eligible for use on January 1).

To meet the reporting requirements of immunization registries, vaccine distribution programs, and reporting systems (eg, Vaccine Adverse Event Reporting System), the exact vaccine product administered should be reported. Multiple codes for a particular vaccine are provided in the CPT codebook when the schedule (number of doses or timing) differs for two or more products of the same vaccine type (eg, hepatitis A, Hib) or the vaccine product is available in more than one chemical formulation, dosage, or route of administration.

Separate codes are available for combination vaccines (eg, DTP-Hib, DtaP-Hib, HepB-Hib). It is not appropriate to code each component of a combination vaccine separately. If a specific vaccine code is not available, code **90749**, *Unlisted vaccine/toxoid,* should be reported until a new code becomes available.

If a significant, separately identifiable Evaluation and Management (E/M) service (eg, office or other outpatient service, preventive medicine service) is performed, then the appropriate E/M service code should be reported in addition to the vaccine and toxoid administration codes.

✓ Check Your Knowledge

1. Is it appropriate to code each component of a combination vaccine separately?

EXAMPLE

A 5-year-old child is seen in the office for diphtheria and tetanus toxoids. The physician counsels the patient and family and administers the injection.

Code **90702** is reported for the DT toxoids and **90460** for the immunization administration.

Gastroenterology

Codes **91034** and **91035** identify nasal insertion of pH catheters (**91034**) or mucosal attachment of telemetry pH electrodes (**91035**) for detection of gastroesophageal reflux disease (GERD). These codes allow for testing of both acid and nonacid reflux.

These codes describe important tests for the diagnosis of GERD. GERD results from the abnormal reflux of stomach contents into the esophagus. This can result in heartburn and other serious problems such as dysphagia, dysphonia, asthma, and Barrett's esophagus. Measuring the level of acid in the esophagus is an important step in the diagnosis of patients with symptomatic GERD and establishing treatment plans. Further, pH monitoring can be used to determine the

Chapter 7

effectiveness of treatment and the potential need for additional medical, pharmacologic, endoscopic, and/or surgical intervention. When performing an esophageal acid reflux test (code **91034**), a catheter with a pH electrode is placed into the esophagus, either through the nares or by swallowing, to measure intraesophageal pH (an indicator of gastric reflux). See Figure 7-1.

FIGURE 7-1 *Esophageal Acid Reflux Test*

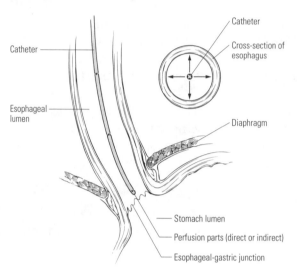

General Ophthalmological Services

Coding Tip

The general ophthalmologic services do not require the E/M three key components of history, examination, and medical decision making, or use of the CMS documentation guidelines, for proper code selection.

The CPT codebook includes codes for intermediate and comprehensive ophthalmologic services, which are special codes that describe the unique nature of ophthalmologic examinations (**92002-92014**). These codes overlap with the general E/M codes (**99201-99215**), depending on the specific services provided to the patient. The E/M and ophthalmology codes may be used by any physician, including ophthalmologists or optometrists, to report an office evaluation. CPT codes **92002-92014** share several definitions with the E/M codes, such as "new" and "established" patient, and may be used to report services rendered in the ophthalmology or optometry office. Differing from the E/M codes, the general ophthalmologic services describe the physician's activity as intermediate and comprehensive in scope and do not require the three key components of history, examination, and medical decision making, or use of the documentation guidelines of the Center for Medicare & Medicaid Services (CMS), to determine the proper code selection.

Routine ophthalmoscopy is part of the general and special ophthalmologic services whenever indicated. It is a nonitemized service and is not reported separately. Figure 7-2 is an illustration of retinal structure to document for comparison with future examinations, as is done with extended ophthalmoscopy (codes **92225**, *Ophthalmoscopy, extended, with retinal drawing (eg, for retinal detachment, melanoma),* *with interpretation and report; initial,* and **92226**, *Ophthalmoscopy, extended, with retinal drawing (eg, for retinal detachment, melanoma), with interpretation and report; subsequent.*

FIGURE 7-2 *Extended Ophthalmoscopy*

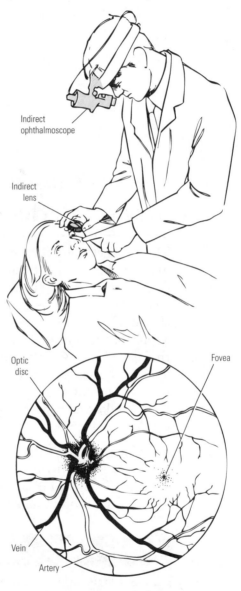

Ophthalmoscopic appearance of retina

Coding Tip

Comprehensive ophthalmological services often include, as indicated, biomicroscopy, examination with cycloplegia or mydriasis, and tonometry and always include initiation of diagnostic and treatment programs.

When performing fluorescein angiography (code **92235**), fluorescein dye is injected in a peripheral vein to enhance imaging. Serial multiframe angiography is performed to evaluate choroidal and retinal circulation. In Figure 7-3, arteries display an even fluorescence, while veins appear striped from the laminar dye flow.

Chapter 7

FIGURE 7-3 *Fluorescein Angiography*

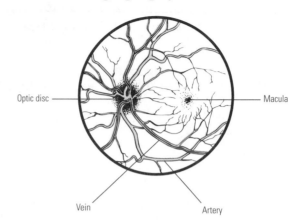

Optic disc — Macula

Vein — Artery

Contact Lens Services and Spectacle Services (Including Prosthesis for Aphakia)

The Contact Lens Services subsection of the CPT code set is unusual because, in addition to the professional services involved in the prescription and fitting of contact lenses, the CPT nomenclature contains a code for the replacement of contact lenses (**92326**) and may include the supply of the contact lens itself as part of the fitting service. The supply of the contact lenses may also be reported separately by using the appropriate supply codes. Reporting requirements for the supply of contact lens materials vary, depending on the specific reporting and reimbursement policies of the individual payers.

The following represent two options for reporting the supply of contact lens materials:

- CPT guidelines allow for reporting of the supply of the lens as part of the service of fitting.
- HCPCS Level II codes are available for reporting of materials, including contact lenses.

✓ Check Your Knowledge

2. Is it true that the supply of contact lenses may be reported separately by using the appropriate supply codes.

Reporting Services for Contact Lenses

The provision of eye care, as well as the mechanisms to report that care, have evolved, with different methods to report many of the

Coding Tip

When reporting codes **92310-92326**, the fitting of contact lenses includes instruction and training of the wearer and incidental revision of the lenses during the training period.

Key Terms

- **Aphakia**
- **Immunotherapy**

Coding Tip

For aural rehabilitation services following cochlear implant, including evaluation of rehabilitation status, see **92626-92633**.

services and materials involved. This can be challenging because reporting requirements vary among third-party payers.

Third-party payers frequently address eye care in the following two categories:

- Eye care covered by vision care insurance, and
- Eye care covered by major medical insurance.

The codes in the Contact Lens Services subsection indicate that the prescription of a contact lens includes specification of optical and physical characteristics (such as power, size, curvature, flexibility, gas permeability), which is not a part of the general ophthalmological services.

Reporting Services for Spectacles

The codes in the Spectacle Services (Including Prosthesis for Aphakia) subsection are differentiated by the presence or absence of aphakia. **Aphakia** is defined as the absence of the crystalline lens of the eye. The most common cause of this condition is surgical removal of the lens due to cataract. Aphakia may also be rarely caused by absorption, degeneration, or congenital absence of the lens. When the fitting of spectacles is provided, it may be reported by codes **92340-92371**. The supply of materials is a separate service component and is not part of the service of fitting spectacles.

Special Otorhinolaryngologic Services

The Evaluative and Therapeutic Services code range (**92601-92700**) includes codes for reporting diagnostic analysis for cochlear implants, evaluation and therapeutic services for augmentative and alternative communication devices, evaluation of oral and pharyngeal swallowing function, motion fluoroscopic evaluation and flexible fiberoptic endoscopic evaluation of swallowing, and laryngeal sensory testing. Parenthetical notes and guidelines are included to instruct the user in the selection of the appropriate code.

Evaluative and Therapeutic Services (92601-92633)

Codes **92601** and **92603** describe postoperative analysis and fitting of previously placed external devices, connection to the cochlear implant, and programming of the stimulator. Codes **92602** and **92604** describe subsequent sessions for measurements and adjustment of the external transmitter and reprogramming of the internal stimulator. Figure 7-4 shows the elements that are addressed in the diagnostic analysis and reprogramming of the cochlear implant procedures **92601-92604**.

FIGURE 7-4 *A View of the Outer Cochlear Implant*

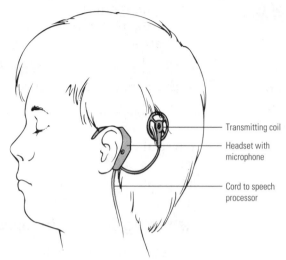

Transmitting coil

Headset with microphone

Cord to speech processor

Key Terms

Aphakia: The absence of the crystalline lens of the eye.

Immunotherapy: The parenteral administration of allergenic extracts as antigens at periodic intervals, usually on an increasing scale, to a dose that is selected as maintenance therapy.

Cardiovascular

The first code in this series is **92950**, *Cardiopulmonary resuscitation (eg, in cardiac arrest)*, for reporting cardiopulmonary resuscitation (CPR). This code is intended to describe CPR to restore and maintain the patient's respiration and circulation after cessation of heartbeat and breathing. Basic CPR consists of assessing the victim, opening the airway, restoring breathing (eg, mouth-to-mouth, bag valve mask), then restoring circulation (eg, closed chest cardiac massage). In most instances, CPR is performed prior to, with continuation during, advanced life support interventions, eg, drug therapy and defibrillation, which would be included by reporting the appropriate critical care services code(s) from the E/M section of the CPT codebook.

Codes **92960** and **92961** are used to report cardioversion. Code **92960** specifically describes elective (nonemergency) external electrical cardioversion using an external electrical stimulator source, such as cardioversion paddles. Elective cardioversion may be used to

Coding Tip

CPR is not included in the reporting of critical care services. If CPR and critical care are both provided, it would be appropriate to separately report these services.

Chapter 7

treat atrial fibrillation and atrial flutter if antiarrhythmic drugs fail to convert the heart back to normal sinus rhythm or if the patient is hemodynamically unstable.

Code **92961** is used to report internal cardioversion. This procedure is most commonly used to convert atrial fibrillation to normal sinus rhythm when external cardioversion is unsuccessful.

Code **92961** is designated as a separate procedure. Internal elective cardioversion is not separately reported when performed as an integral component of another procedure or service, as in an electrophysiologic (EP) study or cardiac catheterization. However, if the internal elective cardioversion is performed independently, unrelated or distinct from other procedure(s) or service(s) provided at that time, it would be appropriate to separately report the internal cardioversion. The parenthetical note that follows this code indicates that it is not appropriate to report internal cardioversion in conjunction with codes **93282-93284**, **93287**, **93289**, **93295**, **93296**, **93618-93624**, **93631**, **93640-93642**, **93650-93652**, and **93662**.

Defibrillation is the delivery of an electrical impulse to the heart. This impulse is intended to interrupt abnormal rhythms (eg, ventricular fibrillation) and allow the normal sinus impulse and electrical conduction to resume. The electrical impulse must be strong enough to cause depolarization (neutralization of the positive and negative electrical charges) of a large percentage of the myocardium. The time of the defibrillation is not synchronized to the cardiac cycle.

No CPT code exists to report defibrillation as a procedure performed in isolation. Defibrillation may be performed as part of critical care services, at the end of open heart surgery, during cardiac catheterization, during cardioverter-defibrillator implantation, or during an EP procedure. In all of these situations, defibrillation is **not** a separately reportable service.

When an intravascular ultrasound (coronary vessel or graft) is performed (code **92978**), a catheter with a transducer at its tip is inserted and threaded through a selected coronary artery(s) or coronary bypass graft(s). See Figure 7-5.

Codes **92980** and **92981** are used to report coronary artery stenting. Coronary angioplasty (**92982**, **92984**) or atherectomy (**92995**, **92996**), in the same artery is considered part of the stenting procedure and is not reported separately. (See Figure 7-6.) Codes **92973** (percutaneous transluminal coronary thombectomy) and **92974** (coronary brachytherapy) are add-on codes for reporting procedures performed in addition to coronary stenting, atherectomy, and angioplasty and are not included in the "therapeutic interventions" in **92980**. Codes **92978** and **92979** are add-on codes for reporting intravascular ultrasound procedures performed in addition to coronary and bypass graft diagnostic and interventional services.

Coding Tip

Code **92974**, *Transcatheter placement of radiation delivery device for subsequent coronary intravascular brachytherapy (List separately in addition to code for primary procedure)*, does not include the calculation or placement of the radioelement. Intravascular radioelement application is reported with codes **77785-77787**.

Key Term

Defibrillation: The delivery of an electrical impulse to the heart.

Chapter 7

FIGURE 7-5 *Intravascular Ultrasound (Coronary Vessel or Graft)*

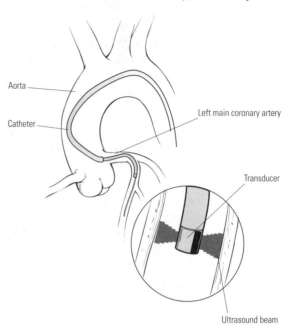

FIGURE 7-6 *Percutaneous Transluminal Coronary Angioplasty (PTCA)*

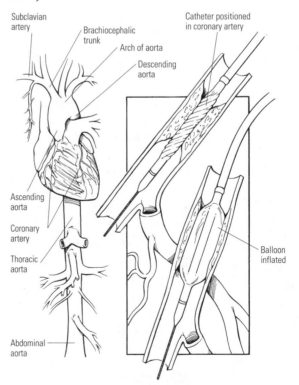

Cardiography and Cardiovascular Monitoring Services

The codes included in the **93000-93278** series are used to report various methods of obtaining cardiographic readings for the heart. The correct code to use for the procedure is dependent on the capabilities of the equipment being used as well as the information that is obtained regarding heartbeat and any irregularities that may occur.

Cardiovascular Monitoring Services

Cardiovascular monitoring services are diagnostic medical procedures using in-person and remote technology to assess cardiovascular rhythm (ECG) data. Holter monitors (codes **93224-93227**) include up to 48 hours of continuous recording. **Mobile cardiac telemetry** monitors (codes **93228**, **93229**) have the capability of transmitting a tracing at any time, always have internal ECG analysis algorithms designed to detect major arrhythmias, and transmit to an attended surveillance center. Event monitors (codes **93268-93272**) record segments of ECGs with recording initiation triggered either by patient activation or by an internal automatic, preprogrammed detection algorithm (or both) and transmit the recorded electrocardiographic data when requested (but cannot transmit immediately based upon the patient or algorithmic activation rhythm) and do not require **attended surveillance**.

Key Terms

Attended surveillance: Immediate availability of a remote technician to respond to rhythm or device alert transmissions from a patient, either from an implanted or wearable monitoring or therapy device, as they are generated and transmitted to the remote surveillance location or center.

Mobile cardiovascular telemetry (MCT): Continuously records the electrocardiographic (ECG) rhythm from external electrodes placed on the patient's body. Segments of the ECG data are automatically (without patient intervention) transmitted to a remote surveillance location by cellular or land-line telephone signal.

Device, single lead: a pacemaker or implantable cardioverter-defibrillator (ICD) with pacing and sensing function in only one chamber of the heart.

Device, dual lead: a pacemaker or implantable cardioverter-defibrillator (ICD) with pacing and sensing function in only two chambers of the heart.

Device, multiple lead: a pacemaker or implantable cardioverter-defibrillator (ICD) with pacing and sensing function in three or more chambers of the heart.

Chapter 7

Implantable cardiovascular monitor (ICM): Implantable cardiovascular device used to assist the physician in the management of non–rhythm-related cardiac conditions such as heart failure. The device collects longitudinal physiologic cardiovascular data elements from one or more internal sensors (such as right ventricular pressure, left atrial pressure, or an index of lung water) and/or external sensors (such as blood pressure or body weight) for patient assessment and management. The data are stored and transmitted to the physician by either local telemetry or remotely to an Internet-based file server or surveillance technician.

Implantable cardioverter-defibrillator (ICD): Implantable device that provides high-energy and low-energy stimulation to one or more chambers of the heart to terminate rapid heart rhythms called *tachycardia* or *fibrillation*. ICDs also have pacemaker functions to treat slow heart rhythms, called *bradycardia*.

Implantable loop recorder (ILR): Implantable device that continuously records the electrocardiographic (ECG) rhythm triggered automatically by rapid and slow heart rates or by the patient during a symptomatic episode. The ILR function may be the only function of the device or it may be part of a pacemaker or implantable cardioverter-defibrillator device (ICD). The data are stored and transmitted to the physician by either local telemetry or remotely to an Internet-based file server or surveillance technician. Extraction of data and compilation or report for physician interpretation is usually performed in the office setting.

Interrogation device evaluation: An evaluation of an implantable device such as a cardiac pacemaker, implantable cardioverter-defibrillator (ICD), implantable cardiovascular monitor (ICM), or implantable loop recorder (ILR). Using an office, hospital, or emergency department (ED) instrument or via a remote interrogation system, stored and measured information about the lead(s) when present, sensor(s) when present, battery and the implanted device function, as well as data collected about the patient's heart rhythm and heart rate are retrieved.

Pacemaker: An implantable device that provides low-energy localized stimulation to one or more chambers of the heart to initiate contraction in that chamber.

Coding Tip

ECG rhythm–derived elements are distinct from physiologic data, even when the same device is capable of producing both. Implantable cardiovascular monitor (ICM) device services are always separately reported from implantable cardioverter-defibrillator (ICD) service.

Implantable and Wearable Cardiac Device Evaluations

Cardiac device evaluation services are diagnostic medical procedures using in-person and remote technology to assess device therapy and cardiovascular physiologic data. Codes **93279-93299** describe this technology and technical/professional physician and service center practice. Codes **93279-93292** are reported per procedure. Codes **93293-93296** are reported no more than once every 90 days. Do not report **93293-93296** if the monitoring period is less than 30 days. Codes **93297**, **93298** are reported no more than once up to every 30 days. Do not report **93297-93299** if the monitoring period is less than 10 days.

The required components that must be evaluated for both remote and in-person interrogations for the various types of implantable cardiac devices include:

- Pacemaker: Programmed parameters, lead(s), battery, capture and sensing function, and heart rhythm.
- Implantable cardioverter-defibrillator (ICD): Programmed parameters, lead(s), battery, capture and sensing function, presence or absence of therapy for ventricular tachyarrhythmias, and underlying heart rhythm.
- Implantable cardiovascular monitor (ICM): Programmed parameters and analysis of at least one recorded physiologic cardiovascular data element from either internal or external sensors.
- Implantable loop recorder (ILR): Programmed parameters and the heart rate and rhythm during recorded episodes from both patient-initiated and device algorithm–detected events, when present.

Echocardiography

A complete transthoracic echocardiogram **without** spectral or color flow Doppler (code **93307**) is a comprehensive procedure that includes two-dimensional and, when performed, selected M-mode examination of the left and right atria, the left and right ventricles, the aortic, mitral, and tricuspid valves, the pericardium, and adjacent portions of the aorta. Multiple views are required to obtain a complete functional and anatomic evaluation, and appropriate measurements are obtained and recorded. A complete transthoracic echocardiogram **with** spectral and color flow Doppler (**93306**) is a comprehensive procedure that includes spectral Doppler and color flow Doppler in addition to the two-dimensional and selected M-mode examinations, when performed. Spectral Doppler (**93320**, **93321**) and color flow Doppler (**93325**) provide information regarding intracardiac blood flow and hemodynamics.

With Transesophageal Echocardiography (TEE) codes **93312-93318**, an endoscopic ultrasound transducer is passed through the mouth into the esophagus and two-dimensional images are obtained from the posterior aspect of the heart. See Figure 7-7.

Cardiac Catheterization

Cardiac catheterization is a diagnostic medical procedure that includes introduction, positioning and repositioning, when necessary, of catheter(s) within the vascular system, recording of intracardiac and/or intravascular pressure(s), and final evaluation

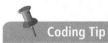

Coding Tip

Echocardiography includes obtaining ultrasonic signals from the heart and great vessels, with real time image and/or Doppler ultrasonic signal documentation, with interpretation and report. When interpretation is performed separately, use modifier 26.

FIGURE 7-7 *Transesophageal Echocardiography (TEE)*

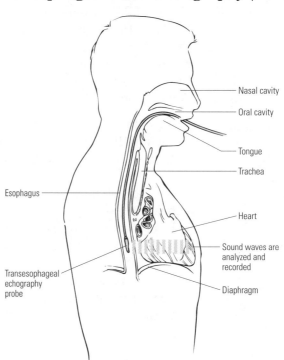

Nasal cavity

Oral cavity

Tongue

Trachea

Esophagus

Heart

Sound waves are
analyzed and
recorded

Transesophageal
echography
probe

Diaphragm

and report of procedure. There are two code families for cardiac catheterization: one for congenital heart disease and one for all other conditions. Anomalous coronary arteries, patent foramen ovale, mitral valve prolapse, and bicuspid aortic valve are to be reported with **93451-93464, 93566-93568**.

Right heart catheterization includes catheter placement in one or more right-sided cardiac chamber(s) or structures (ie, the right atrium, right ventricle, pulmonary artery, pulmonary wedge), obtaining blood samples for measurement of blood gases, and cardiac output measurements (Fick or other method), when performed. Left heart catheterization involves catheter placement in a left-sided (systemic) cardiac chamber(s) (left ventricle or left atrium) and includes left ventricular injection(s) when performed.

Contrast injection to image the access site(s) for the specific purpose of placing a closure device is inherent to the catheterization procedure and not separately reportable. Closure device placement at the vascular access site is inherent to the catheterization procedure and not separately reportable.

With a right heart catheterization procedure (code **93451**), the physician introduces a cardiac catheter into the venous system, and the catheter is directed into the right atrium, right ventricle, and pulmonary artery. The catheter is advanced retrograde through the arterial system to the ascending aorta; pressures are measured in the aortic root; and the catheter is manipulated using fluoroscopic guidance into the ostium of a coronary artery, arterial bypass conduit, or venous coronary bypass graft. See Figure 7-8.

Coding Tip

Modifier **51** should not be appended to **93451**, **93456**, or **93503**.

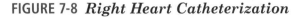

FIGURE 7-8 *Right Heart Catheterization*

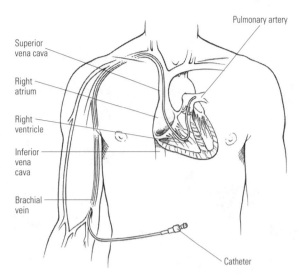

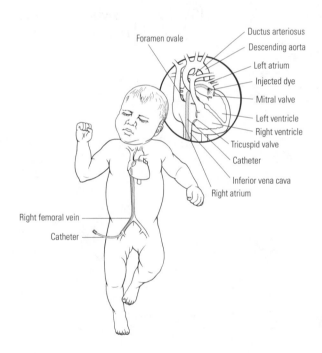

With a left heart catheterization procedure (code **93452**), a catheter is inserted into the arterial system and then into the left ventricle. See Figure 7-9.

When performing coronary angiography without concomitant left heart catheterization (code **93454**), the catheter does not cross the aortic valve into the left ventricle (left heart catheterization). See Figure 7-10.

When performing intravascular distal blood flow velocity (code **93571**), a Doppler guidewire is positioned in a proximal coronary artery with the transducer beam parallel to blood flow to measure blood flow velocity. See Figure 7-11 on page 283.

FIGURE 7-9 *Left Heart Catheterization*

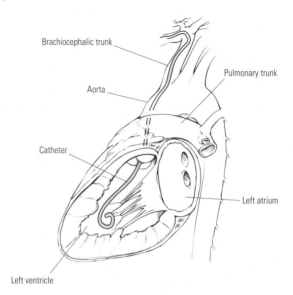

FIGURE 7-10 *Coronary Angiography Without Concomitant Left Heart Catheterization*

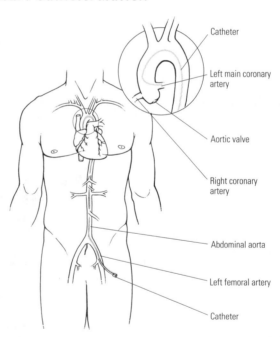

Intracardiac Electrophysiological Procedures/Studies (EPS)

Electrophysiology is a subspecialty of cardiology devoted to the diagnosis and treatment of heart rhythm disturbances. EPS (codes **93600-93662**) are invasive diagnostic medical procedures that include the insertion and repositioning of electrode catheters, recording of electrograms before and during pacing or programmed stimulation of multiple locations in the heart, analysis of recorded information, and report of the procedure. Electrophysiologic studies are most often performed with two or more electrode catheters. Because of the complex nature of EPS testing, it is necessary to understand the normal electrophysiology of the heart. See Figures 7-12 and 7-13, which describe the normal electrical conduction of the heart.

FIGURE 7-11 *Intravascular Distal Blood Flow Velocity*

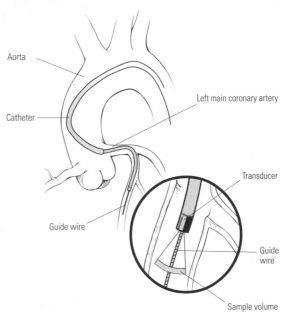

FIGURE 7-12 *Heart Conduction System*

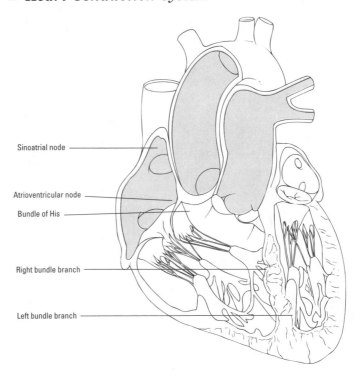

FIGURE 7-13 *Electrical Conduction of the Heart*

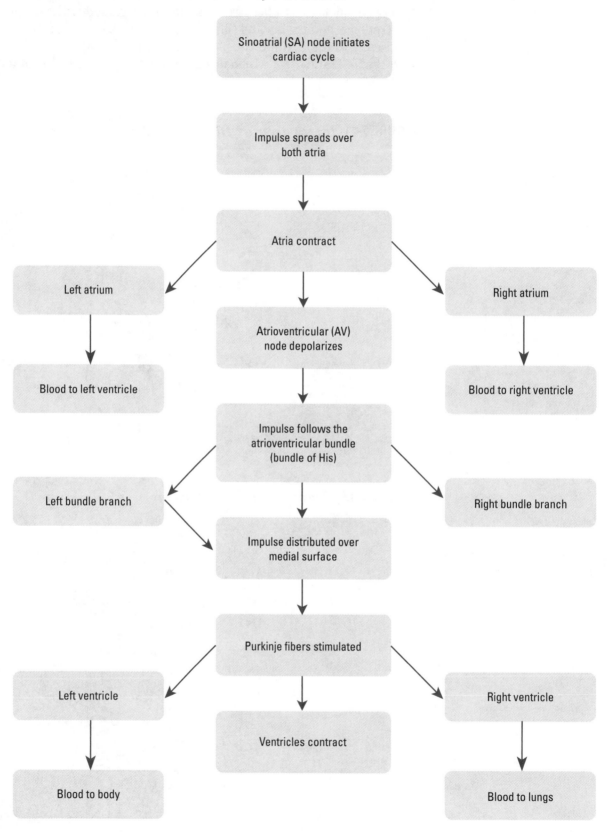

Chapter 7

Pulmonary

Ventilator management is comprised of four codes (**94002-94005**), which describe ventilator assist and management services with initiation of pressure or volume preset ventilators for assisted or controlled breathing. Codes in the **94010-94799** series are used to report various pulmonary services and procedures. These codes include laboratory procedure(s) and interpretation of test results. The term *laboratory* does not refer to the services performed that are reported by codes from the Pathology and Laboratory section of the CPT codebook (**80002-89399** series). Rather, these codes describe diagnostic and therapeutic procedures performed in a pulmonary function testing department, a facility (eg, a hospital), or a pulmonary function laboratory in an office. If the services provided include services described by codes in the Pathology and Laboratory section of the CPT codebook, as well as pulmonary services from the **94010-94799** code series, then it is appropriate to report codes from both sections. If a separately identifiable E/M service is performed, the appropriate E/M code should be reported in addition to code(s) from the **94010-94799** series.

Coding Tip

Code **95027**, *Intracutaneous (intradermal) tests, sequential and incremental, with allergenic extracts for airborne allergens, immediate type reaction, including test interpretation and report by a physician, specify number of tests*, is reported one time per allergen.

Allergy and Clinical Immunology

Allergy sensitivity tests describe the performance and evaluation of selective cutaneous and mucous membrane tests consistent with the history, physical examination, and other observations of the patient. The number of tests performed should be judicious and dependent on the history, physical findings, and clinical judgment of the practitioner.

Immunotherapy (desensitization, hyposensitization) is the parenteral administration of allergenic extracts as antigens at periodic intervals, usually on an increasing scale, to a dose that is selected as maintenance therapy. For medical conferences on the use of mechanical and electronic devices (precipitators, air conditioners, air filters, humidifiers, dehumidifiers), climatotherapy, and physical, occupational, and recreational therapy, see the Evaluation and Management section.

Coding Tip

Do not report modifier **50** in conjunction with code **95865**, *Needle electromyography; larynx*, as this procedure is typically performed on both sides of the larynx. For a unilateral procedure, report modifier **52** in conjunction with code **95865**.

Neurology and Neuromuscular Procedures

Electromyography

Needle electromyographic (EMG) procedures include the interpretation of electrical waveforms measured by equipment that produces both visible and audible components of electrical signals recorded from the muscle(s) studied by the needle electrode. Needle EMG of the larynx, reported with code **95865**, is performed to diagnose laryngeal nerve and muscle disorders, for intraoperative monitoring during procedures performed on the larynx, and during botox injections in the

Chapter 7

laryngeal muscles. Needle EMG of the hemidiaphragm, reported with code **95866**, is performed to diagnose respiratory muscle disorders and, less frequently, for intraoperative monitoring.

EXAMPLE

A 36-year-old male complains of a raspy voice following prolonged intubation.

Code **95865** is reported for laryngeal muscle assessment in which the needle electrode is inserted through the skin into the cricothyroid membrane until muscle activity is located. When the correct muscles are identified, electrodiagnostic properties of the muscle are reviewed, including insertion activity, spontaneous activity, and voluntary activity. Motor unit potentials may be analyzed according to morphology, amplitude, frequency, and recruitment. The needle is withdrawn, and direct pressure to prevent bleeding is applied.

Codes **+95873** and **+95874** are used to report electrical stimulation for guidance with chemodenervation and needle EMG for guidance with chemodenervation. Prior to the chemodenervation procedure, it may be necessary to perform a more precise localization for needle placement before the chemical is injected. Code **+95873** is an add-on code that describes electrical stimulation and **+95874** is an add-on code that describes needle EMG.

Special EEG Tests (95950-95967)

Codes **95950-95953** and **95956** are used per 24 hours of recording. For recording more than 12 hours, do not use modifier **52**. For recording 12 hours or less, use modifier **52**. Codes **95951** and **95956** are used for recordings in which interpretations can be made throughout the recording time, with interventions to alter or end the recording or to alter the patient care during the recordings as needed. See Figure 7-14.

Codes **95961** and **95962** use physician time as a basis for unit of service. Report for each hour of physician attendance. Report **95961** for the first hour of physician attendance. Use modifier **52** with **95961** for 30 minutes or less. Report **95962** for each additional hour of physician attendance.

Neurostimulators, Analysis-Programming

Simple and complex neurostimulator systems are currently available and effective in managing patients with neurological disorders. Neurostimulator codes were established to differentiate the time and effort associated with evaluation, testing, programming, or reprogramming of neurostimulator systems. Deep brain stimulation is used to

FIGURE 7-14 *Electroencephalographic (EEG) Monitoring and Video Recording*

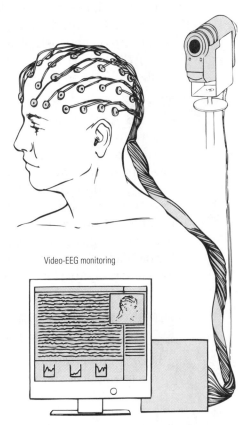

Video-EEG monitoring

treat movement disorders (eg, rigidity, tremors, balance control). For example, with the electrode array placed in the thalamus, stimulation is used for treatment of essential tremor or tremor resulting from Parkinson disease. A deep-brain stimulator can also be placed in the globus pallidus or subthalamic nucleus for Parkinson disease, essential tremor, and other conditions such as multiple sclerosis. With the array placed in these locations, several clinical features such as rigidity, dyskinesia, and/or tremor can be treated. When several clinical features are treated, the evaluation and monitoring of the patient's reaction to each stimulation setting is a complex process. Repeated and very detailed neurologic testing is often required to ascertain the most appropriate stimulation setting. For example, a given setting revision may improve one feature (eg, rigidity) but worsen another (eg, dyskinesia).

CPT guidelines differentiate between a simple and a complex neurostimulator as follows:

- A simple neurostimulator pulse generator/transmitter (**95970, 95971**) is capable of affecting or changing three or fewer of the following features: pulse amplitude, pulse duration, pulse frequency, eight or more electrode contacts, cycling (meaning automatic on and off for different times in microseconds), stimulation train duration, train spacing, number of programs, number of channels, alternating electrode polarities, dose time (stimulation parameters changing in periods of minutes including dose lockout times), and more than one clinical feature (eg, rigidity, dyskinesia, tremor).

- A complex neurostimulator pulse generator/transmitter (**95970, 95972-95975**) is one capable of affecting more than three of the above features.

The stimulation programming codes are based on what the system is capable of affecting and not on what parameters are being used for programming at any given programming session. For example, programming of thalamic deep brain stimulation is considered simple programming. The reason is that only one clinical feature (ie, tremor) is mainly, if not entirely, affected by stimulation in this location. It is true that "tremor" can occur in different body positions at different times and have different forms, etc, but ultimately it is still only one clinical feature being treated. Stimulation in the globus pallidus or subthalamic nucleus, on the other hand, affects multiple clinical features such as tremor, rigidity, and dyskinesia.

✓ Check Your Knowledge

3. CPT guidelines differentiate between a simple and a complex neurostimulator. **True or False?**

Health and Behavior Assessment/ Intervention

Codes **96150-96155** are intended to describe services offered to patients who present with primary physical illnesses, diagnoses, or symptoms and who may benefit from assessments and interventions that focus on the biopsychosocial factors related to the patient's health status. These services do not represent preventive medicine counseling and risk factor reduction interventions.

Health and behavior assessment procedures (**96150** and **96151**) are used to identify the psychological, behavioral, emotional, cognitive, and social factors important to the prevention, treatment, or management of physical health problems.

The focus of the assessment is not on mental health but on the biopsychosocial factors important to physical health problems and treatments. For patients who can benefit from this type of treatment, the assessment may focus on factors related to the patient's physical health, which may include assisting a patient in changing his or her behavioral habits for taking medication, managing and expressing symptoms, or eliminating behaviors that exacerbate the symptoms.

Health and behavior intervention procedures (**96152-96155**) are used to modify the psychological, behavioral, emotional, cognitive, and social factors identified as important to or directly affecting the patient's physiologic functioning, disease status, health, and well-being. The focus of the intervention is to improve the patient's health and well-being by means of cognitive, behavioral, social, and/or psychophysiologic procedures designed to improve specific disease-related problems.

From a CPT coding perspective, codes **96150-96155** may be reported by, but are not limited to, psychologists, advanced practice nurses, clinical social workers, and other nonphysician health care professionals within their scope of practice who have specialty or subspecialty training in health and behavior assessment or intervention procedures. These codes are not intended to be used by physicians. Instead, physicians performing these services may identify their efforts by choosing the E/M codes appropriate to the type and level of service being provided using the key components (ie, history, examination, medical decision making) to identify the level of service provided or, when counseling and/or coordination of care represent 50% or more of the total time spent for the visit, using time for choosing the appropriate E/M code. Because these services are inherently identified as face-to-face services, questionnaires given to the patient without face-to-face contact should not be reported with these codes. In addition, these services do not include neuropsychological testing. Separate codes should be used to identify this service, if performed.

Health and Behavior Assessment/Intervention codes are not intended to represent preventive medicine services, as these services do not identify the comprehensive evaluation services as identified in the Preventive Medicine Services codes. If comprehensive evaluation services are performed, these codes (**99381-99397**) should be used to identify those specific services. These codes should not be reported on the same day in addition to Preventive Medicine Services and/or Counseling Risk Factor Reduction and Behavior Change Intervention services (**99401-99412**).

For patients who require psychiatric services (**90801-90899**) as well as health and behavior assessment/intervention (**96150-96155**), report the predominant service performed. The psychiatry codes (**90801-90899**) refer to psychotherapy, psychological testing, and psychiatric evaluation, and all require a mental health diagnosis. In most cases, difficulties associated with an acute or chronic illness, prevention of a physical illness or disability, and maintenance of health do not meet criteria for a psychiatric diagnosis. Use of the Health and Behavior Assessment/Intervention codes eliminates inappropriate labeling of the patient as having a mental health disorder when the problem is actually a physical illness.

Coding Tip

Health and behavior intervention codes **96150-96155** are not intended to be used by physicians.

Coding Tip

It is not appropriate to report **96150-96155** in conjunction with **90801-90899** on the same date.

✓ Check Your Knowledge

4. For patients who require behavior assessment/intervention (**96150-96155**), along with psychiatric services (**90801-90899**), are codes from both subsections reported? If yes, why. If no, what is reported.

Hydration, Therapeutic, Prophylactic, Diagnostic Injections and Infusions, and Chemotherapy and Other Highly Complex Drug or Highly Complex Biologic Agent Administration

The drug administration codes are grouped into three categories:

1. Hydration (**96360-96361**);
2. Therapeutic, Prophylactic, and Diagnostic Injections and Infusions (excludes Chemotherapy and Other Highly Complex Drug or Highly Complex Biologic Agent Administration) (**96365-96379**); and
3. Chemotherapy and Other Highly Complex Drug or Highly Complex Biologic Agent Administration (**96401-96549**).

Hydration codes are reported with CPT codes **96360-96361** and are intended to report a hydration IV infusion consisting of a prepackaged fluid and electrolytes (eg, normal saline, D5-½ normal saline + 30 mEq KCl/liter). These codes are not used to report the infusion of drugs or other substances.

A therapeutic, prophylactic, or diagnostic IV infusion or injection (**96365-96379**) (other than hydration) is for the administration of substances/drugs. When fluids are used to administer the drug(s), the administration of the fluid is considered incidental hydration and is not separately reportable. These services typically require direct physician supervision for any or all purposes of patient assessment, provision of consent, safety oversight, and intraservice supervision of staff. Typically, such infusions require special consideration to prepare, dose, or dispose of; require practice training and competency for staff who administer the infusions; and require periodic patient assessment with vital sign monitoring during the infusion.

If performed to facilitate the infusion or injection, the following services are included and not reported separately:

- Use of local anesthesia
- IV start
- Access to indwelling IV, subcutaneous catheter, or port
- Flush at conclusion of infusion
- Standard tubing, syringes, and supplies

Coding Tip

When fluids are used to administer the drug(s), the administration of the fluid is considered incidental hydration and is not separately reportable.

Initial, Subsequent, Concurrent, Sequential Injections

When multiple drugs are administered, report the service(s) and the specific materials or drugs for each. When administering multiple

Chapter 7

infusions, injections, or combinations, only one "initial" service code should be reported, unless protocol requires that two separate IV sites must be used. **Modifier 59**, *Distinct procedural service,* may be reported when the protocol requires two separate IV sites. The **initial** code that best describes the key or primary reason for the encounter should always be reported, irrespective of the order in which the infusions or injections occur. The primary service is the key to choosing the initial service code. If an injection or infusion is of a subsequent or concurrent nature, even if it is the first such service within that group of services, then a subsequent or concurrent code from the appropriate section should be reported (eg, the first IV push given subsequent to an initial one-hour infusion is reported using a subsequent IV push code). A "subsequent" service is the infusion or injection of a second or subsequent drug after the initial drug. A "concurrent" infusion service is when multiple infusions are provided simultaneously through the same IV line and reported with code **96368**. Code **96368** is reported only once per encounter. When reporting codes for which infusion time is a factor, use the actual time over which the infusion is administered.

If a significant, separately identifiable E/M service is performed, then the appropriate E/M service code should be reported using **modifier 25** in addition to these codes.

Key Terms

Initial: Describes the key or primary reason for the encounter.

Subsequent: Infusion or injection of a second or subsequent drug after the initial drug.

Concurrent: When multiple infusions are provided simultaneously through the same IV line.

Coding Tip

Multiple substances mixed in one bag are considered to be one infusion and reported as a concurrent infusion. Each substance can be reported separately but only one administration is reported.

Chemotherapy Administration

Chemotherapy administration codes **96401-96549** apply to parenteral administration of nonradionuclide antineoplastic drugs and also to antineoplastic agents provided for treatment of noncancer diagnoses (eg, cyclophosphamide for autoimmune conditions) or to substances such as certain monoclonal antibody agents and other biologic response modifiers. These services can be provided by any physician. Chemotherapy services are typically highly complex and require direct physician supervision for any or all purposes of patient assessment, provision of consent, safety oversight, and intraservice supervision of staff. Typically, such chemotherapy services require advanced practice training and competency for staff who provide these services; special considerations for preparation, dosage, or disposal; and commonly, these services entail significant patient risk and frequent monitoring. Examples are frequent changes in the infusion rate, prolonged presence of the nurse administering the solution for patient monitoring and

Chapter 7

infusion adjustments, and frequent conferring with the physician about these issues.

There are separate codes for each parenteral method of administration when chemotherapy is administered by different techniques. The administration of medications (eg, antibiotics, steroidal agents, antiemetics, narcotics, analgesics) administered independently or sequentially as supportive management of chemotherapy administration are separately reported using **96360**, **96361**, **96365**, **96379**, as appropriate. The specific service as well as code(s) for the specific substance(s) or drug(s) provided are reported. The fluid used to administer the drug(s) is considered incidental hydration and is not separately reportable.

When administering multiple infusions, injections, or combinations, only **one** initial service code should be reported unless protocol requires that two separate IV sites must be used. The initial code that best describes the key or primary reason for the encounter should always be reported, irrespective of the order in which the infusions or injections occur. If an injection or infusion is of a subsequent or concurrent nature, even if it is the first such service within that group of services, a subsequent or concurrent code from the appropriate section should be reported (eg, the first IV push given subsequent to an initial one-hour infusion is reported using a subsequent IV push code). When reporting codes for which infusion time is a factor, use the actual time over which the infusion is administered. If a significant, separately identifiable E/M service is performed, the appropriate E/M service code should be reported using **modifier 25** in addition to **96401-96549**.

Coding Tip

Infusion time is measured when the infusate is actually running; pre- and posttimes are not considered. It is important, therefore, to document infusion start and stop times.

EXAMPLE

A 65-year-old female presents with colon cancer with the appropriate indications for chemotherapy.

Code **96401** is reported for the chemotherapy administration in which the physician provides direct supervision and is immediately available in the office. The physician assesses the patient's response to the treatment.

Physical Medicine and Rehabilitation

Codes in the **97001-97755** series are intended to report a variety of physical medicine and rehabilitation procedures and services. Separate series of codes are available for reporting within this subsection as follows:

- Evaluations
- Modalities (supervised and constant attendance)
- Therapeutic procedures
- Active wound care management
- Tests and measurements
- Orthotic management and prosthetic management

Codes in this series are not restricted to use by a specific specialty group. They may be used by any provider who is qualified to perform the service represented by the specific code. No distinction is made in CPT concerning the licensure or professional credentials of the provider. Licensure varies on a state-by-state basis, and credentialing varies on an institutional or individual provider basis. Relevant state and institutional authorities should be consulted regarding the appropriate provision of these services by health care professionals.

Evaluations

Codes **97001-97004** are used to report physical and occupational therapy evaluation and re-evaluation. These codes identify a dynamic process in which clinical judgments are made on the basis of data gathered. These evaluations result in the development of a plan for management of a patient's problems as they relate to his or her disease or disability. Codes **97005** and **97006** describe athletic training evaluation and re-evaluation, respectively.

Use of the evaluation and re-evaluation codes is dependent on whether the service being provided is a significant, separate service needed to gather objective data from tests and measurements and utilized to guide patient management. Physical therapy evaluation (**97001**) and occupational therapy evaluation (**97003**) should signal the start of an episode of care at each level of care (eg, home health, skilled nursing, outpatient). Determining when to use the re-evaluation codes (**97002, 97004**) depends on the patient's status and the need to identify indicators for modification in the treatment plan. Physical medicine and rehabilitation services include an assessment component as part of the preservice work. Therefore, a re-evaluation (**97002** or **97004**) should not be reported on every date of service.

Modalities

The following are two series of codes for reporting **modalities**:

- Supervised modality codes (**97010-97028**) are for the application of a modality that does not require direct (one-on-one) patient contact by the provider.
- Constant attendance modality codes (**97032-97039**) are for the application of a modality that requires direct (one-on-one) patient contact by the provider.

Although the language in the descriptor for these codes indicates "application of a modality to 1 or more areas," the number of areas of application is not a consideration in the reporting of these codes. For example, if hot packs are placed on the knee and cervical spine, code **97010** is reported once for that patient encounter even though two hot packs were placed. Also, the number of diagnoses is not a determinant of how many units of supervised modalities can be reported.

The descriptor language of the constant attendance modality codes includes a time component that helps define their use. The constant

Key Term

- **Modality**

attendance codes (**97032-97039**) indicate that these codes are reported for each 15 minutes. Therefore, they may be reported once for each 15-minute interval spent providing the service. The supervised modality codes (**97010-97028**) do not include an increment of time in the descriptor; therefore, time is not a component for determining the use of these codes. The code is reported without regard to the length of time spent performing the service. Because time is not a factor in determining the use of the supervised modalities, they are intended to be used only once during an encounter, regardless of the number of areas treated. The descriptor language of the constant attendance modality codes includes a time component that helps define their use. The constant attendance codes indicate that these codes are reported for each 15 minutes. Therefore, they may be reported once for each 15-minute interval spent providing the service. When more than one modality is performed during an encounter, whether supervised or constant attendance or in combination, each modality should be reported separately.

Key Term

Modality: Any physical agent applied to produce therapeutic changes to biologic tissue, including but not limited to thermal, acoustic, light, mechanical, or electric energy.

EXAMPLE

A patient has a lumbosacral sprain with muscle guarding in her dorsal lumbar muscles. The patient is positioned in the prone position, a towel is applied to the lumbar area, and the unit is turned on. The heat agent over the lumbosacral sprain is left in place for 20 minutes. The provider checks the dosage level and skin response at 5 minutes following institution of the treatment and checks patient's response at the end of the 20-minute time period. One unit is reported for this modality. This instance is assigned code **97024**.

A patient has a lateral epicondylitis of the right elbow. The patient is positioned with the elbow resting on a pillow in a comfortable position. The therapist prepares the iontophoresis electrodes, applies them to the skin, attaches the wire leads to the electrodes, and turns on the unit to the appropriate setting. The provider monitors the patient for pain and skin response. The treatment lasts 30 minutes. This instance is assigned code **97033**.

Therapeutic Procedures

The therapeutic procedure codes (**97110-97546**) are intended to report a manner of effecting change through the application of clinical skills and/or services that attempt to improve the patient's functions. When reporting this series of codes, the physician or therapist is required to have direct (one-on-one) patient contact.

Common elements of preservice work include chart reviews, setup of activities and the equipment area, review of previous documentation and medical reports, communication with other health care professionals (eg, social worker or nurse), discussions with the family, and calls to other medical providers for additional information. Upon completion of the therapeutic service, the treatment is recorded and the patient's status including functional progress is documented. Therapeutic procedures may be reported on the same date of service as an evaluation or re-evaluation and should be reflected in the documentation.

Code **97140**, *Manual therapy techniques (eg, mobilization/manipulation, manual lymphatic drainage, manual traction), 1 or more regions, each 15 minutes,* is intended to be reported for manual therapy techniques, based on each 15 minutes of manual therapy provided to one or more regions. This code is not intended to include chiropractic manipulation techniques (CMT). The appropriate CMT procedure code(s) **(98940-98943)** should be reported for those manipulative techniques. This code is also not intended for reporting massage techniques that are reported appropriately with **97124**.

When manual therapy techniques are required in addition to CMT procedure(s), it is appropriate to additionally report the manual therapy techniques (based on each 15-minute interval of service). The documentation should clearly differentiate the two procedures.

Code **97150**, *Therapeutic procedure(s), group (2 or more individuals),* is intended to report therapeutic procedures provided to patients in a group setting. If one or more of the therapeutic procedures in the Physical Medicine and Rehabilitation subsection are performed simultaneously with two or more individuals, then only code **97150** is reported. It is appropriate to report code **97150** for each member of the group.

Code **97542**, *Wheelchair management (eg, assessment, fitting, training) each 15 minutes,* is reported for all services associated with provision of a wheelchair. Typically, this applies to wheelchairs that do not include assistive technology adaptations (eg, sip and puff mobility controls, head switches). Reportable minutes include those needed to assess the patient for the type of wheelchair that is indicated, measurement of the patient to ensure proper fit of the chair, fitting the chair to the patient (eg, adjusting swing-away foot rests and the foot plate angle), and training of the patient and/or caregiver in the mobility of the chair.

Coding Tip

If manual traction is performed to treat a cervical spine injury, and on the same day the chiropractor also performs chiropractic manipulation to the lumbar region, report codes **97140 59** for the manual therapy technique and **98940** for the chiropractic manipulative treatment to the lumbar spine. Modifier **59** is appended to indicate that a distinct procedural service was provided.

Coding Tip

Group therapy procedures involve constant attendance of a physician or therapist; however, by definition, they do not require one-on-one patient contact by the provider. Code **97150** is an untimed code; therefore, only one unit can be reported for each patient in the group per session.

EXAMPLE

A 22-year-old patient with T12 paraplegia requires a manual wheelchair for mobility at home and in the community. The therapist assesses the patient to determine the appropriate type of chair and components that should be ordered. Measurements of the patient are taken so the correct dimensions are ordered. Once the patient receives the chair, the therapist must make any adjustments that are necessary. The therapist trains the patient in the safe operation and management of the wheelchair in order to achieve independent mobility in the home and community environment. This instance is assigned code **97542**.

Active Wound Care Management

Codes **97605** and **97606** describe negative pressure wound therapy, which is a method of wound care management that requires a vacuum (or suctioned pulling force) to remove devitalized wound tissue and tissue exudate (fluid discharge) that inhibits wound healing. Promotion of wound closure with minimal scar formation is a goal of treatment. The vacuum cleanses the wound and stimulates the wound bed, reduces localized edema, and improves local oxygen supply.

Active wound care interventions (**97597-97606**) are performed to remove devitalized and/or necrotic tissue and promote wound healing. These procedures use both selective and nonselective debridement techniques without the use of anesthesia and are not reported in addition to codes **11042-11047**. Direct (one-on-one) contact with the patient is required to report this series of codes. These are not time codes so only one unit can be reported per session. Codes **97597** and **97598** are used to report selective debridement, which is the removal of specific areas of devitalized tissue from a wound. Selective debridement includes the use of sharp instruments (eg, scissors, scalpel, forceps), high-pressure water jet, and autolysis or other selected agents. The techniques for sharp selective debridement include the use of scalpels or scissors to cut along a line of demarcation that separates viable tissue from devitalized necrotic tissue. Selective debridement is distinctly different than nonselective debridement. When selective debridement techniques are performed, no prior preparation of tissue is required.

Code **97602** describes nonselective debridement, which is the gradual removal of loosely adherent devitalized tissue, usually over a number of patient visits. Nonselective debridement is intended to remove loosely adherent necrotic tissue by the use of enzymatic agents, abrasion, or wet to dry dressings.

Because the code descriptor language for code **97602** states "wound(s)" (indicating a single wound site or multiple wound sites), it is not appropriate to report this code for each wound or anatomical area debrided at the same session. However, in the instance that nonselective debridement is performed on separate anatomical sites at two distinctly separate sessions on the same date, it is appropriate to report this code twice (ie, **97602**, **97602 59**). Modifier **59**, *Distinct procedural service,* should be appended to indicate that an additional debridement was performed at a different session on a separate anatomical site on the same date.

Coding Tip

Codes **97597**, **97598**, and **97602** include application of and removal of any protective or bulk dressings. Performance of a dressing change only or in the absence of wound care is not separately reported and is included within the E/M service. These procedures also include any assessment regarding the active wound care management that is necessary. Assessment to determine the type of wound care treatment required is not separately reported.

Coding Tip

Codes **97597**, **97598**, **97605**, and **97606** are reported according to the size of the total surface area of the wounds treated. These codes should be reported once per debridement session regardless of the number of wounds or areas debrided at that specific session.

Tests and Measurements

Code **97750** is intended to report testing and measurement of physical performance of a select area or number of areas. This service is reported in 15-minute units. Examples include functional capacity evaluation, isokinetic testing, and computerized muscle testing. Because this is a time-based code, it should be reported according to the time the provider spent in direct contact providing the service. Code **97755** is intended to report assessment of seating, mobility, and environmental control systems for persons with severe disabilities to facilitate functional independence in such areas as wheeled mobility, activities of daily living (ADLs), and written and oral communication. This type of assistance and assessment may provide opportunities for people with disabilities to fully participate in all aspects of life. This code is not intended for reporting wheelchair management for the less disabled patient requiring typical mobility needs. Both codes **97750** and **97755** require the completion of a separate written report.

The parenthetical note in this section differentiates use of these codes from services that identify evaluation for prescription of nonspeech communication devices (**92605**) and therapeutic services for nonspeech generating devices (**92607**).

Orthotic Management and Prosthetic Management

Codes **97760**-**97762** are used to report orthotic and/or prosthetic management. Orthotic management includes assessing the patient, determining the proper orthotic design in relation to the patient's skin integrity, sensibility, and healing of tissues with or without surgical repair (eg, static vs dynamic, prefabricated vs custom designed, choice of materials such as thermoplastic, pulleys, and elastic tension). This code also includes fitting of the orthotic, training in use, care and wearing time of the orthotic, and brief instructions in exercises that are to be performed while the orthotic is in place. These are time-based codes that are reported once for each 15-minute increment. Materials and supplies may be separately reported with an appropriate supply or material code (eg, CPT code **99070** or HCPCS Level II code).

Code **97760** is used also to report time associated with orthotic modification, training during follow-up visits including exercises performed in the orthotic, instruction in skin care, and orthotic wearing time.

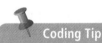

Coding Tip

A parenthetical note appears at the end of the Application of Casts and Strapping subsection in the Musculoskeletal System section to refer the reader to codes **97760-97762** for orthotics management and training. This note is to clarify that casting and strapping codes (eg, **29049**) are not intended to report orthotics fitting and training.

EXAMPLE

A 65-year-old female lacerated the volar side of her left middle finger at the level of the proximal interphalangeal (PIP) joint (flexor tendon zone II) while cutting a bagel. She sustained a full laceration of the flexor digitorum profundus and superficialis tendons and underwent surgical repair of both tendons. The patient was referred to therapy for a custom fabricated dorsal forearm-based orthotic.

Chapter 7

The patient had to be trained in protected and limited range of motion while wearing the orthotic and surgical dressings; skin care; and care of the orthotic. In this instance, code **97760** is assigned.

Code **97762** is intended for established patients who have already received the orthotic or prosthetic device (permanent or temporary). It is important for the health care practitioner to follow up with the patient after he or she has been provided with an orthotic or prosthetic device. The "checkout" visit would include assessing the patient's response to wearing the orthotic or prosthetic device such as possible skin irritation or breakdown; determination if the patient is donning the orthotic or prosthetic device appropriately; need for padding, underwrap, or socks; and tolerance to any dynamic forces being applied. If further training in the use of the orthotic or prosthetic device is required, code **97760** should be reported.

Medical Nutrition Therapy

The codes in the Medical Nutrition Therapy (MNT) subsection (**97802-97804**) include nutritional diagnostic therapy and counseling services provided by a registered dietitian (RD) or licensed nutrition professional for the purpose of managing an acute or chronic condition or disease. A physician referral is frequently required for RDs to provide MNT. RDs and licensed nutrition professionals provide MNT in a variety of settings, such as physicians' offices, outpatient clinics, cardiac rehabilitation units, intensive care units, acute care hospitals, skilled nursing facilities, rehabilitation facilities, long-term care units, home care settings, and the private practices of registered dietitians.

Code **97802** is intended to report the initial MNT assessment and intervention service for an individual patient. Code **97803** is intended to report all subsequent follow-up (re-assessment and intervention) MNT services with individual patients. The codes for individual MNT services are time based and reported for each 15 minutes of service. A typical individual initial visit is 60 to 90 minutes and typical follow-up individual visits are 30 to 45 minutes.

Code **97804** is reported for group MNT services and is reported for each 30 minutes of service. Group MNT sessions are generally 60 minutes. Codes **97803** and **97804** are used in the initial calendar year when reassessment and intervention are provided and also in subsequent follow-up years.

Coding Tip

Orthotic management differs from the purpose of an application of a cast or strapping device, both of which are reported with the casting and strapping codes (**29000** series). Orthotics are used to support a weak or ineffective joint or muscle. In general, they provide support while the patient transitions through treatment. Examples of orthotic devices include ankle-foot orthotics or a spinal support orthotic.

Coding Tip

Reporting requirements for the MNT codes vary among third-party payers. Therefore, it is important to check with your local third-party payer to determine the specific reporting requirements.

EXAMPLE

A 67-year-old male discharged from the hospital with the diagnosis of hypertension and chronic kidney disease is referred to an

RD for MNT services to delay dialysis. This service is described as "nutritional diagnostic therapy and counseling services for the purpose of managing disease." The RD performs the nutrition assessment, nutrition diagnosis, and intervention with the patient to negotiate therapeutic interventions and establish parameters for lifestyle changes. The RD considers factors such as learning style, literacy level, severity of disease, motivation, and interest in determining the MNT intervention. The patient lives alone and frequently eats meals outside the home. The MNT initial intervention targets behavioral or therapeutic and lifestyle factors that include, but are not limited to, new behaviors for food choices, frequency, and preparation. Demonstration and instruction on food portions and appropriate food selection are performed with the patient. The patient is instructed to return in two weeks for MNT reassessment and intervention. In this instance, code **97802** is assigned.

Acupuncture

Codes **97810-97814** describe acupuncture and electroacupuncture services. See Figure 7-15. Acupuncture is reported based on 15-minute increments of personal (face-to-face) contact with the patient. These codes may be reported by any qualified provider according to any state and licensure requirements. However, only one code may be reported for each 15-minute increment, and only one initial code (**97810**, **97813**) is reported per day.

If no electrical stimulation is used during a 15-minute increment, either code **97810** or **97811** should be reported, as appropriate. When electrical stimulation of any needle is used during a 15-minute increment, either code **97813** or **97814** should be reported, as appropriate.

FIGURE 7-15 *Acupuncture, Needle*

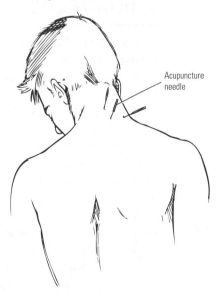

Acupuncture needle

A critical element necessary to understand and appropriately apply the intent of the acupuncture code series pertains to the 15-minute increment. Acupuncture codes are reported based on 15-minute increments of personal (face-to-face) contact with the patient and not the duration of acupuncture needle(s) placement.

If the patient's condition requires a significant, separately identifiable E/M service above and beyond the usual preservice and postservice work associated with the acupuncture services, the E/M service may be reported separately by appending **modifier 25**. It is important to note that the time of the E/M service is not included in the time of the acupuncture service.

EXAMPLE

A 49-year-old female receiving chemotherapy for breast cancer was previously referred for acupuncture to relieve postchemotherapy nausea. This treatment is part of an ongoing series of treatments for this condition. The patient is weak but not faint and has not vomited since chemotherapy was received earlier in the day. In this instance, code **97813** is assigned.

Osteopathic Manipulative Treatment

Osteopathic manipulative treatment (OMT) is reported with codes in the **98925-98929** series. OMT is a form of manual treatment applied by a physician to eliminate or alleviate somatic dysfunction and related disorders. E/M services may be reported separately if the patient's condition requires a significant, separately identifiable E/M service above and beyond the usual preservice and postservice work associated with the procedure. In this case, **modifier 25** would be appended to the E/M code reported. The E/M service may be caused or prompted by the same symptoms or condition for which the OMT service was provided. Therefore, different diagnoses are not required for the reporting of OMT and E/M on the same date.

Chiropractic Manipulative Treatment

Codes **98940-98943** are used to report chiropractic manipulative treatment (CMT). Chiropractic is a health care discipline that emphasizes the inherent recuperative power of the body without the use of drugs or surgery. This is accomplished by focusing on the relationship between structure, primarily of the spine, and function, as coordinated by the nervous system, as that relationship may affect the preservation and restoration of health.

   CMT is a form of manual treatment to influence joint and neurophysiologic function and can be accomplished through the use of a variety of techniques. Chiropractic adjustment is a therapeutic procedure that uses: (1) controlled force, (2) leverage, (3) direction, (4) amplitude, and (5) velocity directed at specific joints or anatomical regions. CMT takes into account a variety of factors including subluxation. Subluxation is a motion segment in which the alignment, movement integrity, and/or physiologic function are altered although contact between joint surfaces remains intact. For purposes of CMT, there are spinal and extraspinal regions to consider. The five spinal regions referred to include the following:

1. Cervical region (includes atlanto-occipital joint)
2. Thoracic region (includes costovertebral and costotransverse joints)
3. Lumbar region
4. Sacral region
5. Pelvic (sacroiliac joint) region

The five extraspinal regions referred to include the following:

1. Head (including temporomandibular joint, excluding the atlanto-occipital region)
2. Lower extremities
3. Upper extremities
4. Rib cage (excluding costotransverse and costovertebral joints)
5. Abdomen

Education and Training for Patient Self-Management

Codes **98960-98962** are used to report educational and training services prescribed by a physician and provided by a qualified nonphysician health care professional using a standardized curriculum to an individual or a group of patients for the treatment of established illness/disease [eg, asthma, diabetes] or to delay comorbidity. Education and training for patient self-management may be reported with these codes only when using a standardized curriculum. This curriculum may be modified as necessary for the clinical needs, cultural norms, and health literacy of the individual patient.

The purpose of the educational and training services is to teach the patient and/or caregiver(s) how to effectively self-manage the patient's illness/disease or delay disease comorbidity in conjunction with the patient's professional health care team. Education and training related to subsequent reinforcement of previously instructed information or due to changes in the patient's condition or treatment plan are reported in the same manner as the original education and training. The type of education and training provided for the patient's clinical condition will be identified by the appropriate diagnosis code(s) reported.

The qualifications of the nonphysician health care professionals and the content of the educational and training program must be consistent with the guidelines or standards established or recognized by a physician society, nonphysician health care professional society/association, or other appropriate source. When counseling and education services are provided by a physician to an individual, the appropriate evaluation and management code(s) should be reported. If counseling and education are provided by a physician to a group, code **99078** should be reported. Counseling and/or risk factor reduction interventions provided by a physician should be reported using a code from the **99401-99412** series. Codes **97802-97804** should be reported when medical nutrition therapy services are performed, and codes **96150-96155** should be reported when health and behavior assessments or interventions that are not part of a structured curriculum are performed.

> ### EXAMPLE
>
> A 56-year-old female patient and a 62-year-old male patient, both with type I diabetes, have been observed by their endocrinologist for several years. They are referred to the endocrinologist's diabetes educator for group intensive insulin therapy training under an approved curriculum. Despite changes to their insulin regimens, they continue to have uncontrolled blood glucose levels with frequent hypoglycemia. Decisions are made to convert them to subcutaneous insulin pump therapy.
>
> In this instance, code **98961**, *Education and training for patient self-management by a qualified, nonphysician health care professional using a standardized curriculum, face-to-face with the patient (could include caregiver/family) each 30 minutes; Education and training for patient self-management by a qualified, nonphysician health care professional using a standardized curriculum, face-to-face with the patient (could include caregiver/family) each 30 minutes; 2–4 patients,* is assigned.

Moderate (Conscious) Sedation

Codes **99143-99150** are used to report moderate (conscious) sedation. Moderate (conscious) sedation is a drug-induced depression of consciousness during which patients respond purposefully to oral commands, either alone or accompanied by light tactile stimulation. No interventions are required to maintain a patent airway, and spontaneous ventilation is adequate. Cardiovascular function is usually maintained. Moderate sedation does not include minimal sedation (anxiolysis), deep sedation, or monitored anesthesia care (**00100-01999**).

When providing moderate sedation, the following services are included and may not be reported separately:

- Assessment of the patient (not included in intraservice time);
- Establishment of IV access and fluids to maintain patency, when performed;
- Administration of agent(s);
- Maintenance of sedation;
- Monitoring of oxygen saturation, heart rate, and blood pressure; and
- Recovery (not included in intraservice time).

Intraservice time begins with the administration of the sedation agent(s), requires continuous face-to-face attendance, and ends at the conclusion of personal contact by the physician providing the sedation.

When a second physician other than the health care professional performing the diagnostic or therapeutic services provides moderate sedation in the facility setting (eg, hospital, outpatient hospital/ambulatory surgery center, skilled nursing facility) for the procedures listed in Appendix G, the second physician reports **99148-99150**. However, for the circumstances in which these services are performed by the second physician in the nonfacility setting (eg, physician office, freestanding imaging center), codes **99148-99150** are not reported.

✓ Check Your Knowledge Answers

1. No
2. True
3. True
4. No, for patients who require psychiatric services (**90801-90899**) as well as health and behavior assessment/intervention (**96150-96155**), report the predominant service performed.

Chapter Exercises

Check your answers in Appendix B.

True or False

1. Many services and procedures provided by nonphysician health care providers are also located in the Medicine section. **True or False**
2. There are three basic types of subsections: those that are procedure oriented, those that are service oriented, and those that refer to particular medical specialties. **True or False**
3. Codes in a specialty subsection, such as gastroenterology, are limited to use by gastroenterologists. **True or False**
4. A 19-year-old female patient presented to the physician's office for tetanus immune globulin to be administered intramuscularly. No other service was provided at this encounter. Code **90389** is the only code reported. **True or False**
5. A 23-year-old female patient presented to the physician's office for IV normal saline for dehydration. No other infusion service was provided that day. Because no infusions of drugs or other substances were administered, this service cannot be reported. **True or False**
6. The Injection and Intravenous Infusion Chemotherapy codes (**96401-96549**) are reported only for treatment of cancer diagnoses. **True or False**

7. Acupuncture is reported based on the duration of acupuncture needle(s) placement. **True or False**
8. When providing moderate sedation, it is appropriate to report the administration of the agent(s) separately. **True or False**

Choose the correct code for the following procedure report

9. A 64-year-old male patient presented to the physician's office for antibiotic infusion because of a prolonged illness. The patient received two simultaneous antibiotics over the course of one hour. He became nauseated and received an IV push of an antiemetic. How is this procedure reported?
10. A 35-year-old established patient was seen in the office for her annual general ophthalmological examination with mild blurring of vision. The ophthalmologist provided a general evaluation of the complete visual system over the course of two sessions. This service included history, general medical observation, external and ophthalmoscopic examinations, gross visual fields, and basic sensorimotor examination. How is this procedure reported?

Answer the Question

11. The visual function screening code **99172** is located in the CPT codebook index, and the coder cannot find the code in the E/M section. Where should the coder look and why?

Category II Codes

Chapter Objectives

- Define and understand the usage of Category II, Performance Measurement codes

- Recognize the code format and exclusion modifiers for Category II codes

Category II CPT codes are a set of *optional* codes developed primarily to support performance measurement. These Category II codes are intended to help collect data by encoding specific services and/or test results that have an evidence base for contributing to positive health outcomes and quality patient care. The measure has to be shown to be well known throughout the country as a practice that contributes to positive patient outcomes when done and has been tested or surveyed ("vetted") to prove this to be true. These codes describe the performance of clinical components that are usually included in an Evaluation and Management (E/M) service or other part of a service. Consequently, Category II codes do not have a relative value or dollar amount associated with them and are not reimbursed.

Remember, the use of these codes is optional and *not* required for correct coding.

The decision to develop Category II codes was based on a desire to standardize the collection of data for performance measurement, a response consistent with current Health Insurance Portability and Accountability Act (HIPAA) guidelines. Former methods of capturing performance data were based on detailed chart review, data abstraction, or site surveys—processes that are costly for physicians and health plans. Measurement based upon data received from claims was limited to process measures with specific Category I or HCPCS Level II codes. Coding data elements of performance measures on a claim provides an opportunity for the administrative data system to allow physicians to supply information on performance measures directly to health plans.

Development of Category II Codes

The CPT Editorial Panel develops CPT codes (including Category II codes) but does not develop measures. Instead, Category II codes that are released via the efforts of the CPT Editorial Panel and the Performance Measures Advisory Group (PMAG) are based on specific measures that are developed by certain designated national organizations. These organizations develop broadly accepted measures that are currently used in health care performance improvement, and include the following:

- The National Committee for Quality Assurance (NCQA)
- The Agency for Healthcare Research and Quality (AHRQ)
- The Joint Commission on Accreditation of Healthcare Organizations (JCAHO)
- The American Medical Association–convened Physician Consortium for Performance Improvement® (referred to as the Consortium or PCPI)

✓ Check Your Knowledge

1. In order to accurately code a claim, are Category I service and procedure codes reported in conjunction with Category II codes?

Code Format

A Category II code consists of five characters with the letter **"F"** as the last character (eg, **1234F**) to distinguish it from Category I and Category III CPT codes. Category II codes are located in the codebook immediately following the final Category I subsection (Medicine). Introductory language in the section explains the purpose of these codes. Similar to codes contained in the Category I section of the CPT codebook, Category II codes are defined by specific code numbers with corresponding descriptor language and include parenthetical notes to guide coders in the use of these codes. When codes are deleted, cross-references may be added to identify replacement codes when they exist. In some instances, certain codes may be deleted without replacement, usually due to changes in the measure.

An alphabetic listing of performance measures is included on the CPT Web site to assist users in identifying all measures related to a given clinical condition or topic. The description for each measure also describes the organization that developed the measure(s), the associated Category II code(s), and a synopsis of the use of Category II codes for a given measure.

Consistent with the arrangement of codes in other sections of the book and to facilitate flexible code number assignment for future codes, Category II codes are grouped into predefined categories based on

Chapter 8

established subjective-objective-assessment-plan (SOAP) guidelines for clinical documentation. Category II codes are grouped according to the following nine predefined categories (definitions for each category are included in the codebook):

- **Composite Measures (0001F-0015F):** Facilitate reporting of a group of services when all components are met.
- **Patient Management (0500F-0526F):** Describe utilization measures or measures of patient care provided for specific clinical purposes (eg, prenatal care, presurgical and postsurgical care, referrals).
- **Patient History (1000F-1137F):** Describe aspects of patient history and review of systems.
- **Physical Examination (2000F-2044F):** Describe aspects of physical examination.
- **Diagnostic or Screening Processes or Results (3006F-3354F):** Describe results of clinical laboratory tests, radiological, or other procedural examination.
- **Therapeutic, Preventive, or Other Interventions (4000F-4250F):** Describe pharmacologic, procedural, or behavioral therapies, including preventive services such as patient education and counseling.
- **Follow-up or Other Outcomes (5005F-5062F):** Describe review and communication of test results to patients, patient satisfaction or experience with care, patient functional status.
- **Patient Safety (6005F-6045F):** Describe patient safety practices.
- **Structural Measures (7010F-7025F):** Address the setting or system of the care delivery and aspects of the capabilities of the organization or health care professional providing the care.

Each code descriptor also includes a *suffix* or an abbreviated clinical topic listing at the end of the descriptor to cross-reference the code to the specific clinical topic(s) and measure(s) in which that code is included. The translations for these suffix listings can be found in the Alphabetic Listing of Performance Measures in alphabetical order next to the full name for that abbreviation on the CPT Web site.

Performance Measurement Exclusion Modifiers

Occassionally reasons may exist that warrant the exclusion of a certain group of patients from a given measure. Three modifiers are available for reporting these situations. These modifiers report circumstances identified in a performance measure for services that were considered but not provided because of medical, patient, or system reasons documented in the medical record. These reasons are identified as *exclusions*, meaning that they identify a population of patients for whom the ordinary measure requirements do not apply. For the services being measured for these patients, one of three exclusion modifiers is appended to the Category II code to note the special circumstance for the service, procedure, or criteria being measured.

- **Modifier 1P identifies exclusions for medical reasons.** For example, nonprescription of medication noted in the measure due to patient allergies or absence of the organ or limb identified by the measure.
- **Modifier 2P identifies exclusions for patient reasons.** For example, patient exclusions due to patient refusal of services, religious reasons, or economic reasons.
- **Modifier 3P identifies exclusions for system reasons.** For example, lack of availability of resources for the procedures or services, lack of insurance coverage, or payer-related issues.

Note that exclusion modifiers should be appended only to Category II codes and should not be used with Category I codes.

The following is the only Category II modifier that is not used as an exclusion modifier:

- **Modifier 8P serves as a reporting modifier.** For example, when provision of services to a patient that are unrelated to the measure (eg, treatment of a broken leg for a patient with diabetes where the diabetes is being managed by another physician). This includes *any* nonmedical, patient, or system reasons for not meeting measure requirements.

✓ Check Your Knowledge

2. Can modifiers listed in Appendix A of the CPT codebook and exclusion modifiers listed in the Category II section of the CPT codebook all be appended to the service and procedure codes listed in Category I of the CPT codebook?

✓ Check Your Knowledge Answers

1. No. The use of Category II codes is optional and **not** required for correct coding.

2. No. The exclusion modifiers should be appended only to Category II codes and should not be used with Category I codes.

Chapter Exercises

Check your answers in Appendix B.

1. Why were Category II codes created?

True or False

2. The following organizations are involved in the development of Category II Performance Measurement codes.

- The National Committee for Quality Assurance (NCQA) **True or False**
- The Agency for Healthcare Research and Quality (AHRQ) **True or False**
- The Joint Commission on Accreditation of Healthcare Organizations (JCAHO) **True or False**
- The AMA Physician Consortium for Performance Improvement® (the Consortium or PCPI) **True or False**

3. The code format for Category II codes consists of five characters with the letter P as the last character. **True or False**

Answer the Question

4. Where are the Category II codes located in the CPT codebook?

Category III Codes

Chapter Objectives

- Understand the difference between Category I and Category III codes
- Understand the use of Category III codes
- Know the implementation dates for the Category III codes

Category III (Emerging Technology) CPT codes are a set of temporary codes for emerging technology, services, and procedures. Category III CPT codes allow data collection for these services and procedures. These codes are intended to be used for data collection purposes or to substantiate widespread usage in the Food and Drug Administration (FDA) approval process. Because Category III CPT codes are intended to be used for data collection purposes, they are not intended for services or procedures that are not accepted by the CPT Editorial Panel because the proposal was incomplete, more information is needed, or the Advisory Committee did not support the proposal.

Category III codes were developed to provide an alternative for the addition of codes because of the length of time required to develop a CPT code and the requirements for approval of a CPT code. These factors in the development of a Category I code in the CPT process conflicted with the needs of researchers for coded data to track emerging technology services throughout the research process. For a procedure to be approved as a Category I code, the CPT Editorial Panel at a minimum requires all of the following:

- Services or procedures be performed by many health care professionals across the country
- FDA approval be documented or be imminent within a given CPT cycle
- The service or procedure has proven clinical efficacy

As such, the Category III CPT codes may not conform to these usual CPT code requirements. For services and procedures to be eligible for Category III codes, the service or procedure must have relevance for research, either ongoing or planned.

✓ Check Your Knowledge

1. What are some of the criteria for Category III codes?

Category I CPT codes are restricted to clinically recognized and generally accepted services, not emerging technologies, services, and procedures. Another important consideration in the development of Category III codes was the elimination of local codes under HIPAA. The August 17, 2000, Final Rule supported the elimination of local codes and the transition to national standard code sets. Many of the local codes were temporary codes used by payers until services and procedures were more fully substantiated through research and received a CPT code. On December 31, 2003, CMS eliminated the local codes for reporting. Thus, Category III codes can take the place of temporary local codes used for this purpose.

As with Category I CPT codes, inclusion of a descriptor and its associated code number in CPT nomenclature does not represent endorsement by the AMA of any particular diagnostic or therapeutic procedure or service. Inclusion or exclusion of a procedure or service does not imply any health insurance coverage or reimbursement policy.

Category III codes are alphanumeric, consisting of four numeric digits followed by the letter **"T"** in the fifth field.

EXAMPLE

0019T	Extracorporeal shock wave involving musculoskeletal system, not otherwise specified, low energy
0019	= four digits
T	= alpha character

These codes are located in a separate section of the CPT codebook, after the Category II code section. Introductory language in this Code Section explains the purpose of these codes.

To get new CPT Category III codes into the field as soon as possible, once they have been approved by the CPT Editorial Panel, the newly added Category III codes are made available on a semiannual basis via electronic distribution on the AMA CPT Web site (www.ama-assn.org/go/cpt). The full set of Category III codes is then included in the next published edition for that CPT cycle. Such an early release is possible for Category III codes because payment is based on the policies of payers and not on a yearly fee schedule. The AMA's CPT Web site features updates of the CPT Editorial Panel actions and early release of the Category III codes in July and January in a given CPT nomenclature cycle.

The dates for early release correspond with the CPT Editorial Panel meetings for each CPT cycle (February, June, and October).

Category III CPT codes are not referred to the AMA/Specialty RUC for evaluation because no relative value units are assigned to these codes. Payment for these services and procedures is based on the policies of payers and not on a yearly fee schedule.

These codes are archived after five years if the code has not been accepted for placement in the Category I section of the CPT codebook, unless it is demonstrated that a Category III code is still needed. These archived codes are not reused.

Implementation Dates for Category III and Other CPT Codes

Category III CPT codes and Category I vaccine codes are typically "early-released" for reporting on either January 1 or July 1 of a given CPT cycle.

Category II codes are typically released one month after the CPT Editorial Panel meeting at which they were accepted and implemented three months later.

For federal programs, January 1 of each year is generally the effective date for using the new CPT Category I codes. The AMA prepares each annual update so that the new CPT codebooks are available in late fall of each year preceding their implementation. However, other third-party payers might not implement the new codes on the same date. It is important to be familiar with individual payer policies for implementation schedules of new codes each year.

✓ Check Your Knowledge

2. When do Category III codes get released?

✓ Check Your Knowledge Answers

1. Services or procedures be performed by many health care professionals across the country, FDA approval be documented or be imminent within a given CPT cycle, and the service or procedure has proven clinical efficacy

2. Either January 1 or July 1 of a given CPT cycle.

Chapter 9 Exercises

Check your answers in Appendix B.

1. What are Category III codes?
2. How many characters do Category III codes have?
3. When are Category III codes released?
4. After how many years are Category III codes archived?

True or False

5. Use of unlisted codes offer the opportunity for collection of specific data. **True or False**
6. Category III codes endorse clinical efficacy. **True or False**
7. Category III codes are not temporary codes. **True or False**

Multiple Choice

8. Which of the following is a Category III code?

   a. 96999, Unlisted special dermatological service or procedure
   b. 2000F, Blood pressure measured (CAD, CKD, HF, HTN) (DM)
   c. 3006F, Chest X-ray results documented and reviewed (CAP)
   d. 0058T, Cryopreservation; reproductive tissue, ovarian

9. Which of the following uses Category III codes?

   a. health services researchers
   b. health policy experts
   c. other qualified health care providers
   d. all of the above

10. When are Category III codes published in the CPT codebook?

    a. semi-annually
    b. annually
    c. quarterly
    d. once every three months.

Modifiers

Chapter Objectives

- Understand how to select the appropriate modifiers to append to procedures and services
- Comprehend usage of modifiers for various circumstances
- Recognize which modifiers are reported in the global period of a procedure

Modifiers are essential tools in the coding process. They enhance a code narrative to describe the circumstances of each procedure or service and how it individually applies to the patient. They are also essential ingredients to effectively communicate between providers and payers. While some modifiers may increase reimbursement, other modifiers are only informational and the rules for using them vary. A modifier provides the means to indicate that a service or procedure that has been performed has been altered by some specific circumstance but not changed in its definition or code. Modifiers also enable health care professionals to respond effectively to payment policy requirements established by other entities. This chapter reviews the two-digit numeric modifiers found in the CPT code set and in Appendix A of the CPT codebook. (Discussion of the anesthesia physical status modifiers can be found in Chapter 3 of this book.)

Modifiers may be used in many instances, such as to report the following:

- A service or procedure was performed bilaterally.
- A service was mandated by a third-party payer.
- Only the professional component of a procedure or service was performed.
- Multiple procedures were performed at the same session by the same provider.
- Assistant surgeon services.
- A portion of a service or procedure was reduced or eliminated at the physician's discretion.
- A service or procedure was performed by more than one physician.

To report a modifier, the modifier is appended to the procedure code. If the computer system being used allows seven or more digits to report a service on a single line, the two-digit modifier may be appended as **49500 50**.

The following examples will show when a modifier would be applicable.

> **EXAMPLE**
>
> The physician performs arthrocentesis, injection of the small joint or bursa of both right and left toes.
>
> CPT code reported: **20600 50**.
>
> **20600** Arthrocentesis, aspiration and/or injection; small joint or bursa (eg, fingers, toes)

Appending modifier **50**, *Bilateral procedure,* in the above Example indicates that the procedure was performed bilaterally. Appending modifier **50** at the end of the code does not change the original definition of the procedure, but it indicates that the procedure was performed on both sides.

Please note, some third-party payers may require a 1- or 2-line item with the modifier **50**.

Coding Tip

The procedures described by codes **20600-20610** are unilateral procedures. In the instance when injections are performed bilaterally, modifier **50**, *Bilateral procedure,* may be appended.

> **EXAMPLE**
>
> A neurosurgeon and an otolaryngologist work together to perform a transsphenoidal excision of a pituitary neoplasm. Each physician performs a distinct part of the procedure.
>
> CPT code reported: **61548 62**.
>
> **61548** Hypophysectomy or excision of pituitary tumor, transnasal or transseptal approach, nonstereotactic

In this example, modifier **62**, *Two surgeons,* indicates to the insurance carrier (or third-party payer) that two surgeons performed specific parts to the procedure, but it does not change the original definition of the code.

In addition to the CPT modifiers listed in Appendix A of the CPT codebook, Health Care Common Procedure Coding System (HCPCS) Level II modifiers are available for reporting purposes. HCPCS Level II modifiers are updated by the Centers for Medicare & Medicaid Services (CMS). (Refer to Appendix C of this book for further discussion of the HCPCS Level II codes.) Some payers may require HCPCS Level II modifiers and/or CPT modifiers.

Modifier 22

Increased Procedural Services

When the work required to provide a service is substantially greater than typically required, it may be identified by adding modifier **22**,

Increased procedural services, to the usual procedure code. Documentation must support the substantial additional work and the reason for the additional work (ie, increased intensity, time, technical difficulty of procedure, severity of patient's condition, physical and mental effort required). **Note:** This modifier should not be appended to an evaluation and management (E/M) service.

The word *procedural* in the descriptor of modifier **22** is intended to indicate that modifier **22** may be used with any procedure but is not used with the E/M codes. When the E/M service provided is prolonged or otherwise greater than that usually required for the highest level of E/M service within a given category, codes **99354-99357** are reported.

> ### EXAMPLE
>
> A physician excises a lesion located in a crease of the neck of a very obese person. The obesity makes the excision more difficult. The physician indicates the complexity of the removal of the lesion by appending modifier **22** to the code used to report the removal of the lesion. When reporting this service to a third-party payer, it may be helpful to include a copy of the operative report to demonstrate the increased procedural services provided.

Modifier 23

Unusual Anesthesia

Occasionally a procedure, which usually requires either no anesthesia or local anesthesia because of unusual circumstances must be done under general anesthesia. This circumstance may be reported by adding modifier **23**, *Unusual anesthesia*, to the procedure code of the basic service.

The guidelines in the Surgery section of the CPT codebook for the CPT Surgical Package Definition indicate that a given CPT surgical code includes, on a procedure-by-procedure basis, a variety of services. In addition to the operation, one of the services included is local infiltration, metacarpal/metatarsal/digital block, or topical anesthesia, when used. Certain codes in the CPT nomenclature represent services performed under anesthesia (eg, **57410**, *Pelvic examination under anesthesia [other than local]*); for these codes, modifier **23** would not be appended.

Procedures that generally do not require general anesthesia may, in some cases, require general anesthesia because of the extent of the service or other circumstances. In these cases, modifier **23** is appended to the procedure code reported.

The physical condition of some patients—such as patients who are mentally retarded, extremely apprehensive, or living with particular physical conditions (eg, tremors, spasticity)—may require the use of general anesthesia to perform certain procedures that would normally not require anesthesia. When these cases are reported, modifier **23** is appended to the procedure code.

Chapter 10

Modifier 24

Unrelated Evaluation and Management Service by the Same Physician During a Postoperative Period

The physician may need to indicate that an E/M service was performed during a postoperative period for reason(s) unrelated to the original procedure. This circumstance may be reported by adding modifier **24**, *Unrelated evaluation and management service by the same physician during a postoperative period*, to the appropriate level of E/M service.

Modifier **24** is used when a physician provides a surgical service related to one problem and then, during the period of follow-up care for the surgery (global period), provides an E/M service unrelated to the problem requiring the surgery. In this circumstance, diagnosis code selection is particularly critical to indicate the reason for the additional E/M service.

EXAMPLE

An orthopedic surgeon performs a hip replacement on Mrs. Jones. During the normal, uncomplicated postoperative period related to the hip surgery, she falls and sprains her wrist. The orthopedic surgeon reports the E/M service (related to the sprained wrist) performed in the office using the established patient, office or other outpatient service codes. The level of E/M service reported is based on the services provided related to the sprained wrist. Appending modifier **24** to the E/M service indicates to the third-party payer that the E/M service provided in the global period is for the sprained wrist, and not related to the hip replacement surgery.

Modifier 25

Significant, Separately Identifiable Evaluation and Management Service by the Same Physician on the Same Day of the Procedure or Other Service

It may be necessary to indicate that on the day a procedure or service identified by a CPT code was performed, the patient's condition required a significant, separately identifiable E/M service above and beyond the other service provided or beyond the usual preoperative and postoperative care associated with the procedure that was performed. A significant, separately identifiable E/M service is defined or substantiated by documentation that satisfies the relevant criteria for the respective E/M service to be reported (see Evaluation and Management Services Guidelines for instructions on determining level of E/M service). The E/M service may be prompted by the symptom or condition for which the procedure and/or service was provided. As such, different diagnoses are not required for reporting an E/M service on the same date. This circumstance may be reported by adding modifier **25**, *Significant, separately identifiable evaluation and management service by the same physician on the same day of the procedure or other service*, to the appropriate level of E/M service.

Note: This modifier is not used to report an E/M service that resulted in a decision to perform surgery (see modifier **57**). For significant, separately identifiable non-E/M services, see modifier **59**.

For significant, separately identifiable E/M services, by the same physician on the same day of the procedure or other service, modifier **25** is appended to the appropriate level of E/M service.

Modifier **25** is not restricted to a specific level of E/M service and may be reported with the appropriate code for the level of service supported by documentation in the medical record.

Modifier **25** is used to indicate that a significant, separately identifiable E/M service is performed by the same physician on the day of a procedure. As stated in the definition, the E/M service must be "above and beyond" the other service or "beyond" the usual preoperative and postoperative care associated with the procedure. CPT guidelines do not require different diagnoses for an E/M service and the procedure/service performed to be separately reported. However, the E/M service must either meet the key components (ie, history, examination, medical decision making) or be selected on the basis of time when counseling and/or coordination of care dominates (more than 50%) the physician-patient and/or physician-family encounter (face-to-face time in the office or other outpatient setting or floor or unit time in the hospital or nursing facility) of that level of E/M service, including medical record documentation.

Coding Tip

For significant, separately identifiable *non-E/M services*, modifier **59** is appended to *non-E/M services*.

Chapter 10

EXAMPLE

A physician examines a patient exhibiting a fever, headache, vomiting, and stiff neck and performs a spinal tap, as well as the services described in code 99214. To report this patient encounter, the physician appends modifier **25** to code 99214 and separately reports code 62270, Spinal puncture, lumbar, diagnostic, to indicate that both a significant E/M service and a procedure were performed on the same day.

✓ Check Your Knowledge

1. When a significant, separately identifiable E/M service is performed on the same date that a procedure and/or service was provided, are different diagnoses required for reporting an E/M service on the same date?

Modifier 26

Professional Component

Properly reporting the technical and professional components for procedures is a complex process. Because CPT codes are intended to represent physician and other health care practitioner services, the CPT code set does not contain a coding convention to designate the technical component for a procedure or service. CPT coding guidelines do not specifically address billing for the technical component of a procedure or service. CPT coding does provide modifier **26** for separately reporting the professional (or physician) component of a procedure or service. Certain procedures are a combination of a physician professional component and a technical component. For procedures with both a technical and a professional component, modifier **26** is used to indicate that the professional component of the procedure is being reported separately.

However, many third-party payers have established modifiers and/or specific reporting policies for reporting the technical component of a procedure. For example, Medicare established the **TC** modifier for reporting the technical component. Other payers may also require the use of the **TC** modifier, or they may have developed their own method for such reporting. When reporting the technical component of a procedure or service, one should become familiar with the various reporting requirements of individual insurance companies in one's area, because reporting and reimbursement policies vary among insurance companies.

In general, if a procedure is composed of both a technical and a professional component and is performed on facility-owned equipment, it may be necessary for the physician to indicate that he or she is reporting only the professional component by appending modifier **26** to the procedure code(s) reported. This is because a hospital or other facility may be reporting the technical component of the procedure.

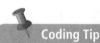

Coding Tip

Modifier **26**, *Professional component*, is not appended to the cardiac catheterization injection procedure codes (eg, **93451-93461**), as these are solely performed by the physician.

Coding Tip

Unmodified CPT codes are intended to describe **both** the technical and professional components of a service. The professional and technical components together are referred to as the "global service." If the technical and professional components of the service are performed by the same provider, it is not appropriate or necessary to report the components of the service separately.

EXAMPLE

Sometimes a physician performs a complex cystometrogram in his or her office, while other times he or she may only interpret the results of a complex cystometrogram. When the physician only interprets the results and/or operates the equipment, the professional component modifier **26** is appended. The guidelines for reporting urodynamic studies, found preceding code **51725**, indicate that all procedures in that section imply that these services are performed by or under the direct supervision of a physician and that all instruments, equipment, fluids, gases, probes, catheters, technician's fees, medications, gloves, trays, tubing, and other sterile supplies are provided by the physician. Thus, when the physician only interprets the results and/or operates the equipment and does not provide the equipment, supplies, technicians, etc, modifier **26** is used to identify the physician's services.

Modifier 32

Mandated Services

Services related to mandated consultation and/or related services (eg, third-party payer, governmental, legislative, or regulatory requirement) may be identified by adding modifier **32**, *Mandated services*, to the basic procedure.

Coding Tip

Modifier **32** should not be appended to an E/M service when a patient or family member requests a second opinion.

Modifier 33

Preventive Service

Providers can identify to insurance payers that the service was preventive under applicable laws, and that patient cost-sharing does not apply by appending the modifier **33**. This modifier assists in the identification of preventive services in payer-processing systems to indicate where it is appropriate to waive the deductible associated with copayment or coinsurance and may be used when a service was initiated as a preventive service, which then resulted in a conversion to a therapeutic service.

The most notable example of this is screening colonoscopy (code **45378**), which results in a polypectomy (code **45383**). CPT modifier **33** should be appended to codes representing the preventive services, unless the service is inherently preventive, eg, a screening mammography or immunization. If multiple preventive medicine services are provided on the same day, the modifier is appended to the codes for **each** preventive service rendered on that day. Please note that Medicare has created HCPCS Level II codes for some of these preventive medicine services.

Modifier 47

Anesthesia by Surgeon

Regional or general anesthesia provided by the surgeon may be reported by adding modifier **47**, *Anesthesia by surgeon*, to the basic service. (This does not include local anesthesia.) **Note:** Modifier **47** would not be used as a modifier for the anesthesia procedures.

If a physician personally performs the regional or general anesthesia for a surgical procedure he or she also performs, modifier **47** would be appended to the surgical code, and no codes from the Anesthesia section would be used.

EXAMPLE

A surgeon performs a regional nerve block prior to performing surgery to decompress the nerve at the carpal tunnel. To report this, the physician uses code **64721**, *Neuroplasty and/or transposition; median nerve at carpal tunnel*, with modifier **47** appended. Code **64415**, *Injection, anesthetic agent; brachial plexus, single*, would also

Chapter 10

Chapter 10

Coding Tip

Under no circumstance should modifier **47** be appended to the anesthesia procedure codes **00100-01999**.

Coding Tip

Modifier **50** is not appended to CPT codes described as bilateral services or procedures.

be reported to describe the regional nerve block performed. Use of modifier **47** alerts the third-party payer that the surgeon personally performed the anesthesia. Listing the code for the anesthesia (in this case, a nerve block) indicates specifically which nerve was blocked.

Modifier 50

Bilateral Procedure

Unless otherwise identified in the listings, bilateral procedures that are performed at the same operative session should be identified by adding modifier **50**, *Bilateral procedure*, to the appropriate five-digit CPT code.

This modifier is used to report bilateral procedures that are performed at the same operative session. The use of this modifier is applicable only to services or procedures performed on identical anatomic sites, aspects, or organs (eg, arms, legs, eyes). The intent is for the modifier to be appended to the appropriate unilateral code as a one-line entry on the claim form to indicate that the procedure was performed bilaterally.

Furthermore, when a procedure is reported with modifier **50** appended to the code, the units-box on the claim form (see Figures 10-1 and 10-2) should indicate that "1" unit of service was provided, because one procedure is being performed bilaterally.

Although the intended reporting of modifier **50** is that the code be listed only once, third-party payer reporting guidelines may require that the code be listed twice, with modifier **50** appended to the first or second line entry. The coder may want to contact the various payers regarding their preferred method of reporting bilateral procedures.

EXAMPLE

A physician repairs bilateral reducible inguinal hernias on a two-year-old. The physician reports code **49500**, *Repair initial inguinal hernia, age 6 months to younger than 5 years, with or without hydrocelectomy; reducible*, with modifier **50** appended (**49500 50**).

Note that, although the text of this modifier refers to "operative session," these words are used in a broad context. Diagnostic as well as therapeutic procedures may require the use of the bilateral modifier if the anatomic structures are found bilaterally and the identical procedure is performed on both sides.

✓ Check Your Knowledge

2. Would modifier **50** be appended to code **76645**, *Ultrasound, breast(s) (unilateral or bilateral), real time with image documentation*? Explain why or why not.

FIGURE 10-1 *Claim Form: Example 1*

	24. A. DATE(S) OF SERVICE From MM DD YY	To MM DD YY	B. PLACE OF SERVICE	C. EMG	D. PROCEDURES, SERVICES, OR SUPPLIES (Explain Unusual Circumstances) CPT/HCPCS	MODIFIER	E. DIAGNOSIS POINTER	F. $ CHARGES	G. DAYS OR UNITS	H. EPSDT Family Plan	I. ID. QUAL.	J. RENDERING PROVIDER ID. #
1					49500	50					NPI	
2											NPI	
3											NPI	
4											NPI	
5											NPI	
6											NPI	

25. FEDERAL TAX I.D. NUMBER	SSN EIN	26. PATIENT'S ACCOUNT NO.	27. ACCEPT ASSIGNMENT? (For govt. claims, see back)	28. TOTAL CHARGE	29. AMOUNT PAID	30. BALANCE DUE
	☐ ☐		☐ YES ☐ NO	$	$	$

PHYSICIAN OR SUPPLIER INFORMATION

FIGURE 10-2 *Claim Form: Example 2*

	24. A. DATE(S) OF SERVICE From MM DD YY	To MM DD YY	B. PLACE OF SERVICE	C. EMG	D. PROCEDURES, SERVICES, OR SUPPLIES (Explain Unusual Circumstances) CPT/HCPCS	MODIFIER	E. DIAGNOSIS POINTER	F. $ CHARGES	G. DAYS OR UNITS	H. EPSDT Family Plan	I. ID. QUAL.	J. RENDERING PROVIDER ID. #
1					49500						NPI	
2					49500	50					NPI	
3											NPI	
4											NPI	
5											NPI	
6											NPI	

25. FEDERAL TAX I.D. NUMBER	SSN EIN	26. PATIENT'S ACCOUNT NO.	27. ACCEPT ASSIGNMENT? (For govt. claims, see back)	28. TOTAL CHARGE	29. AMOUNT PAID	30. BALANCE DUE
	☐ ☐		☐ YES ☐ NO	$	$	$

PHYSICIAN OR SUPPLIER INFORMATION

Modifier 51

Multiple Procedures

When multiple procedures, other than E/M services, physical medicine and rehabilitation services, or provision of supplies (eg, vaccines) are performed at the same session by the same provider, the primary procedure or service may be reported as listed. The additional procedure(s) or service(s) may be identified by appending modifier **51**, *Multiple procedures*, to the additional procedure or service code(s).

Historically, payers and providers have used modifier **51** in varying ways. To alleviate confusion about the intent of the modifier, the definition includes language to indicate that it is not appended to add-on codes (listed in Appendix D of the CPT codebook), E/M codes, or codes designated as modifier **51**–exempt (listed in Appendix E of the CPT codebook). (Refer to Appendix E in the CPT codebook for further discussion of modifier **51**–exempt add-on codes.)

Also, the language "by the same provider" is included in the definition to indicate that this modifier is not to be appended to procedures performed and reported by another physician at the same session.

Modifier **51** has four applications to identify the following:

- Multiple medical procedures performed at the same session by the same provider
- Multiple, related operative procedures performed at the same session by the same provider
- Operative procedures performed in combination at the same operative session by the same provider, whether through the same or another incision or involving the same or different anatomy
- A combination of medical and operative procedures performed at the same session by the same provider

Coding Tip

Modifier **51** may be appended to the same related family of codes when multiple surgical endoscopic, laparoscopic, or arthroscopic procedures are reported. This modifier should not be appended to designated add-on codes (see Appendix D of the CPT codebook).

Modifier 52

Reduced Services

Under certain circumstances, a service or procedure is partially reduced or eliminated at the physician's discretion. Under these circumstances, the service provided can be identified by its usual procedure number and the addition of modifier **52**, *Reduced services*, signifying that the service is reduced. This provides a means of reporting reduced services without disturbing the identification of the basic service. **Note:** For hospital outpatient reporting of a previously scheduled procedure or service that is partially reduced or cancelled as a result of extenuating circumstances or those that threaten the well-being of the patient prior to or after administration of anesthesia, modifiers **73**, *Discontinued Out-Patient Hospital/Ambulatory Surgery Center (ASC) Procedure Prior to the Administration of Anesthesia*, and **74**, *Discontinued Out-Patient Hospital/Ambulatory Surgery Center (ASC) Procedure After Administration of Anesthesia*.

Chapter 10

EXAMPLE

Procedure performed:

93923 Complete bilateral noninvasive physiologic studies of upper or lower extremity arteries, 3 or more levels (eg, for lower extremity: ankle/brachial indices at distal posterior tibial and anterior tibial/dorsalis pedis arteries plus segmental blood pressure measurements with bidirectional Doppler waveform recording and analysis, at 3 or more levels, or ankle/brachial indices at distal posterior tibial and anterior tibial/dorsalis pedis arteries plus segmental volume plethysmography at 3 or more levels, or ankle/brachial indices at distal posterior tibial and anterior tibial/dorsalis pedis arteries plus segmental transcutaneous oxygen tension measurements at 3 or more levels,or single level study with postural provocative functional maneuvers (eg, measurements with postural provocative tests, or measurements with reactive hyperemia)

If an extremity arterial study is performed on a patient who previously had an above-the-knee amputation, modifier **52** would be appended to code **93923** to indicate that this study was not performed in its entirety.
Reported as: **93923 52**.

Modifier 53

Discontinued Procedure

Under certain circumstances, the physician may elect to terminate a surgical or diagnostic procedure. Due to extenuating circumstances or those that threaten the well-being of the patient, it may be necessary to indicate that a surgical or diagnostic procedure was started but discontinued. This circumstance may be reported by adding modifier **53**, *Discontinued procedure*, to the code reported by the physician for the discontinued procedure. **Note:** This modifier is not used to report the elective cancellation of a procedure prior to the patient's anesthesia induction and/or surgical preparation in the operating suite. For outpatient hospital or **Ambulatory Surgery Center** (ASC) reporting of a previously scheduled procedure/service that is partially reduced or cancelled as a result of extenuating circumstances or those that threaten the well-being of the patient prior to or after administration of anesthesia, see modifiers **73** and **74**. (See Appendix A in the CPT codebook for modifiers approved for ASC hospital outpatient use.)

Modifier **53** is used for physician reporting purposes. It is used to report circumstances when patients experience unexpected responses (eg, arrhythmia, hypotensive or hypertensive crisis) that cause the procedure to be terminated. Modifier **53** differs from **52** (which describes a procedure that was reduced at the physician's discretion) in that a patient's life-threatening condition precipitates the discontinued procedure. Modifier **53** is not used to report elective cancellation of procedures prior to anesthesia induction or surgical preparation in the surgical suite, including situations in which cancellation is due to patient instability.

✓ **Check Your Knowledge**

3. After anesthesia induction, the patient experiences an arrhythmia that causes the procedure to be terminated. Which modifier should the physician append to the code reported for the planned procedure? Modifier **52** or **53**?

Modifiers 54, 55, and 56

Modifier 54, *Surgical Care Only*

When one physician performs a surgical procedure and another provided preoperative and/or postoperative management, surgical services may be identified by adding modifier **54**, *Surgical care only*, to the usual procedure number.

Modifier 55, *Postoperative Management Only*

When one physician performed the postoperative management and another physician performed the surgical procedure, the postoperative component may be identified by adding modifier **55**, *Postoperative management only*, to the usual procedure number.

Modifier 56, *Preoperative Management Only*

When one physician performed the preoperative care and evaluation and another physician performed the surgical procedure, the preoperative component may be identified by adding modifier **56**, *Preoperative management only*, to the usual procedure number.

EXAMPLE

In certain locations or types of practice, a surgeon may be asked to perform a surgical procedure while another physician(s) performs the preoperative and postoperative services associated with a particular service. The operating surgeon reports the surgical procedure performed and appends modifier **54** to the surgical procedure code. The physician who provides the preoperative and postoperative management appends modifiers **55** and **56** to the surgical procedure code.

For example, a patient travels to a medical center for specialized surgery and subsequently receives postoperative care from his or her local physician. The surgeon, in this case, reports the preoperative management and the surgical procedure code (ie, reports the surgical procedure with modifiers **54** and **56**). The physician who performed the postoperative management reports the operative procedure code with modifier **55** appended. Reporting the postoperative management indicates that the physician performed all of the postoperative care.

Modifier 57

Decision for Surgery

An E/M service that resulted in the initial decision to perform the surgery may be identified by adding modifier **57**, *Decision for surgery*, to the appropriate level of E/M service.

Modifier **57** provides a means of identifying the E/M services that result in the initial decision to perform the surgery. The modifier, supported by documentation that the decision for surgery was made at the time of the visit, may allow separate payment for the E/M service if covered by the payer. Many variations and coverage interpretations can exist among payers regarding this modifier.

EXAMPLE

A physician is consulted to determine whether surgery is necessary for a patient with abdominal pain. The physician's services meet the criteria necessary to report a consultation (ie, documents findings, communicates by written report to the requesting physician). The requesting physician agrees with the consultant's findings and requests that the consultant assume the case and discuss his findings with the patient.

The patient consents to undergo surgery to repair a perforated ulcer; the operation is performed later that same day. To code this, the surgeon reports the E/M services (consultation) by means of the appropriate consultation code and appends modifier **57**. The surgeon also reports the appropriate code for the specific surgery (without a modifier) in addition to the E/M service.

It is incorrect to append modifier **25** to the consultation code for the decision to perform surgery. Appending modifier **57** to the consultation described previously indicates to the third-party payer that the consultation is not part of the global surgical procedure.

Modifier 58

Staged or Related Procedure or Service by the Same Physician During the Postoperative Period

It may be necessary to indicate that the performance of a procedure or service during the postoperative period was:

- Planned or anticipated (staged),
- More extensive than the original procedure, or
- For therapy following a surgical procedure.

This circumstance may be reported by adding modifier **58**, *Staged or related procedure or service by the same physician during the postoperative period*, to the staged or related procedure. **Note:** For treatment of a problem that requires a return to the operating or procedure room (eg, unanticipated clinical condition), see modifier **78**.

Use of modifier **58** indicates that the reported procedure is related to the original procedure, is intended to be performed sometime in the future as a "staged" procedure, and may represent one or more of the following circumstances (it is not necessary to meet all of the following criteria to qualify for use of modifier **58**):

- A procedure performed by the original surgeon or provider
- A follow-up surgery more extensive than the original procedure
- A therapy following a diagnostic surgical procedure
- The time frame for the performance of the "staged" procedure may occur during the postoperative period (ie, "global period") associated with the original surgery

Note that the modifier **58** descriptor indicates that modifier **58** is not to be used to report the treatment of a problem that requires an unanticipated trip to the operating room for a clinical condition.

EXAMPLE

A surgeon performs a mastectomy on a patient. During the postoperative global period, the surgeon inserts a permanent prosthesis (**11970**). The surgeon reports the code for the permanent prosthesis insertion with modifier **58** to indicate that the service was related to the mastectomy (staged to occur at a time after the initial surgery). If the physician did not append modifier **58**, a third-party payer could reject the claim because the surgery occurred during the postoperative period associated with the mastectomy.

In a second case, a diabetic patient with advanced circulatory problems has three gangrenous toes removed from her left foot (**28820, 28820 51, 28820 51**). During the postoperative period, it becomes necessary to amputate the patient's left foot. To report this, modifier **58** would be appended to the code for the amputation of the foot (**28805 58**).

Because the amputation is related to the reason for the previous amputation of the toes (diabetic gangrene), modifier **58** is used (rather than modifier **78**) even though the use of an operating room is necessary. The amputation of the foot was **not** due to a complication of the first surgery but was due to the underlying disease process.

Modifier 59

Distinct Procedural Service

Under certain circumstances, it may be necessary to indicate that a procedure or service was distinct or independent from other non-E/M services performed on the same day. Modifier **59**, *Distinct procedural service*, is used to identify procedures/services, other than E/M services, that are not normally reported together but are appropriate under the circumstances. Documentation may support a different session, different procedure or surgery, different site or organ system, separate incision/excision, separate lesion, or separate injury (or area of injury in extensive injuries) not ordinarily encountered or performed on the same day by the same individual. However, when another already-established modifier is appropriate, it should be used rather than modifier **59**. Only if no more descriptive modifier is available and the use of modifier **59** best explains the circumstances should modifier **59** be used.

Modifier **59** is also intended to assist in the reporting of codes with the *separate procedure* designation. Some of the codes in the CPT code set have been identified with the term *separate procedure* in the code descriptor.

When a procedure or service that is designated as a separate procedure is carried out independently or considered unrelated or distinct from other procedures or services provided at that time, it may be reported by itself or in addition to other procedures/services by appending modifier **59** to the specific separate procedure code reported. This indicates that the procedure is not considered a component of another procedure but is a distinct, independent procedure, such as a different session, different site or organ system, separate incision/excision, separate lesion, or treatment of a separate injury (or area of injury in extensive injuries).

Codes designated as separate procedures may not be additionally reported when the procedure/service is performed as an integral component of another procedure or service.

Modifier 62

Two Surgeons

When two surgeons work together as primary surgeons performing distinct part(s) of a procedure, each surgeon should report his or her distinct operative work by adding modifier **62**, *Two surgeons*, to the procedure code and any associated add-on code(s) for that procedure as long as both surgeons continue to work together as primary surgeons. Each surgeon should report the co-surgery once using the same procedure code. If additional procedure(s) (including add-on procedure(s)) are performed during the same surgical session, separate code(s) may also be reported with modifier **62** added.

Note: If a co-surgeon acts as an assistant in the performance of additional procedure(s) during the same surgical session, those services may be reported using separate procedure code(s) with modifier **80** or modifier **82** added, as appropriate.

Co-surgery may be required because of the complexity of the procedure(s), the patient's condition, or both. The additional surgeon is not acting as an assistant at surgery in these circumstances but is performing a distinct portion of the procedure.

The approach surgeon and the spine surgeon must discuss, before a scheduled surgery, what portion of the operation each is expected to perform on the basis of the case's complexity. If, because of the complexity of the procedure, the approach surgeon is needed as a co-surgeon (both the spine and approach surgeon serve as primary surgeons) to

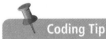
Coding Tip

Modifier **59** should **not** be appended to an E/M service. To report a separate and distinct E/M service with a non–E/M service performed on the same date, modifier **25** may be used.

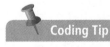
Coding Tip

Modifier **62** should not be appended to the bone graft codes **20900-20938** and spinal instrumentation codes **22040-22855**. Documentation to establish medical necessity for both surgeons is required for some services.

Chapter 10

also perform additional procedures, modifier **62** may be appended to these agreed-on procedures.

When an approach surgeon opens and closes only, modifier **62** is appended to the distinct principal procedure along with any additional levels that require approach work by only the approach surgeon.

Modifier **62** may be added to additional procedural codes only if both surgeons agree to continue to work together as primary surgeons on the basis of the complexity of the case.

Modifier **80**, *Assistant surgeon* (discussed later in this chapter), may be appended to additional procedural code(s) by the approach surgeon, provided both surgeons agree that the approach surgeon is needed to continue to work as an assistant to the spine surgeon.

The following are case examples for when to append modifiers **62** and/or **80**:

EXAMPLES

Anterior Thoracic Two-Level Arthrodesis; Anterior Single-Level Discectomy; Anterior Plate Instrumentation, Structural, Autograft Iliac Crest Bone Graft

Case 1

Procedure: Approach surgeon performs approach and closure only

Surgeon performing approach only reports:

22556 62

22585 62

Surgeon performing the spine procedure reports:

22556 62

22585 62

63077 51

22845

20938

Case 2

Procedure: Approach surgeon performs as co-surgeon with spine surgeon for entire case

Surgeon performing approach and serving as co-surgeon for the entire case reports:

22556 62

22585 62

63077 62 51

Surgeon performing the spine procedure reports:

22556 62

22585 62

63077 62 51

22845

20938

Case 3

Procedure: Approach surgeon performs approach and closure and performs rest of case as assistant to spine surgeon

Surgeon performing approach and serving as an assistant for the entire case reports:

22556 62

22585 62

63077 80 51

Surgeon performing the spine procedure reports:

22556 62

22585 62

63077 51

22845

20938

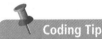

Coding Tip

Modifier **63** is intended to be used only with invasive surgical procedures and reported only for those invasive procedures performed on neonates and infants up to the 4-kg cutoff. Modifier **63** represents the significant increase in work intensity required in this population of patients. The factors related to this increase in work intensity include difficulties in maintenance of temperature control, obtaining intravenous access (which may require upward of 45 minutes), and the performance of the procedure itself, which is technically more difficult, especially with regard to maintenance of homeostasis.

Modifier 63

Procedure Performed on Infants less than 4 kg

Procedures performed on neonates and infants up to a present body weight of 4 kg may involve significantly increased complexity and physician work commonly associated with these patients. This circumstance may be reported by adding modifier **63**, *Procedure performed on infants less than 4 kg*, to the procedure number. **Note:** Unless otherwise designated, this modifier may only be appended to procedures/services listed in the **20000-69990** code series. Modifier **63** should not be appended to CPT codes listed in the Evaluation and Management Services, Anesthesia, Radiology, Pathology/Laboratory, or Medicine sections.

There are many procedures with which it would be inappropriate to report modifier **63**. These procedures are those performed solely on the very young patient, for which the difficulty of the procedure has already been considered in the establishment of the code. Procedures that include the work inherent in modifier **63** and that would not be reported in addition to this modifier are denoted with a parenthetical statement. The following is an example:

44055 Correction of malrotation by lysis of duodenal bands and/or reduction of midgut volvulus (eg, Ladd procedure)
(Do not report modifier 63 in conjunction with 44055)

CPT procedure codes to which modifier **63** would be appropriately appended include:

44120 Enterectomy, resection of small intestine; single resection and anastomosis

44140 Colectomy, partial; with anastomosis

33820 Repair of patent ductus arteriosus; by ligation

EXAMPLE

A physician performs a patent ductus arteriosus repair on a three-week-old, 800-g, 28-week premature neonate. Special services required in performing this procedure include maintenance of the operating suite temperature at an appropriately hot level, establishment of adequate venous access, careful positioning of the patient on the Bovie grounding plate, and placement of appropriate barriers for prevention of heat loss. The patent ductus arteriosus repair is subsequently completed. The patient is placed into the isolate and transferred to the neonatal intensive care unit (NICU), still on the ventilator. This surgery is often further complicated by the fact that the procedure is performed in the NICU, relocating the operating team and equipment to the NICU to lessen the risk of the transfer to the operating suite in these delicate neonates.

Surgeon performing the cardiac procedure codes:

33820 63

Modifier 66

Surgical Team

Under some circumstances, highly complex procedures (requiring the concomitant services of several physicians, often of different specialties, plus other highly skilled, specially trained personnel, and various types of complex equipment) are carried out under the surgical team concept. Such circumstances may be identified by each participating physician with the addition of modifier **66**, *Surgical team*, to the basic procedure number used for reporting services.

In certain CPT codes, one major procedure is listed without indicating the various components of that service (eg, code **33945**, *Heart transplant, with or without recipient cardiectomy*). This code lists one major service that combines the work of several physicians and other specially trained personnel.

EXAMPLE

Generally, each physician on a heart transplant team performs the same portion of the surgery each time. Perhaps one surgeon opens the chest and inserts the chest tubes while another surgeon prepares the great vessels for anastomosis to the donor heart. Each surgeon reports the same code with the same modifier, in this case code **33945 66**. It is important that all the physicians on the surgical team jointly provide a description of each physician's general role on the heart transplant team, and send the report to each third-party payer, to indicate each physician's role in the performance of the surgery.

If one surgeon assists another surgeon with a procedure, modifiers **80**, *Assistant surgeon*; **81**, *Minimum assistant surgeon*; or **82**, *Assistant surgeon (when qualified resident surgeon not available)*, may be more appropriate to report than modifier **66**.

Modifiers 76, 77, 78, and 79

Modifier 76, *Repeat Procedure or Service by Same Physician or Other Qualified Health Care Professional*

When a procedure or service is repeated by the same physician subsequent to the original procedure or service by the same physician, this circumstance may be reported by adding modifier **76**, *Repeat procedure or service by same physician or other qualified health care professional*, to the repeated procedure or service.

Modifier 77, *Repeat Procedure or Service by Another Physician or Other Qualified Health Care Professional*

When a basic procedure or service performed by **another** physician had to be repeated, it may be reported by adding modifier **77**, *Repeat procedure or service by another physician or other qualified health care professional*, to the repeated procedure or service.

Modifier 78, *Unplanned Return to the Operating/ Procedure Room by the Same Physician or Other Qualified Health Care Professional Following Initial Procedure for a Related Procedure During the Postoperative Period*

It may be necessary to indicate that another procedure was performed during the postoperative period of the initial procedure (unplanned procedure following initial procedure). When this procedure is related to the first and requires the use of an operating/procedure room, it may be reported by adding modifier **78**, *Unplanned return to the operating/ procedure room by the same physician or other qualified health care professional following initial procedure for a related procedure during the postoperative period to the related procedure.*

Modifier 79, *Unrelated Procedure or Service by the Same Physician During the Postoperative Period*

The physician may need to indicate that the performance of a procedure or service was performed during the postoperative period was unrelated to the original procedure. This circumstance may be reported by using modifier **79**, *Unrelated procedure or service by the same physician during the postoperative period*. For repeat procedures on the same day, see modifier **76**.

EXAMPLE

A physician performs a femoral-popliteal bypass graft in the morning. Later that day, the graft clots, and the entire procedure is repeated by the same physician. The initial procedure is reported with code **35556**, *Bypass graft, with vein; femoral-popliteal*. The repeat procedure is reported as code **35556 76**. Appending modifier **76** alerts the third-party payer that code **35556** has not accidentally been reported twice. Documentation supporting the reoperation should be provided to the third-party payer when these services are reported.

Following is the same example with two different surgeons involved. The patient has a femoral-popliteal graft in the morning and it clots later that day. However, Physician A performs the surgery in the morning but is not available to perform the repeat operation later that day. A second surgeon, Physician B, performs the same procedure later that night. Physician A reports code **35556**, and Physician B reports code **35556 77**.

Physician B is not affected by Physician A's global service. Physician B's performance of a surgical service (**35556**) will begin a global package related to the repeat surgical procedure. Again, documentation should be provided to the third-party payer to clarify that a repeat procedure was performed by another surgeon.

To expand on this coding example, the patient who had the repeat femoral-popliteal graft (**35556**) goes home and the incision and graft heal well. However, the patient develops acute renal failure a week after returning home and is hospitalized within the postoperative period of the bypass procedure. The patient does not respond to medical treatment of the renal failure. Hemodialysis is indicated, and Physician B inserts a cannula for hemodialysis: code **36810**, *Insertion of cannula for hemodialysis, other purpose (separate procedure); arteriovenous, external (Scribner type)*.

Physician B's services for the insertion of the cannula for hemodialysis are reported as code **36810 79**, because this service (**36810**) is unrelated to the femoral-popliteal bypass graft (**35556**) performed during the previous hospitalization. If modifier **79** is not appended to this procedure, the third-party payer may not know that this service is unrelated to the femoral-popliteal graft (ie, the computer program used by the third-party payer may not be able to distinguish that this service is not related to the previous surgery and may automatically reject this claim). One must provide documentation to the third-party payer to indicate that this service is unrelated to the first procedure.

In another case, if a patient's operative site bleeds after an initial surgery and requires a return to the operating room to stop the bleeding, the same procedure is not repeated. Thus, a different code, **35860**, *Exploration for postoperative hemorrhage, thrombosis or infection; extremity*, would be reported with modifier **78** appended. Because the same procedure is not repeated, modifier **76** would not be appropriate to use.

> Modifier **78** is appended to procedures that are performed during the postoperative period that require a patient to return to the operating or procedure room and are directly associated with the performance of the initial operation.

Modifiers 80, 81, and 82

Modifier 80, *Assistant Surgeon*

Although the intent of the assistant surgeon modifiers is to report physician services, many users report these modifiers for a variety of nonphysician surgical assistant services. The most common misinterpretation of the assistant surgeon modifiers is to report physician assistant or nurse practitioner assistant surgical services. Although from a CPT perspective, the assistant surgeon modifiers are not intended to be reported for physician assistant or nurse practitioner assistant surgical services, some third-party payers consider this an acceptable means of reporting these services during surgery. Many have established their own guidelines for reporting assistant surgeon services.

Coding Tip

The assistant surgeon reports the same CPT code as the operating surgeon, with modifier **80** appended.

EXAMPLE

Case 1

Primary operating surgeon performs approach and closure and assistant surgeon assists during entire surgical case

Procedure:

Closure of Intestinal Cutaneous Fistula

Surgeon performing approach and closure reports:

44640

Assistant surgeon reports:

44640 80

One physician may assist another physician in performing a procedure. If an assistant surgeon assists a primary surgeon and is present for the entire operation or a substantial portion of the operation, the assisting physician reports the same procedure code as the operating surgeon. The operating surgeon does not append a modifier to the procedure code that he or she reports. The assistant surgeon reports the same CPT code as the operating physician, with modifier **80** appended. The individual operative report submitted by each surgeon should indicate the distinct service(s) provided by each surgeon.

Modifier 81, *Minimum Assistant Surgeon*

Minimum surgical assistant services are identified by adding modifier **81**, *Minimum assistant surgeon*, to the usual procedure number.

While a primary operating physician may plan to perform a surgical procedure alone, during an operation circumstances may arise that require the services of an assistant surgeon for a relatively short time. In this instance, the second surgeon provides minimal assistance for which he or she reports the surgical procedure code with modifier **81** appended.

Modifier 82, *Assistant Surgeon (When Qualified Resident Surgeon not Available)*

The unavailability of a qualified resident surgeon is a prerequisite for use of modifier **82**, *Assistant surgeon (when qualified resident surgeon not available)*, appended to the usual procedure code number(s).

In certain programs (eg, teaching hospitals), the physician acting as the assistant surgeon is usually a qualified resident surgeon. However, there may be times (eg, during rotational changes) when a qualified resident surgeon is not available and instead another surgeon assists in the operation. In these instances, the services of the nonresident assistant surgeon are reported with modifier **82** appended to the appropriate code. This indicates that another surgeon is assisting the operating surgeon instead of a qualified resident surgeon.

Modifier 90

Reference (Outside) Laboratory

When laboratory procedures are performed by a party other than the treating or reporting physician, the procedure may be identified by adding modifier **90**, *Reference (outside) laboratory*, to the usual procedure number. This modifier is used by a physician or clinic when the laboratory tests performed for a patient are performed by an outside or reference laboratory. This modifier is used to indicate that, although the physician is reporting the performance of a laboratory test, the actual testing component was a service from a laboratory.

EXAMPLE

Dr J, an internist, performs an examination of a patient and as part of the examination orders a complete blood count. Dr J does not perform in-office laboratory testing. He has an arrangement with a laboratory to bill him for the testing procedure, and in turn he bills the patient. Dr J's staff performs the venipuncture. Dr J may report an appropriate E/M code as well as code **36415**, *Collection of venous blood by venipuncture*, and also reports that the laboratory analysis of the specimen was performed by an outside laboratory, for example, code **85025 90**, *Blood count; complete (CBC), automated (Hgb, Hct, RBC, WBC and platelet count) and automated differential WBC count.*

Modifier 91

Repeat Clinical Diagnostic Laboratory Test

In the course of treatment of the patient, it may be necessary to repeat the same laboratory test on the same day to obtain subsequent (multiple) test results. Under these circumstances, the laboratory test performed can be identified by its usual procedure number and the addition of modifier **91**, *Repeat clinical diagnostic laboratory test*. This modifier may not be used when tests are rerun to confirm initial results, because of testing problems with specimens or equipment, or for any other reason when a normal, one-time, reportable result is all that is required. This modifier may not be used when other codes describe a series of test results (eg, glucose tolerance tests, evocative/suppression testing). This modifier may be used only for laboratory test(s) performed more than once on the same day on the same patient.

Modifier 92

Alternative Laboratory Platform Testing

When laboratory testing is being performed with the use of a kit or transportable instrument that wholly or in part consists of a single-use, disposable analytical chamber, the service may be identified by adding modifier **92**, *Alternate laboratory platform testing*, to the usual laboratory procedure code (HIV testing, reported with the code series **86701-86703**). The test does not require permanent dedicated space and hence by its design may be hand carried or transported to the vicinity of the patient for immediate testing at that site, although location of the testing is not in itself determinative of the use of this modifier.

Modifier 99

Multiple Modifiers

Under certain circumstances two or more modifiers may be necessary to completely delineate a service. In such situations, modifier **99**, *Multiple modifiers*, should be added to the basic procedure, and other applicable modifiers may be listed as part of the description of the service.

This modifier is used to alert third-party payers that several modifiers are being used to report a service.

EXAMPLE

A surgical procedure is performed by using an assistant surgeon (modifier **80**), and, at the physician's discretion, a portion of the procedure is reduced or eliminated (modifier **52**). The service provided by the assistant surgeon would be reported in one of the following ways:

43510 99

43510 99 80 52

✓ Check Your Knowledge Answers

1. No. Different diagnoses are not required for reporting an E/M service on the same date.

2. No. The code descriptor lists "unilateral or bilateral," therefore the procedure may be performed bilaterally and should not be appended with the modifier **50**.

3. Modifier **53** is not used to report elective cancellation of procedures prior to anesthesia induction or surgical preparation in the surgical suite, including situations in which cancellation is due to patient instability. Modifier **53** differs from **52** (which describes a procedure that was reduced at the physician's discretion) in that a patient's life-threatening condition precipitates the discontinued procedure.

Chapter Exercises

Check your answers in Appendix B.

True or False

1. The American Medical Association maintains and updates the Health Care Common Procedure Coding System (HCPCS) Level II (national) codes. **True or False**

2. Local infiltration, metacarpal/metatarsal/digital block, or topical anesthesia are included in a given CPT surgical code and these services are always included in addition to the operation per se. **True or False**

3. It is appropriate to append modifier **23** to certain codes in the CPT nomenclature that represent services performed under anesthesia. **True or False**

4. Modifier **25** should not be used to report an E/M service that results in a decision to perform surgery. **True or False**

Short Answer

5. Indicate the appropriate code(s) for reporting a bilateral arthrocentesis, injection of the small joint or bursa of both right and left toes.

6. Which modifier is used to indicate that an E/M service was performed during a postoperative period for reason(s) unrelated to the original procedure?

7. Multiple, related operative procedures performed at the same session by the same provider are identified by means of which CPT modifier?

8. When the same laboratory test is repeated to obtain subsequent (multiple) test results, which modifier is appended to the laboratory code reported?

9. When two surgeons work together to perform a procedure, which modifier is appended to represent their distinct part of the procedure?

Appendixes

Chapter Objectives

This chapter will assist in accomplishing the following objectives:

- Understand the use of the appendixes within the CPT codebook
- Understand the application of appropriate CPT coding

The appendixes, which are placed in the latter section of the CPT codebook, complement the CPT code set by providing invaluable guidance on the appropriate use of CPT codes. They were introduced to the CPT codebook with the intent of providing supplementary information to users of the CPT code set. As the CPT code set has evolved over the years, especially with advancements in the medicine and technology fields, so too have the appendixes. Following is an overview of each appendix.

Appendix A: Modifiers

Appendix A, the first appendix implemented to the CPT codebook, is a complete listing of the CPT modifiers, their definitions, and guidelines for their use. The modifiers are arranged in numeric ascending order and, based upon CPT guidelines, should be appended to the respective CPT code(s), as appropriate. This appendix also provides a complete listing of modifiers approved for Ambulatory Surgery Centers (ASC) Hospital Outpatient Use, in addition to Level II (HCPCS/National) Modifiers that have been approved by the National Uniform Billing Committee for hospital outpatient reporting.

Appendix B: Summary of Additions, Deletions, and Revisions

Appendix B provides a comprehensive summary of additions, deletions, and revisions applicable to the current annual edition of the CPT codebook. New procedure codes, developed for each edition of the CPT codebook, are identified with the ● symbol placed before the code number. In instances in which a code revision has resulted in an altered code descriptor, the ▲ symbol is placed before the code number. All deleted codes are identified with a strikethrough.

Coding Tip

The Clinical Examples found in Appendix C of the CPT codebook provide a deeper understanding of the services encompassed in the E/M codes and are intended to be used as a tool for reporting E/M services. However, the clinical examples are just examples, and do not encompass the entire scope of the medical practice.

Appendix C: Clinical Examples

Appendix C illustrates a unique in-depth look at various clinical examples related to the CPT codes for Evaluation and Management (E/M) services. The explanatory paragraphs preceding the clinical examples contain critical information regarding the use of these clinical examples. The clinical examples, when used with the E/M Services code descriptors found in the full text of the CPT codebook, are intended to be used as a tool for reporting services provided to patients. It is essential for users of the CPT E/M services codes to take the time to understand the intent of these clinical examples. The examples can lead to a deeper understanding of the services encompassed in the E/M codes, but it is important to note that the clinical examples are just that: *examples*. They do not encompass the entire scope of medical practice.

Appendix D: Summary of CPT Add-on Codes

Appendix D provides a summary of the codes designated as CPT add-on codes for the current edition of the CPT codebook. These codes are also identified throughout the text of the CPT codebook with the ✚ symbol placed before the code for quick and easy reference.

Appendix E: Summary of CPT Codes Exempt From Modifier 51

The codes in the listing that appears in this appendix are exempt from the use of modifier **51** but have not been designated as CPT add-on codes. These codes are identified throughout the text of the CPT codebook with the ⊘ symbol placed before the code.

Appendix F: Summary of CPT Codes Exempt From Modifier 63

The codes listed in Appendix F are exempt from the use of modifier **63**, *Procedure Performed on Infants.* These codes are identified throughout the text of the CPT codebook with the parenthetical instruction, "(Do not report modifier **63** in conjunction with . . .)."

✓ Check Your Knowledge

1. Where do the modifiers appear in the CPT codebook?

EXAMPLE

(Do not report modifier **63** in conjunction with code **30540, 30545**)

Appendix G: Summary of CPT Codes That Include Moderate (Conscious) Sedation

The procedure codes listed in this appendix include conscious sedation as an inherent part of providing the procedure. These codes are identified throughout the text of the CPT codebook with a ⊙ symbol placed before the code. This indicates that it would not be appropriate to separately report conscious sedation in addition to the procedure code, as it is already included in the procedure code.

Appendix H: Alphabetical Clinical Topics Listing (AKA – Alphabetical Listing)

Appendix H provides an alphabetic index of performance measures categorized by clinical condition or topic. Prior to reporting a code, the user must review the complete description of the code in the Category II section of the CPT codebook and the complete description of its associated measure by accessing the measure developer's Web site provided in the footnoted reference of the table. It should be noted that some measures may apply to more than one condition and, as a result, may appear more than one time within Appendix H.

Appendix I: Genetic Testing Code Modifiers

Appendix I provides CPT users with a listing of genetic testing modifiers intended to be reported in conjunction with molecular laboratory procedures related to genetic testing. Appendix I allows for the opportunity to address advances in technology, capture specific data for tracking utilization, and provide diagnostic granularity and specific information to allow payers to adjudicate claims for such analyses. This numeric-alphabetic modifier coding system is arranged in a hierarchical system with the first (numeric) character indicating the disease type and the second (alphabetic) character indicating the disease or gene. These modifiers should be used in conjunction with CPT and HCPCS codes in order to provide granularity of service to enable providers to submit complete and precise genetic testing information without altering test descriptors. This system presents a viable solution to the expected growth of molecular genetics testing in clinical practice over the next decade while the technology and nomenclature system mature.

Appendix J: Electrodiagnostic Medicine Listing of Sensory, Motor, and Mixed Nerves

This appendix was added to provide users of the CPT codebook with two coding references: a list of nerve families and a table of the type of study and maximum number of studies. The nerve families list provides nerve branches included within a nerve family and is intended to assist in selecting the appropriate assignment of codes for nerve conduction studies (**95900**, **95903**, **95904**).

The maximum number of studies table summarizes the recommended maximum number of studies per diagnostic category necessary for a physician to arrive at a diagnosis in 90% of patients with that final diagnosis, when performing needle electromyography (EMG) tests (codes **95860-95864** and codes **95867-95870**); nerve conduction studies (codes **95900**, **95903**, **95904**); and other EMG studies (codes **95934**, **95936**, **95937**). Each column represents the number of studies recommended. The numbers in the table should be utilized as a tool to detect outliers to assist in appropriate reporting. Each number in the table constitutes one study or unit. The maximum numbers are designed to apply to a diverse range of practice styles as well as practice types, including those at referral centers where more complex testing is frequently necessary. In simple, straightforward cases, fewer tests will be necessary. This is particularly true when results of the most critical tests are normal. In complex cases, the maximum numbers in the table will be insufficient for the physician to arrive at a complete diagnosis. In cases in which there are borderline findings, additional tests may be required to determine if the findings are significant.

The appropriate number of studies to be performed should be left to the judgment of the physician performing the electrodiagnostic (EDX) evaluation. However, in the small number of cases that require testing in excess of the numbers listed in the table, the physician should be able to provide supplementary documentation to justify the additional testing. Such documentation should explain what other differential diagnostic problems needed to be ruled out in that particular situation. In some patients, multiple diagnoses will be established by EDX testing, and the recommendations listed in the table for a single diagnostic category will not apply. It should be noted that in some situations it is necessary to test an asymptomatic contralateral limb to establish normative values for an individual patient. Normal values based on the general population alone are less sensitive than this approach; therefore, restrictions on contralateral asymptomatic limb testing will reduce the sensitivity of electrodiagnostic tests.

Appendix K: Product Pending FDA Approval

Appendix K contains a list of vaccine product codes pending approval from the Food and Drug Administration (FDA). For example, some vaccine products have been assigned a CPT Category I code in anticipation of future approval from the FDA. Code **90668** is a vaccine product code pending FDA approval status that is identified in the codebook with the ⁄ symbol.

Appendix L: Vascular Families

Appendix L provides a Vascular Families table that identifies the applicable vessels within a vascular family. This table is provided as a useful resource to assist in the assignment of procedure codes based upon the vascular family and the order of the vessel within the family from the point of origin. The assignment of branches to first, second, and third order in this table makes the assumption that the starting point is catheterization of the aorta. This categorization would not be accurate, for example, if a femoral or carotid artery were catheterized directly in an antegrade direction.

Appendix M: Deleted CPT Codes

Appendix M provides a crosswalk of deleted codes and descriptors that have been renumbered. When substantial revisions are made to the CPT codebook, they will be addressed (crosswalked) in this appendix. This appendix will include revisions, deletions, and renumbered codes as well as subheadings that are added to provide more appropriate code sections for more meaningful, logical location of the codes in the CPT codebook.

> ✓ **Check Your Knowledge Answer**
>
> 1. Appendix A of the CPT codebook provides a complete list of CPT modifiers, their definitions, and guidelines for their use.

Chapter Exercises

Check your answers in Appendix B.

Matching

Match the correct appendix with the proper description.

a. Appendix L
b. Appendix A
c. Appendix M
d. Appendix C
e. Appendix K
f. Appendix B
g. Appendix D
h. Appendix I
i. Appendix G
j. Appendix E
k. Appendix F
l. Appendix H
m. Appendix J

1. This appendix has numeric-alphabetic modifiers used for reporting molecular laboratory procedures related to genetic testing.
2. This appendix provides users with a table of the type of study and maximum number of EDX studies.
3. This appendix provides users with a table that shows the assignment of vascular branches to first, second, and third order.
4. This appendix provides a listing of codes exempt from the use of the modifier that identifies procedures performed on infants.
5. This appendix provides a listing of codes identified throughout the text of the CPT codebook with the ✚ symbol placed before the code.
6. This appendix provides examples related to the CPT codes for Evaluation and Management (E/M) services.
7. This appendix contains a listing of modifiers, their definitions, and guidelines for use.
8. This appendix provides a listing of codes that have not been designated as CPT add-on codes and are exempt from the use of multiple procedures modifier.
9. This appendix provides a summary of codes identified with the ● symbol and ▲ symbol placed before the code number.

10. This appendix provides users with an indication that it would not be appropriate to separately report conscious sedation in addition to the procedure code.
11. This appendix provides users with an alphabetic index of performance measures categorized by clinical condition or topic.
12. This appendix provides a list of vaccine product codes pending FDA approval status.

Billing and Reimbursement

Although CPT codes and guidelines do not address reimbursement or third-party payer policy issues, this Appendix will provide a general overview of how the coding lessons taught in this publication apply to real-life situations of coding claims and obtaining reimbursement. It is important to note that CPT coding guidelines may differ from third-party payer guidelines. Eligibility for payment, as well as coverage policy, is determined by each individual insurer or third-party payer. Information provided by the American Medical Association (AMA) does not constitute clinical advice nor dictate a third-party payer's reimbursement policy. In all cases, the practitioner performing a procedure is responsible for the correct coding of the procedure, and information provided by the AMA is not a substitute for the professional judgment of the practitioner involved. For reimbursement or third-party payer policy issues, it is best to contact third-party payers directly.

For the purposes of this book, the term **third-party payers** represents all health insurance carriers, both private (eg, Blue Cross and Blue Shield) and public (ie, Medicare and Medicaid). Coding a claim correctly is the first step in receiving accurate payment from third-party payers. Submitting what is often referred to as a *clean claim* is the first step. A **clean claim** is an accurately coded claim that contains the appropriate patient demographic information and all required fields on the claim form are appropriately completed. A clean claim is a complete and error-free claim submitted to the health insurer on the health insurer's claim form.

Key Terms

- **Third-party payers**
- **Clean claim**

Medical Record Documentation

The patient's symptom(s) and condition(s) should be thoroughly documented in the patient's medical record (chart) along with the diagnosis, procedures and services performed on that date of service, and the treatment plan. An appropriately documented medical record is a crucial step in selecting the correct codes and obtaining the appropriate reimbursement for the services provided. The patient's medical records serve as a legal document to verify the care provided. Remember that if it's not documented in the medical records, it didn't happen.

The **claims management process** is the internal workflow for preparing and submitting claims and collecting payment on the claims. The process begins when the necessary patient and insurance information (demographics) is obtained and ends when the appropriate payment is received for the services rendered.

A **super bill**, also referred to as an *encounter form* or *patient charge slip*, is a form that physician practices and other facilities use to record services rendered by a physician or health care professional during the patient encounter. (See Figure AA-1.) This form is generally only one page long and lists the most common diagnostic codes (ICD-9) and service and procedural codes (CPT) performed in the practice or facility. This can be a helpful tool for physicians and coders to use. Physicians may select the procedures performed and services rendered along with the diagnosis on these forms. Coders are then able to verify the appropriate coding by reviewing the documentation in the patient's medical record along with the code selection on the super bill to make certain that the physician has identified and coded all the services rendered. The coder may need to append the appropriate modifiers to the CPT codes, as deemed necessary.

Key Terms

Third-party payers: Insurance carriers, both private and public (ie, Medicare and Medicaid) that provide medical coverage to their members.

Clean claim: A paper claim that is submitted and meets all of the health insurer's standard submission requirements and that the health insurer has accepted for processing. When an electronic claim is submitted, and it is covered by the Health Insurance Portability and Accountability Act of 1996 (HIPAA), then this clean claim meets all the HIPAA submission requirements and is in compliance with that Act.

Claims management process: The internal workflow for preparing and submitting claims and collecting payment on the claims.

Super bill: The form that physician practices and other facilities use to record services rendered by a physician or health care professional during the patient encounter.

CMS-1500: The universal claim form that physicians and other health care professionals use to submit claims to Medicare; also, the claim form most health insurers accept.

Clearinghouse: An entity that submits electronic claims on behalf of providers while maintaining the health insurer requirements for claim submission specified by each payer.

FIGURE AA-1 *Sample Encounter Form (Super Bill)*

Jane Doe, M.D.
Internal Medicine
300 Practitioner Road
Smallville, State 99999

Telephone: (555) 555-1212

DATE:

LAST NAME	FIRST	ACCOUNT#	DOB	☐ Male ☐ Female
INSURANCE		PLAN#	SUBSCRIBER#	GROUP#

OFFICE CARE

√ DESCRIPTION	CPT-MOD		
NEW PATIENT			
Focused	99201		
Expanded	99202		
Detailed	99203		
Comprehensive-Mod.	99204		
Comprehensive-High	99205		
ESTABLISHED PATIENT			
Minimal	99211		
Focused	99212		
Expanded	99213		
Detailed	99214		
Comprehensive-Mod.	99215		
Comprehensive-High	99216		
CONSULTATION OFFICE			
Focused	99241		
Expanded	99242		
Detailed	99243		
Comprehensive-Mod.	99254		
Comprehensive-High	99265		
Dr.			
Post-op Exam	99024		
EVALUATION/MANAGEMENT			
Brief - 30 minutes	99361		
Intermediate - 60	99362		
Telephone-Brief	99371		
Telephone-Intermed.	99372		
Telephone-Complex	99373		

PROCEDURES

√ DESCRIPTION	CPT-MOD		
Treadmill	93015		
24 Hour Holter	93224		
Recording only	93225		
Interp. & Report	93227		
EKG and interp.	93000		
EKG (Medicare)	93005		
Sigmoidoscopy	45300		
Sigmoidoscopy (flex)	45330		
Sigmoid (flex) w/bx	45331		

DIAGNOSIS

052.9	Chickenpox, NOS	266.2	B12 deficiency w/o anemia	309.9	Adjustment reaction, unspecified
111.9	Dermatomycosis, unspecified	276.5	Dehydration	305.00	Alcohol abuse, unspecified
009.1	Gastroenteritis, infectious	250.91	Diabetes mellitus, I, compl	303.90	Alcoholism, unspecified
007.1	Giardiasis	250.01	Diabetes mellitus, I, uncompl	331.0	Alzheimers
098.0	Gonorrhea, acute, lower GU	250.90	Diabetes mellitus, II, compl	307.1	Anorexia nervosa
054.9	Herpes simplex, any site	250.00	Diabetes mellitus, II, uncompl	300.00	Anxiety state, unspecified
053.9	Herpes zoster, NOS	250.13	Diabetic ketoacidosis	314.01	Attention deficit, w/ hyperactivity
042	HIV Disease	271.9	Glucose intolerance		
V08	HIV positive, asymp	240.9	Goiter, unspecified	314.00	Attention deficit, w/o hyperactivity
136.9	Infectious/parasitic dis unspec	274.9	Gout, unspecified		
487.1	Influenza w/ upper resp sx	275.42	Hypercalcemia	307.51	Bulimia
007.9	Intestinal protozoa, NOS	276.7	Hyperkalemia	312.90	Conduct disorder, unspecified
088.81	Lyme disease	276.0	Hypernatremia	311	Depressive disorder, NOS
055.9	Measles, NOS	252.0	Hyperparathyroidism	305.90	Drug abuse, unspecified

DIAGNOSIS			☐ Cash
RETURN APPT	REFERRING MD	SIGNATURE	☐ Check ☐ Credit

Source: American Medical Association. *Mastering the Reimbursement Process.* 3rd Ed. Chicago, IL: AMA Press; 2000.

Appendix A

Claim Forms

The billing staff is responsible for accurately reporting and billing ICD-9 and CPT codes and fees as they appear on the super bill. Once the codes from the super bill and medical record have been selected and verified, it is now time to enter the codes onto the claim form. When completing a claim form, whether on paper (**CMS-1500** form, see Figure AA-2) or electronic, it is important to include the appropriate CPT codes (the most comprehensive CPT code is generally listed first), linked with the appropriate ICD-9 codes to the highest level of specificity, and any HCPCS codes (discussed in Chapter 1).

Once the billing staff generates a claim, it is sent either by mail or electronically transmitted to the health insurer through a **clearinghouse** or other electronic submission provider. It is important to review each claim before submission to ensure all the required fields have been completed.

Key Terms

- **Explanation of benefits (EOB)**

- **Remittance advice (RA)**

- **Clearinghouse**

What Happens to My Claim Once I Submit It?

After the claim has been accurately coded, listing all of the procedures and services rendered, and sent to the third-party payer, what happens to the claim? Each third-party payer processes claims differently. The information in this Appendix is intended to be a brief overview and is only a general list of steps insurers may take once a claim is received, and it is not meant to be a comprehensive or inclusive list of steps that insurers always take in processing claims.

If a claim is lacking required information, such as the patient's date of birth, or a valid current CPT code, the claim will not be processed and will be rejected, and the provider will be notified. The claim will then need to be corrected and resubmitted by the billing staff. However, once a clean claim is received by the third-party payer, the patient's eligibility and benefit level are first assessed. Meaning, if the patient's insurance coverage terminated prior to the date of service, the claim will be denied, and the **explanation of benefits (EOB)** or **remittance advice (RA)** will be sent to the provider explaining so.

The health insurer will process the claim and, if approved for payment, a payment will be routed to the physician along with an EOB or RA. Another EOB is sent to the patient. The EOB is an explanation of the third-party payers' allowed and covered charges, the amount the patient may owe (from their deductible, coinsurance, or copayment amount), and any contractual adjustments (amounts not covered by the insurer that the patient is not responsible to pay). The EOB also includes the patient name, insurer member identification number, group number, dates of service, and charges with fees. An RA is similar to an EOB with similar information, and it outlines the reimbursement data for single or multiple patient claims, but is generally electronic.

If the patient is found to be eligible for insurance coverage, the processing of the claim continues. Third-party payers may apply what is

FIGURE AA-2 *CMS 1500 Form*

PLEASE
DO NOT
STAPLE
IN THIS
AREA

CARRIER →

[ ] [ ] PICA

HEALTH INSURANCE CLAIM FORM

PICA [ ] [ ]

1. MEDICARE	MEDICAID	CHAMPUS	CHAMPVA	GROUP HEALTH PLAN	FECA BLK LUNG	OTHER	1a. INSURED'S I.D. NUMBER	(FOR PROGRAM IN ITEM 1)
(Medicare #)	(Medicaid #)	(Sponsor's SSN)	(VA File #)	(SSN or ID)	(SSN)	(ID)		

2. PATIENT'S NAME (Last Name, First Name, Middle Initial)

3. PATIENT'S BIRTH DATE MM | DD | YY   SEX   M [ ] F [ ]

4. INSURED'S NAME (Last Name, First Name, Middle Initial)

5. PATIENT'S ADDRESS (No., Street)

6. PATIENT RELATIONSHIP TO INSURED   Self [ ] Spouse [ ] Child [ ] Other [ ]

7. INSURED'S ADDRESS (No., Street)

CITY   STATE

8. PATIENT STATUS   Single [ ] Married [ ] Other [ ]

CITY   STATE

ZIP CODE   TELEPHONE (Include Area Code) ( )

Employed [ ] Full-Time Student [ ] Part-Time Student [ ]

ZIP CODE   TELEPHONE (INCLUDE AREA CODE) ( )

9. OTHER INSURED'S NAME (Last Name, First Name, Middle Initial)

10. IS PATIENT'S CONDITION RELATED TO:

11. INSURED'S POLICY GROUP OR FECA NUMBER

a. OTHER INSURED'S POLICY OR GROUP NUMBER

a. EMPLOYMENT? (CURRENT OR PREVIOUS)   YES [ ] NO [ ]

a. INSURED'S DATE OF BIRTH MM | DD | YY   SEX   M [ ] F [ ]

b. OTHER INSURED'S DATE OF BIRTH MM | DD | YY   SEX   M [ ] F [ ]

b. AUTO ACCIDENT?   PLACE (State)   YES [ ] NO [ ]

b. EMPLOYER'S NAME OR SCHOOL NAME

c. EMPLOYER'S NAME OR SCHOOL NAME

c. OTHER ACCIDENT?   YES [ ] NO [ ]

c. INSURANCE PLAN NAME OR PROGRAM NAME

d. INSURANCE PLAN NAME OR PROGRAM NAME

10d. RESERVED FOR LOCAL USE

d. IS THERE ANOTHER HEALTH BENEFIT PLAN?   YES [ ] NO [ ] *If yes*, return to and complete item 9 a-d.

READ BACK OF FORM BEFORE COMPLETING & SIGNING THIS FORM.

12. PATIENT'S OR AUTHORIZED PERSON'S SIGNATURE I authorize the release of any medical or other information necessary to process this claim. I also request payment of government benefits either to myself or to the party who accepts assignment below.

SIGNED _____   DATE _____

13. INSURED'S OR AUTHORIZED PERSON'S SIGNATURE I authorize payment of medical benefits to the undersigned physician or supplier for services described below.

SIGNED _____

14. DATE OF CURRENT: MM | DD | YY   ◄ ILLNESS (First symptom) OR INJURY (Accident) OR PREGNANCY(LMP)

15. IF PATIENT HAS HAD SAME OR SIMILAR ILLNESS. GIVE FIRST DATE MM | DD | YY

16. DATES PATIENT UNABLE TO WORK IN CURRENT OCCUPATION MM | DD | YY   FROM   TO   MM | DD | YY

17. NAME OF REFERRING PHYSICIAN OR OTHER SOURCE

17a. I.D. NUMBER OF REFERRING PHYSICIAN

18. HOSPITALIZATION DATES RELATED TO CURRENT SERVICES MM | DD | YY   FROM   TO   MM | DD | YY

19. RESERVED FOR LOCAL USE

20. OUTSIDE LAB?   YES [ ] NO [ ] $ CHARGES

21. DIAGNOSIS OR NATURE OF ILLNESS OR INJURY. (RELATE ITEMS 1,2,3 OR 4 TO ITEM 24E BY LINE)

1. |___.___| 3. |___.___|

2. |___.___| 4. |___.___|

22. MEDICAID RESUBMISSION CODE   ORIGINAL REF. NO.

23. PRIOR AUTHORIZATION NUMBER

24. A DATE(S) OF SERVICE From MM DD YY To MM DD YY	B Place of Service	C Type of Service	D PROCEDURES, SERVICES, OR SUPPLIES (Explain Unusual Circumstances) CPT/HCPCS	MODIFIER	E DIAGNOSIS CODE	F $ CHARGES	G DAYS OR UNITS	H EPSDT Family Plan	I EMG	J COB	K RESERVED FOR LOCAL USE
1											
2											
3											
4											
5											
6											

25. FEDERAL TAX I.D. NUMBER   SSN [ ] EIN [ ]

26. PATIENT'S ACCOUNT NO.

27. ACCEPT ASSIGNMENT? (For govt. claims, see back)   YES [ ] NO [ ]

28. TOTAL CHARGE $

29. AMOUNT PAID $

30. BALANCE DUE $

31. SIGNATURE OF PHYSICIAN OR SUPPLIER INCLUDING DEGREES OR CREDENTIALS (I certify that the statements on the reverse apply to this bill and are made a part thereof.)

SIGNED _____   DATE _____

32. NAME AND ADDRESS OF FACILITY WHERE SERVICES WERE RENDERED (If other than home or office)

33. PHYSICIAN'S, SUPPLIER'S BILLING NAME, ADDRESS, ZIP CODE & PHONE #

PIN#   GRP#

(APPROVED BY AMA COUNCIL ON MEDICAL SERVICE 8/88)   *PLEASE PRINT OR TYPE*   APPROVED OMB-0938-0008 FORM CMS-1500 (12-90), FORM RRB-1500,
APPROVED OMB-1215-0055 FORM OWCP-1500,   APPROVED OMB-0720-0001 (CHAMPUS)

PATIENT AND INSURED INFORMATION

PHYSICIAN OR SUPPLIER INFORMATION

Appendix A

called **claim edits** that affect the claim payment during their claim processing. The health insurer then generates an EOB or RA and sends that to the provider along with any payment.

Once EOBs and RAs are received, billers and coders should carefully review them to be sure that the codes submitted for the services and procedures performed were appropriately processed and paid by checking for inappropriately denied or bundled procedures. Claims may need to be corrected and resubmitted, or an appeal for the denied or bundled procedures may need to be sent requesting further payment from the insurer.

Key Terms

Explanation of benefits (EOB): An explanation of the health insurer's allowed and covered charges, the amount the patient may owe (from their deductible, coinsurance, or copayment amount), and any contractual adjustments (amounts not covered by the insurer that the patient is not responsible to pay).

Remittance advice (RA): A report, generally electronic, that outlines reimbursement data for single or multiple patient claims. It generally includes the patient name, insurer member identification number, group number, dates of service, charges with fees, the covered amount (or allowed charges), the noncovered amount (due to contractual agreements [patient is not responsible for] or not covered for policy exclusion or other reasons, as well as the portion (eg, deductible, coinsurance, copayment) that patient is responsible for, and the amount the insurer will pay.

Claim edits: A set of business rules that the health insurer establishes to ensure that specific fields are completed and CPT codes are paid in accordance with the health insurer's business design.

Health Insurance Portability and Accountability Act (HIPAA): A law requiring, among other things, all third-party payers to use and accept CPT codes and modifiers for procedure coding and ICD-9-CM for diagnosis coding.

HIPAA

All third-party payers follow certain procedures when a claim is received. There are many differences in the way third-party payers process and pay claims. For example, some may reimburse for the least expensive, similar procedure if conflicting information is reported.

Effective October 16, 2003, the Department of Health and Human Services (HHS) required that all claims be submitted electronically to Medicare unless a waiver is obtained. Since then, the standard transaction or electronic claim form is the 837. This replaced the CMS 1500 format for professional claims and the UB-92 form for institutional claims. Additional information can be obtained at the Centers for Medicare & Medicaid Services (CMS) Web site at www.hhs.gov.

The **Health Insurance Portability and Accountability Act (HIPAA)** requires, among other things, all third-party payers to use and accept CPT codes and modifiers for procedure coding, and ICD-9-CM for diagnosis coding. Payers can no longer generate their own codes.

Most claims-related transactions are electronic in nature. This paperless transmission eliminates many of the problems of mailed claims and allows for faster payment. The electronic health care transactions standard is a federal law. All HIPAA-covered entities must comply with this law. HIPAA electronic transactions promote better communication among providers, payers, and patients through the use of a designated set of codes to identify services, procedures, and other information related to the delivery of health care.

Upcoming Changes Impacting Claims Submissions

ICD-10

HHS announced that starting on October 1, 2013, ICD-10 will replace ICD-9 as the HIPAA-adopted code set for use in inpatient settings for coding diagnoses, inpatient hospital procedures, and in physicians' offices and other outpatient settings for diagnoses. Please note that CPT will remain in place to identify procedural services in physician offices and outpatient settings.

HHS is requiring the move from ICD-9 to ICD-10 because they, and others in the health care community, believe the current ICD-9 code set is outdated and lacks room for new codes, and that ICD-10 provides greater code specificity and will provide better data for public health surveillance and research initiatives.

CMS is the agency within HHS that will oversee the adoption of ICD-10. The National Center for Health Statistics (NCHS) maintains the ICD-10-CM code set for diagnoses. You can access information and the code set files on the NCHS Web site at www.cdc.gov/nchs/icd.htm.

HIPAA 5010

The current version of the electronic transactions named in HIPAA is Version 4010 and is used to electronically submit transactions, such as checking a patient's eligibility, filing a claim, or receiving a remittance advice. Within the current HIPAA 4010, numerous technical issues were identified within the transactions and were corrected, and changes were made to accommodate new business needs. As a result, a newer version of each transaction, named Version 5010, will be required for use by physicians and others on January 1, 2012. CMS is the agency within HHS charged with overseeing compliance with the standards.

Appendix A

Answers to Chapter Exercises

Chapter 1 – Introduction to CPT Coding

1. There are eight sections in the CPT codebook.

2. Evaluation and Management, Anesthesia, Surgery, Radiology, Pathology and Laboratory, Medicine, Category II, Category III codes.

3. The Appendixes are located in the back of the CPT codebook.

4. From a historical perspective, procedures and services have been placed in the CPT codebook in general sections according to where physicians will most conveniently find them. The CPT code set is not a strict classification system; there may be some procedures that appear in sections other than those in which the user might expect to find them.

5. Unlisted procedure codes provide the means of reporting and tracking services and procedures until a more specific code is established in the CPT code set.

6. Modifiers are appended to CPT codes to indicate that a performed service or procedure has been altered or modified by some specific circumstance, but not changed in its definition.

7. Following are some examples of modifier use:

   - To report only the professional component of a procedure or service.
   - To report a service mandated by a third-party payer.
   - To indicate that a procedure was performed bilaterally.
   - To report multiple procedures performed at the same session by the same provider.
   - To report that a portion of a service or procedure is reduced or eliminated at the physician's discretion.
   - To report assistant surgeon services.

8. The format of the terminology was originally developed as stand-alone descriptions of medical procedures. However, to conserve space and avoid having to repeat common terminology, some of the procedure descriptors in the CPT codebook are not printed in

their entirety, but rather refer back to a previous code that shares a portion of the procedure descriptor.

9. The index is located after the appendixes in the CPT codebook.

10. i

11. j

12. h

13. f

14. d

15. c

16. a

17. e

18. b

19. g

20. a

21. b

22. f

23. c

24. d

25. e

Chapter 2 – Evaluation and Management

1. d

Rationale for Code Selection: The counseling physician may perform the evaluation of the patient, initiate diagnostic services, and initiate therapy at the same encounter. This activity assumes that the consultation has been requested and that the consulting physician provides and documents it and communicates the consulting opinion and any services provided in a written report to the requesting physician. The service may be coded as a consultation with codes **99241-99245**.

2. **99238** **Hospital discharge day management;** 30 minutes or less or 99239 more than 30 minutes

3. **99392** **Periodic comprehensive preventive** medicine reevaluation and management of an individual including an age and gender appropriate history, examination, counseling/anticipatory guidance/risk factor reduction interventions, and the ordering of appropriate laboratory/diagnostic procedures, established patient; early childhood (age 1 through 4 years)

   ● **90460** Immunization administration through 18 years of age via any route of administration, with counseling by physician or other qualified health care professional; first vaccine/toxoid component

➕ ● **90461**   each additional vaccine/toxoid component (List separately in addition to code for primary procedure)

▶ (Use 90460 for each vaccine administered. For vaccines with multiple components [combination vaccines], report 90460 in conjunction with 90461 for each additional component in a given vaccine) ◀

▶ (90465-90468 have been deleted. To report, see 90460, 90461, 90471-90474) ◀

90700   Diphtheria, tetanus toxoids, and acellular pertussis vaccine (DTaP), when administered to individuals younger than 7 years, for intramuscular use

Rationale for Code Selection: As an uneventful well-child visit for an established patient between the ages of one and four years, the visit is reported with code **99392**. If the child were a new patient, the visit would be reported with code **99382**.

In addition, the diphtheria, tetanus toxoids, and acellular pertussis vaccine (DTaP) immunization merits code **90700**. The corresponding administration codes are **90460** and **90461**.

4. 99402   **Preventive medicine counseling** and/or risk factor reduction intervention(s) provided to an individual (separate procedure); approximately 30 minutes

Rationale for Code Selection: The focus of this encounter is in providing counseling, specifically risk-factor reduction and patient education, so an evaluation and management (E/M) code should be submitted. The patient's lack of a chief complaint or symptom rules out the use of a standard office visit code. Instead, the appropriate code to submit is **99402**. According to CPT coding guidelines, preventive medicine codes **99401** to **99412** are to be used for services provided "at a separate encounter for the purpose of promoting health and preventing illness or injury" for patients without symptoms or established illness. These codes may be used to describe counseling, anticipatory guidance, or risk factor–reduction interventions provided separately from or without a preventive service examination.

5. 99285   Emergency department visit for the evaluation and management of a patient, which requires these 3 key components within the constraints imposed by the urgency of the patient's clinical condition and/or mental status
- **A comprehensive history;**
- **A comprehensive examination; and**
- **Medical decision making of high complexity.**

Counseling and/or coordination of care with other providers or agencies are provided consistent with the nature of the problem(s) and the patient's and/or family's needs.

Usually, the presenting problem(s) are of high severity and pose an immediate significant threat to life or physiologic function.

Rationale for Code Selection: Although the patient's medical condition might appear to meet the criteria for critical care, the physician did not provide services for a sufficient length of time to be eligible to report critical care services code **99291**. Code **99291** requires a minimum of 30 minutes of critical care services provision, in total, for the patient by the physician on any one date. Therefore, the appropriate emergency department E/M service should be reported.

It seems evident that the nature of the patient's presenting problem is consistent with code **99285**. Whereas it is noted that the medical history and physical examination available and/or performed are insufficient to satisfy the criteria for the key components of code **99285**, the descriptor for code **99285** allows the criteria for the key components to be waived when appropriate (ie, ". . . within the constraints imposed by the urgency of the patient's clinical condition and/or mental status"). Such waiver of criteria for key components is allowable only with code **99285** in the emergency department E/M code set.

6. Emergency department services code (**99281-99285**) appropriate to service performed and documented in medical record.

99291   Critical care, evaluation and management of the critically ill or critically injured patient; first 30–74 minutes

93010   Electrocardiogram, routine ECG with at least 12 leads; interpretation and report only

31500   Intubation, endotracheal, emergency procedure

92950   Cardiopulmonary resuscitation (eg, in cardiac arrest)

93010 76   Electrocardiogram, routine ECG with at least 12 leads; interpretation and report only

93042   Rhythm ECG, 1–3 leads; interpretation and report only

Rationale for Code Selection: Code **99291**: For most ED patients, critical care services can be reported in addition to other E/M services provided on the same date. The patient was critically ill for 80 minutes, during which the attending ED physician was providing services. However, the time spent in separately reportable services performed during critical care (eg, codes **92950**, **31500**, **93010**, **93042**, etc) cannot be counted in determining the total physician-provided critical care service time. In this instance, code **92950** comprised 20 minutes. The performance of the other separately reportable services would consume some additional time, leaving a total assessable physician-provided critical care service time as the physician documented at 44 minutes.

Code **93010**: Because the electrocardiogram (ECG) was performed in the hospital by hospital-employed (rather than physician-employed) staff using hospital-owned equipment, only the interpretation and report is reported by the physician.

Code **31500**: Endotracheal intubation is not included in the cardiopulmonary resuscitation service, which encompasses basic cardiopulmonary resuscitation activities only. The endotracheal intubation is also not included in critical care services and is therefore reported separately. However, the time spent in providing the endotracheal intubation service cannot be counted when the total physician-provided critical care service time is determined for coding purposes.

Code **92950**: Basic cardiopulmonary resuscitation consists of assessing the patient, opening the airway, restoring breathing (eg, mouth-to-mouth, bag valve mask), then restoring circulation (eg, closed-chest cardiac massage). In most instances, cardiopulmonary resuscitation is performed first, sometimes with continuation during advanced life support interventions (eg, drug therapy and defibrillation) that would be included by reporting the appropriate critical care service code(s). Also, when endotracheal intubation is performed, it is appropriate to separately report code **31500**.

Code **93010 76**: ECG interpretation is not included in critical care or the cardiopulmonary resuscitation service. Because the ECG was performed in the hospital by hospital-employed (rather than physician-employed) staff using hospital-owned equipment, only the interpretation and report is reported by the physician. Also, because the ECG service (**93010**) was performed subsequent to the initial ECG service (**93010**) on the same date for the same patient by the same physician, this additional procedure may be identified by appending **modifier 76**, *Repeat procedure by same physician.*

Code **93042**: Rhythm ECG is not included in critical care and in cardiopulmonary resuscitation. Because the rhythm ECG was performed in the hospital by hospital-employed (rather than physician-employed) staff using hospital-owned equipment, only the interpretation and report are reported by the physician.

7. **99214** **Office or other outpatient visit** for the evaluation and management of an established patient, which requires at least 2 of these 3 key components:
   - **A detailed history;**
   - **A detailed examination;**
   - **Medical decision making of moderate complexity.**

   Counseling and/or coordination of care with other providers or agencies are provided consistent with the nature of the problem(s) and the patient's and/or family's needs.

   Usually, the presenting problem(s) are of moderate to high severity. Physicians typically spend 25 minutes face-to-face with the patient and/or family.

   99354 Prolonged physician service in the office or other outpatient setting requiring direct (face-to-face) patient contact beyond the usual service; first hour (List separately in addition to code for office or other outpatient **Evaluation and Management** service)

Rationale for Code Selection: Prolonged service codes are reported when the service for direct patient contact exceeds the usual time spent for the patient encounter. The code is reported in addition to the E/M code for the patient visit (consultation, new patient, or established patient). The basis for billing is time and not history, physical examination, or medical decision making. Documentation of the reason for the prolonged service must be included in the record. In this case, the neurologist spent 75 minutes face-to-face with the patient, because of the extended amount of outside records and complexity of the case.

The base E/M code in this scenario is **99214**, which typically requires 25 minutes face-to-face with the patient. The prolonged services code **99354** is reported for the first hour of prolonged outpatient service beyond the E/M service typical time. An hour is defined as 31 to 74 minutes. In this case, the face-to-face time was 25 plus 50 minutes. Thus, codes **99214** and **99354** are reported. If the physician spent 90 minutes face-to-face, then the appropriate coding would be **99214** plus prolonged services codes **99354** and **99355** once each. The code **99355** is for each additional half hour beyond the 74-minute limit defined for code **99354**.

8. **99291** Critical care, evaluation and management of the critically ill or critically injured patient; first 30–74 minutes

   99292   each additional 30 minutes

   (Report code **99291** once and code **99292** three times.)

   Rationale for Code Selection: Critical care codes **99291** and **99292** are used to report the total duration spent by a physician providing critical care services to a critically ill or critically injured patient, even if the time spent by the physician on that date is not continuous. For any given period of time spent providing critical care services, the physician must devote full attention to the patient and, therefore, cannot provide services to any other patient during the same period. In this scenario, the neurologist spent two and one half hours (150 minutes) providing critical care services on the same date. Therefore, code **99291** should be reported once, and code **99292** should be reported three times.

9. A

   99363 Anticoagulant management for an outpatient taking warfarin, physician review and interpretation of International Normalized Ratio (INR) testing, patient instructions, dosage adjustment (as needed), and ordering of additional tests; initial 90 days of therapy (must include a minimum of 8 INR measurements)

   Rationale for Code Selection: Codes **99363** and **99364** are intended to report physician management of patients receiving long-term anticoagulant therapy (eg, warfarin) in the office or outpatient setting, including domiciliary, rest home, or home settings in 90-day increments. Code **99363** is used to report the initial 90 days of therapy and requires that a minimum of eight international normalized ratio (INR) tests are reviewed. Subsequent therapy sessions after the initial therapy period are reported with code **99364** and must include at least three INR measurements. To report either of these 90-day increment codes, the physician manages the patient on anticoagulation therapy for at least 60 continuous days. Therefore, the physician should report code **99363** for the initial 90 days of therapy and requires that a minimum of eight INR tests are reviewed.

10. B

   99339 Individual physician supervision of a patient (patient not present) in home, domiciliary or rest home (eg, assisted living facility) requiring complex and multidisciplinary

Appendix B

care modalities involving regular physician development and/or revision of care plans, review of subsequent reports of patient status, review of related laboratory and other studies, communication (including telephone calls) for purposes of assessment or care decisions with health care professional(s), family member(s), surrogate decision maker(s) (eg, legal guardian) and/or key caregiver(s) involved in patient's care, integration of new information into the medical treatment plan and/or adjustment of medical therapy, within a calendar month; 15–29 minutes

Rationale for Code Selection: Code **99339** is intended to report care plan oversight services of children and adults with special health care needs and chronic medical conditions provided by primary care physicians who coordinate the medical care management with other medical and nonmedical service providers and family. This code may encompass oversight of work or school programs the patient may be attending where therapy is provided. Therefore, the physician should report code **99339** for the 15 minutes of the care plan oversight service.

Chapter 3 – Anesthesia

1. True. Based on the Anesthesia Guidelines, anesthesia time begins when the anesthesiologist begins to prepare the patient for induction of anesthesia, and ends when the patient is safely placed under postoperative supervision. Therefore, the correct answer is True.

2. False. It is not appropriate to report add-on code **99116** as a stand alone code. Add-on codes are always performed in addition to the primary service or procedure and must never be reported as a stand alone code. Therefore, the correct answer is False.

3. True. The phrases "requiring anesthesia," or "with anesthesia" in their descriptors indicate that the work involved in performing that procedure requires anesthesia, whether it is general anesthesia, regional anesthesia, or monitored anesthesia care (MAC). The appropriate anesthesia code may be reported separately. Therefore, the correct answer is True.

4. True. Moderate (conscious) sedation is a drug-induced depression of consciousness during which patients respond purposefully to verbal commands, either alone or accompanied by light tactile stimulation. Therefore, it is not an anesthesia service because the patient cannot be aroused, even by painful stimulation. The correct answer is True.

5. False. The physical status modifiers are identified with the initial letter "P." Therefore the correct answer is False.

6. True. There may be times when other CPT modifiers may be appended with an anesthesia procedure code and a physical status modifier. Therefore, the correct answer is True.

7. P2

8. P5

9. P1

10. P6

11. P3

Chapter 4 – Surgery: Integumentary System

1. True

2. False. The margins refer to the *narrowest* margin required to adequately excise the lesion, based on the physician's judgment.

3. True

4. True

5. False. Codes **19100-19499** are **not** considered bilateral procedures.

6. c

7. e

8. d

9. a

10. f

11. b

12. b

13. a

14. c

15. c

16. b

Chapter 4 – Surgery: Musculoskeletal System

1. False. The codes for trigger point injections, **20552** and **20553**, are intended to be reported once per session, regardless of the number of trigger points or muscles injected.

2. True

3. True

4. False. Fracture reduction and bone biopsy are incidental to code **22523** and should not be reported separately.

5. True.

6. c

7. a

8. d

9. e

10. b

11. c

12. b

13. b

14. a

15. c

16. a

17. b

18. c

19. b

Chapter 4 – Surgery: Respiratory System

1. False. Surgical sinus endoscopy codes **do** include sinusotomy and diagnostic endoscopy.

2. False. The code descriptor for **31231** includes both the termsunilateral or bilateral. Therefore, if performed either unilaterally or bilaterally it would not be appended with the modifier **50**.

3. False. Bronchoscopy codes **31615-31629**, **31634**, **31635**, and **31645-31656** include conscious sedation as an inherent component of the procedure, and therefore, conscious sedation would not be reported separately. These codes are identified in the CPT codebook with the conscious sedation symbol ⊙.

4. False. Code **32855**, *Backbench standard preparation of cadaver donor lung allograft prior to transplantation, including dissection of allograft from surrounding soft tissues to prepare pulmonary venous/ atrial cuff, pulmonary artery, and bronchus; unilateral*, is reported for a unilateral procedure, while code **32856**, *Backbench standard preparation of cadaver donor lung allograft prior to transplantation, including dissection of allograft from surrounding soft tissues to prepare pulmonary venous/atrial cuff, pulmonary artery, and bronchus;*

bilateral, is reported when the procedure is performed bilaterally. When both a unilateral and bilateral code for a procedure are available, it would not be appropriate to report the bilateral procedure with the modifier **52**, *Reduced services.* Therefore, the correct code for the actual procedure performed (**32855**) would be selected.

5. When performed bilaterally, surgical endoscopy code **31237** is reported with the modifier **50** appended.

6. No. Code 31505 is for an indirect diagnostic larynoscopy. To select the appropriate code, choose from the direct diagnostic larynoscopy codes **31520**, **31525**, and **31526**.

7. Code **31628** is reported for the transbronchial biopsy in the right lower lobe. Even though three to six biopsies were obtained, code **31628** is reported only once, as the descriptors specify biopsy or biopsies, which indicates that this code is reported for one or multiple transbronchial biopsies. Also, fluoroscopic guidance is not reported separately, since it is included in this procedure.

31628 Bronchoscopy, rigid or flexible, with or without fluoroscopic guidance, when performed; with transbronchial lung biopsy(s), single lobe

8. Code **31636** is reported for the bronchoscopy with placement of the bronchial stent in the left lower lobe bronchus

31636 Bronchoscopy, rigid or flexible, with or without fluoroscopic guidance, when performed; with placement of bronchial stent(s) (includes tracheal/bronchial dilation as required), initial bronchus

Chapter 4 – Surgery: Cardiovascular System

1. True. According to CPT coding guidelines, if removal and replacement procedures are performed, then both procedures are reported separately.

2. False. Procurement of the upper-extremity vein is not included when a coronary artery bypass graft (CABG) or lower-extremity bypass procedure is reported. Code **35500** is separately reported in addition to the grafting procedure for the harvest of a single vein segment for use in a lower-extremity bypass or CABG procedure.

3. A dual-chamber pacemaker system involves the insertion of electrodes into both the atrium and the right ventricle that are then connected to a pulse generator capable of pacing and sensing both the atrium and the ventricle. If removal and replacement procedures are performed, both procedures are reported separately. Code **33208** is reported for the insertion of the permanent pacemaker and electrodes in the atrium and ventricle. Codes **33233** and **33235** are reported for the removal of the pulse generator (battery) and transvenous electrodes, dual-lead system.

33208   Insertion of permanent pacemaker with transvenous electrode(s); atrial and ventricular

33233   Removal of permanent pacemaker pulse generator

33235   Removal of transvenous pacemaker electrode(s); dual lead system

4. Code **35600** is intended to report the harvest of an upper extremity artery for use in coronary artery bypass grafting (CABG). This includes the procurement, implantation, and management of the free radial artery graft. Use of other arteries listed in the Coronary Artery Bypass guidelines is included within the CABG procedure.

35600   Harvest of upper extremity artery, 1 segment, for coronary artery bypass procedure (List separately in addition to code for primary procedure)

5. Code **33533** is reported for the single arterial graft, left internal mammary artery to left anterior descending artery. Add-on code **33517** is reported for the single venous graft, saphenous vein graft to the right coronary artery. Because this was a reoperation with the original CABG two years ago, add-on code **33530** is reported for the reoperation procedure. Code **33530** is reported to reflect the increased difficulty associated with the coronary artery bypass reoperation procedure.

33533   Coronary artery bypass, using arterial graft(s); single arterial graft

+33517   Coronary artery bypass, using venous graft(s) and arterial graft(s); single vein graft (List separately in addition to code for primary procedure)

+33530   Reoperation, coronary artery bypass procedure or valve procedure, more than 1 month after original operation (List separately in addition to code for primary procedure)

6. An arterial nonselective access code is used with the radiological supervision and interpretation (RS&I) code to describe the study of the abdominal aorta. Additional views of the abdominal aorta (ie, lateral, oblique, or rotational) are not separately coded because they are considered inclusive of the RS&I of the aortogram.

36200   Introduction of catheter, aorta

75625   Aortography, abdominal, by serialography, radiological supervision and interpretation

7. The right and left pulmonary arteries are each first-order selective catheter placements, and because these are bilateral, the first-order selective **36014** is used with modifier **50** appended to indicate the bilateral study. The RS&I code (**75743**) is used to describe the bilateral pulmonary arteriograms.

36014 50   Selective catheter placement, left or right pulmonary artery (bilateral)

75743   Angiography, pulmonary, bilateral, selective, radiological supervision and interpretation

8. Each physician performed distinct parts of the procedure; therefore, using the component coding convention, each physician reports the codes describing the individual services performed. Additionally, the two physicians also worked as cosurgeons to perform one total procedure (**34803**, *Endovascular repair of infrarenal abdominal aortic aneurysm or dissection; using modular bifurcated endoprosthesis [2 docking limbs]*). Physician A performed the open femoral artery exposure via bilateral femoral cutdowns. This work is reported with **34812** with modifier **50** appended. Physician B placed the catheters into the aorta from the bilateral femoral exposure sites. This work is reported with **36200** with modifier **50** appended. Physician B also reports code **75952** to describe the RS&I performed for the endovascular repair of the infrarenal abdominal aortic aneurysm (AAA).

Both physicians report code **34803** with modifier **62** appended. Modifier **62** is appended to **34803** because two physicians performed the work included in one total procedure (**34803**, *Endovascular repair of infrarenal abdominal aortic aneurysm or dissection; using modular bifurcated prosthesis [2 docking limbs]*), reportable with a single code. Each surgeon should report the same endovascular repair code with modifier **62** appended. In separate operative reports, both physicians would document their level of involvement in the surgery. Each should include a copy of his or her notes when reporting the service to the third-party payer. If one surgeon does not use modifier **62**, the third-party payer may assume that the physician reporting the procedure without the modifier performed the entire procedure, despite the second physician reporting the procedure with modifier **62**.

Codes for Physician A

34803 62 Endovascular repair of infrarenal abdominal aortic aneurysm or dissection; using modular bifurcated prosthesis (2 docking limbs)

34812 50 Open femoral artery exposure for delivery of endovascular prosthesis, by groin incision, bilateral

Codes for Physician B

34803 62 Endovascular repair of infrarenal abdominal aortic aneurysm or dissection; using modular bifurcated prosthesis (2 docking limbs)

36200 50 Introduction of catheter, aorta (bilateral)

75952 Endovascular repair of infrarenal abdominal aortic aneurysm or dissection, radiological supervision and interpretation

9. Codes **36200**, *Introduction of catheter, aorta,* and **75630** should be reported for the diagnostic angiogram of the aorta and bilateral iliofemoral arteries performed from the left common femoral artery puncture site. Code **75630** represents the RS&I of the diagnostic angiography to detect the site of the endoleak. Because a more selective catheterization is subsequently performed from the same

puncture site (selection of the left hypogastric artery for angiography and embolization), code **36200** is not submitted, because the work of this nonselective catheter placement is included in code **36245**, which is the appropriate code to be submitted. (See continuing rationale following.)

Codes **35473** and **75962** should be reported for the angioplasty of the left common iliac artery to attempt to treat the endoleak filling the inferior aspect of the aneurysmal sac. Code **75962** represents the RS&I associated with the angioplasty procedure (**35473**). (If ballooning had been done *only* to secure the graft extension, **35473** and **75962** would not be coded, because the work of ballooning the new extension is included in the work of code **34825**.)

Codes **37204** and **75894, 75898, 36245,** and **75736** should be reported for the hypogastric artery selective diagnostic angiogram and subsequent embolization procedure.

Codes **34825** and **75953** should be reported to describe placement of an extension graft from the left common iliac artery limb of the endovascular graft across the origin of the hypogastric artery into the left external iliac artery. The angiogram postextension placement and angioplasty to fully open and seat the graft extension are considered inclusive of **34825** and not separately reportable. Because the extension prosthesis is placed subsequent to the postoperative global period (90 days) and is not considered a staged/planned procedure, it would not be necessary to append modifier **58**.

34825	Placement of proximal or distal extension prosthesis for endovascular repair of infrarenal abdominal aortic or iliac aneurysm, false aneurysm, or dissection; initial vessel
36245	Selective catheter placement, arterial system; each first order abdominal, pelvic, or lower extremity artery branch, within a vascular family
75630	Aortography, abdominal plus bilateral iliofemoral lower extremity, catheter, by serialography, radiological supervision and interpretation
75894	Transcatheter therapy, embolization, any method, radiological supervision and interpretation
37204	Transcatheter occlusion or embolization (eg, for tumor destruction, to achieve hemostasis, to occlude a vascular malformation), percutaneous, any method, non-central nervous system, non-head or neck
⊙● **37220**	Revascularization, endovascular, open or percutaneous, iliac artery, unilateral, initial vessel; with transluminal angioplasty
⊙● **37227**	with transluminal stent placement(s) and atherectomy, includes angioplasty within the same vessel, when performed
75898	Angiography through existing catheter for follow-up study for transcatheter therapy, embolization or infusion
75736	Angiography, pelvic, selective or supraselective, radiological supervision and interpretation
75953	Placement of proximal or distal extension prosthesis for endovascular repair of infrarenal aortic or iliac artery aneurysm, pseudoaneurysm, or dissection, radiological supervision and interpretation

75962 Transluminal balloon angioplasty, peripheral artery other than cervical carotid, renal or other visceral artery, iliac, or lower extremity, radiological supervision and interpretation

G0629 Percutaneous closure device

10. Occasionally, prosthesis is necessary during the postoperative follow-up care when the presence of an endoleak becomes evident. The endovascular components shift, creating the threat of an endoleak, or the aneurysm grows or extends distally. Under these circumstances, the placement of further distal prosthesis extensions to extend coverage of the original components is reported using **33886**. The imaging for endovascular thoracic aorta prosthesis placement is reported using **75959**. The endograft extension requires a large-bore sheath to deliver, typically performed through an open exposure of the femoral or iliac artery. In this case, **34812** is used to describe open exposure of the femoral artery. Catheters are placed into the aorta from both femoral arteries (percutaneous on the contralateral side), coded with **36200** using modifier **50** to signify bilateral. The ballooning done to secure the graft and the roadmapping, contrast injections, and final angiograms are included in the work of **33886**.

33886 Placement of distal extension prosthesis(s) delayed after endovascular repair of descending thoracic aorta

75959 Placement of distal extension prosthesis(s) (delayed) after endovascular repair of descending thoracic aorta, as needed, to level of celiac origin, radiological supervision and interpretation

34812 Open femoral artery exposure for delivery of endovascular prosthesis, by groin incision, unilateral

36200 50 Introduction of catheter, aorta (bilateral)

Chapter 4 – Surgery: Digestive System

1. b

2. a

3. c

4. False. When the endoscopy procedures are reported, the surgical endoscopy **does** include the diagnostic endoscopy.

5. True

Chapter 4 – Surgery: Urinary System

1. c

2. a

3. b

4. d

5. True

6. True. When two distinct endoscopic procedures are performed on the same day or at the same session, it is appropriate to report these procedures separately.

7. CPT code **52647** describes laser coagulation of the prostate. This code is intended to describe laser procedures that primarily heat the prostate and require sloughing (the separation of necrosed tissue from living tissue) for the treatment to be complete. This code should be used even if an incision or small amount of vaporization is done in combination with the coagulation. In this case, it is not appropriate to separately report code 52648 for the small amount of vaporization performed.

> **52647** Laser coagulation of prostate, including control of postoperative bleeding, complete (vasectomy, meatotomy, cystourethroscopy, urethral calibration and/or dilation, and internal urethrotomy are included if performed)

Chapter 4 – Surgery: Female Genital System

1. **57456** Colposcopy of the cervix including upper/adjacent vagina; with endocervical curettage

> **56821 51** Colposcopy of the vulva; with biopsy(s) (multiple procedures)

Rationale for Code Selection: Code **57456** describes the examination indicated by the abnormal Pap smear. Code **56821** describes endoscopic examination, magnification, and biopsy of the vulva to evaluate for viral lesions, neoplasia, or malignancy. If multiple biopsies are performed on the vulva during the same session, code **56821** should be reported only one time, as indicated by the optional plural form of biopsy or biopsies. Modifier **51** is appended to indicate that this is an additional biopsy.

2. **58760 50** Fimbrioplasty (bilateral)

Rationale for Code Selection: Because this was an open procedure, code **58760** was selected. Modifier **50**, *Bilateral procedure,* is appended to indicate that the fimbrioplasty was performed on both the right and left sides. Chromotubation is considered an inherent part of this procedure and is not reported separately.

3. **58180** Supracervical abdominal hysterectomy (subtotal hysterectomy), with or without removal of tube(s), with or without removal of ovary(s)

> **57268 59** Repair of enterocele, vaginal approach (separate procedure) (distinct procedural service)

Rationale for Code Selection: The repair of the enterocele is considered a distinct procedural service from the hysterectomy. Therefore, modifier **59** is appended to code **57268** to indicate this.

4. **58550** Laparoscopy, surgical, with vaginal hysterectomy, for uterus 250 g or less

   51990 51 Laparoscopy, surgical; urethral suspension for stress incontinence (multiple procedures)

Rationale for Code Selection: Because the uterus weighed less than 250 g, code **58550** was selected. Because vaginal and laparoscopic hysterectomy codes are differentiated by uterine weight, it is important that the uterine weight be documented in the medical record.

5. **58662** Laparoscopy, surgical; with fulguration or excision of lesions of the ovary, pelvic viscera, or peritoneal surface by any method

   58558 51 Hysteroscopy, surgical; with sampling (biopsy) of endometrium and/or polypectomy, with or without D & C (multiple procedures)

Rationale for Code Selection: A laparoscopy and hysteroscopy are not bundled.

6. **56620** Vulvectomy, simple; partial

Rationale for Code Selection: A simple or partial vulvectomy may include removal of part or all of the labia majora and the labia minora on one side and the clitoris.

7. **99214** **Office or other outpatient visit** for the evaluation and management of an established patient, which requires at least 2 of these 3 key components:
   - **A detailed history;**
   - **A detailed examination;**
   - **Medical decision making of moderate complexity.**

   Counseling and/or coordination of care with other providers or agencies are provided consistent with the nature of the problem(s) and the patient's and/or family's needs.

   Usually, the presenting problem(s) are of moderate to high severity. Physicians typically spend 25 minutes face-to-face with the patient and/or family.

   57260 Combined anteroposterior colporrhaphy

Rationale for Code Selection: Code **99214** is reported for the E/M service (initial office visit) selected based on time spent counseling the patient. This office visit is outside the global surgical package. However, the preoperative visit that occurs the day before the surgery is included in the global surgical package and is not reported separately.

Code **57260** (combined anteroposterior colporrhaphy) is reported for the procedure. The culdoplasty is not separately reported because it was prophylactic.

8. **99202 25** **Office or other outpatient visit** for the evaluation and management of a new patient, which requires these 3 key components:
   - **An expanded problem focused history;**
   - **An expanded problem focused examination;**
   - **Straight forward medical decision making.**

Counseling and/or coordination of care with other providers or agencies are provided consistent with the nature of the problem(s) and the patient's and/or family's needs.

Usually, the presenting problem(s) are of low to moderate severity. Physicians typically spend 20 minutes face-to-face with the patient and/or family.

57454 Colposcopy of the cervix including upper/adjacent vagina; with biopsy(s) of the cervix and endocervical curettage

58110 Endometrial sampling (biopsy) performed in conjunction with colposcopy (List separately in addition to code for primary procedure)

Rationale for Code Selection: Code **99202 25** is reported for the office visit. Modifier **25** indicates that this was a significant, separately identifiable E/M service on the same day as a procedure.

Code **57454** and code **58110** are reported for the procedures performed. Modifier **51** is not appended to code **58110** because it is an add-on code.

9. **99203** **Office or other outpatient visit** for the evaluation and management of a new patient, which requires these 3 key components:
   - **A detailed history;**
   - **A detailed examination;**
   - **Medical decision making of low complexity.**

   Counseling and/or coordination of care with other providers or agencies are provided consistent with the nature of the problem(s) and the patient's and/or family's needs.

   Usually, the presenting problem(s) are of moderate severity. Physicians typically spend 30 minutes face-to-face with the patient and/or family.

   58150 Total abdominal hysterectomy (corpus and cervix), with or without removal of tube(s), with or without removal of ovary(s);

Rationale for Code Selection: Code **99203** is reported for the E/M service (office visit) selected based on time spent counseling the patient. No modifier is needed since this visit was two weeks before the surgery and therefore outside the global package. Procedure code **58150** is reported for the total abdominal hysterectomy. The weight of the specimen does not affect the coding in cases of abdominal hysterectomies.

10. **99243 57** Office consultation for a new or established patient, which requires these 3 key components:
    - **A detailed history;**
    - **A detailed examination;**
    - **Medical decision making of low complexity.**

    Counseling and/or coordination of care with other providers or agencies are provided consistent with the nature of the problem(s) and the patient's and/or family's needs.

    Usually, the presenting problem(s) are of moderate severity. Physicians typically spend 40 minutes face-to-face with the patient and/or family.

58950 Resection (initial) of ovarian, tubal or primary peritoneal malignancy with bilateral salpingo-oophorectomy and omentectomy

Rationale for Code Selection: Code **99243 57** is reported for the consultation based on time spent counseling the patient. Modifier **57** indicates that the decision for surgery was made during this visit and that the visit was during the preoperative global surgical period. Code **58950** is reported for the procedure.

Chapter 4 – Surgery: Maternity Care and Delivery

1. **59515** Cesarean delivery only; including postpartum care

   59426 Antepartum care only; 7 or more visits

   Rationale for Code Selection: Code **59515** is reported by the obstetrician, as this physician provided the cesarean delivery and postpartum care services. Code **59426** is reported by the family physician, as this physician provided only 12 antepartum visits.

   The family physician may report the admission at a level of service for the management of labor (**99281-99285**) that he or she provided, in addition to code **59426**. The obstetrician may report a consultation (**99241-99245**) appended by modifier **57** to indicate the decision for surgery for the evaluation that led to the decision to perform a cesarean. The obstetrician would report code **59515** for the cesarean delivery.

2. **59812** Treatment of incomplete abortion, any trimester, completed surgically

   Rationale for Code Selection: Code **59812** is used to report the dilation and curettage performed by the physician for the surgical management of an incomplete abortion when the uterus is not entirely emptied of the products of conception. The physician removes the remaining tissue by sharp or suction curettage.

3. **59410** Vaginal delivery only (with or without episiotomy and/or forceps); including postpartum care

   Rationale for Code Selection: Code **59410** describes a vaginal delivery and postpartum care when both are provided by the same physician or the same physician group.

4. **59510** Routine obstetric care including antepartum care, cesarean delivery, and postpartum care

   Rationale for Code Selection: Code **59510** is reported for the cesarean delivery of Twin B and code **59409** with modifier **51** appended is reported for the vaginal delivery of Twin A when the global obstetric care is provided by the same physician or same physician group. Note that code **59510** addresses the antepartum and postpartum care. The use of forceps during a vaginal delivery is included and does not warrant separate identification. Also, the diagnosis code for multiple gestations should be indicated.

In this situation, the primary service is the cesarean section, even though it happened second and vaginal delivery was intended. The global code for the cesarean is reported because it is the primary procedure. The "vaginal only" code is reported because there was only one antepartum period and one postpartum period, even though there were two babies.

5. **99202** **Office or other outpatient visit** for the evaluation and management of a new patient, which requires these 3 key components:
   - **An expanded problem focused history;**
   - **An expanded problem focused examination;**
   - **Straightforward medical decision making.**

   Counseling and/or coordination of care with other providers or agencies are provided consistent with the nature of the problem(s) and the patient's and/or family's needs.

   Usually, the presenting problem(s) are of low to moderate severity. Physicians typically spend 20 minutes face-to-face with the patient and/or family.

Rationale for Code Selection: E/M service code **99202** is reported for the first visit. The other antepartum visits are included in the global obstetric package, because she was seen for a total of 13 visits. If the patient had been seen for 14 antepartum visits, the visit at six weeks would be reported separately.

6. **76805** Ultrasound, pregnant uterus, real time with image documentation, fetal and maternal evaluation, after first trimester (> or = 14 weeks 0 days), transabdominal approach; single or first gestation

   76810 each additional gestation (List separately in addition to code for primary procedure)

   59025 Fetal non-stress test

   59510 Routine obstetric care including antepartum care, cesarean delivery, and postpartum care

   59409 51 Vaginal delivery only (with or without episiotomy and/or forceps) (multiple procedures)

Rationale for Code Selection: Codes **76805** and **76810** are reported for ultrasounds performed for the first gestation and for each additional gestation after the first trimester, respectively. No modifier is appended to code **76810** because this is an add-on code.

Code **59025** with a unit of 2 on the claim form is reported for the fetal nonstress tests beginning at 32 weeks.

Code **59510** is reported for the cesarean section delivery of the second twin, and code **59409 51** is reported for the vaginal delivery of the first twin.

7. **59400** Routine obstetric care including antepartum care, vaginal delivery (with or without episiotomy, and/or forceps) and postpartum care

Rationale for Code Selection: The first physician reports the global obstetric package using code **59400**. The assumption is that the two physicians cover for each other.

8. **59425** Antepartum care only; 4–6 visits

59812 Treatment of incomplete abortion, any trimester, completed surgically

Rationale for Code Selection: Code **59425** is reported for the five antepartum visits. Code **59812** is reported for surgical treatment of the incomplete abortion.

Chapter 4 – Surgery: Nervous System

1. True

2. True. Because a lead array contains at least 4 to 8 electrodes, the plural use of the term *electrodes* occurs in the descriptors of the peripheral nerve neurostimulator codes (**64553-64565**). There are multiple electrode contacts on the catheter, plate, or paddle type of electrode array used in brain, spinal cord, sacral, and peripheral nerve stimulation. However, reporting is **per** insertion of either a *single* electrode array or a *single* plate or paddle. Again, it is **not** appropriate to report based on the number of contact electrodes on a single catheter, plate, or paddle surface.

3. False. The fluoroscopic guidance (eg, codes **76000**, **77003**) is considered inherent in the performance of the percutaneous implantation of the neurostimulator electrode array in the epidural space code **63650**, *Percutaneous implantation of neurostimulator electrode array, epidural*. Therefore, the correct answer is False, as it would not be appropriate to additionally report the fluoroscopic guidance used.

4. False. The codes for destruction by neurolytic agent, paravertebral facet joint nerve (**64622-64627**), are considered unilateral procedures. When both right side and left side injections are performed, the bilateral modifier **50** is appended to the appropriate code (eg, **64622 50**).

5. Each surgeon reports only the CPT code for the specific procedure performed. Dr A would report both the approach and definitive procedures performed, and Dr B would report the reconstruction/repair procedure performed. Since Dr A performed more than one procedure (both approach and definitive, then the modifier **51**, *Multiple procedures,* should be appended to the secondary additional procedure.

6. The cranium is divided into the anterior, middle, and posterior fossae.

7. The skull base procedures are categorized into approach procedure(s), definitive procedure(s), and reconstruction/repair.

8. **64614** Chemodenervation of muscle(s); extremity(s) and/or trunk muscle(s) (eg, for dystonia, cerebral palsy, multiple sclerosis)

Code **64614** is reported once, even though multiple injections are performed in sites along a particular muscle (several muscles are typically injected).

9. **62282** Injection/infusion of neurolytic substance (eg, alcohol, phenol, iced saline solutions), with or without other therapeutic substance; epidural, lumbar, sacral (caudal)

   77003 Fluoroscopic guidance and localization of needle or catheter tip for spine or paraspinous diagnostic or therapeutic injection procedures (epidural, subarachnoid, or sacroiliac joint), including neurolytic agent destruction

Code **62282** is reported for the injection of contrast material and the neurolytic substance. Fluoroscopic guidance for needle placement and to confirm that the needle tip is in the exact level for injection to affect the desired nerve, nerve root, or level of spinal cord is reported with **77003**.

Chapter 4 – Surgery: Eye and Ocular Adnexa

1. False. The orbital bones are ordinarily considered part of the musculoskeletal system, but incision and excision of bone(s) of the orbit are described here in the Eye and Ocular Adnexa subsection for convenience of the user of the CPT codebook. Treatments of fractures of the orbital bones are described and coded in the Musculoskeletal System subsection.

2. False. When photodynamic therapy is performed on the second eye at a single session, the bilateral add-on code + **67225** is reported in conjunction with code **67221**. Modifier **50** is not appended to code **67221**.

3. False. When this phrase "one or more sessions" appears in a code descriptor, the code should be reported only once for the entire defined treatment period, regardless of the number of sessions necessary to complete the treatment. In other words, the code would not be reported for each session in which the patient was seen if it was a visit included in a defined treatment period.

4. **67400-67599**

5. No. Code **66710**, *Ciliary body destruction; cyclophotocoagulation, transscleral*, is not reported for an endoscopic approach for ciliary body destruction by cyclophotocoagulation. Code **66711**, *Ciliary body destruction; cyclophotocoagulation, endoscopic,* describes endoscopic photocoagulation of the ciliary body for the treatment of glaucoma. This technique requires a surgical incision for insertion of the endoscope through the anterior segment to provide direct visualization of the tissue to be coagulated. The photocoagulation procedure described by **66710** is performed externally (or transsclerally) without an incision.

Appendix B

6. b. The guidelines above code **67145** explain that the codes that follow them are repetitive services. The guidelines also state that the services are often performed in multiple sessions or groups of sessions, and therefore the descriptors include all sessions in a defined treatment period. Code **67145** is reported only once for the three sessions.

7. m

8. j

9. d

10. b

11. a

12. n

13. h

14. e

15. k

16. c

17. o

18. l

19. s

20. t

21. f

22. i

23. g

24. p

25. q

26. r

Chapter 4 – Surgery: Auditory

1. True

2. The external ear (**69000-69399**) consists of the auricle or pinna and the external auditory meatus or ear canal. The middle ear (**69400-69799**) consists of several parts: the malleus, incus, stapes, and tympanic cavity. The inner ear (**69801-69949**) is also called the *labyrinth* and includes the cochlea, vestibule, and semicircular canal, as primary terms used in the CPT nomenclature.

3. **69436 50** Tympanostomy (requiring insertion of ventilating tube), general anesthesia

4. **69718** Replacement (including removal of existing device), osseointegrated implant, temporal bone, with percutaneous attachment to external speech processor/cochlear stimulator; with mastoidextomy

5. **69210** Removal of impacted cerumen (separate procedure), 1 or both ears

6. **69399** Unlisted procedure, external ear

   69799 Unlisted procedure, middle ear

   69949 Unlisted procedure, inner ear

Chapter 5 – Radiology

1. True

2. True

3. b

4. a

5. contrast material

6. six

7. **73630** Radiologic examination, foot; complete, minimum of 3 views

8. **72148** Magnetic resonance (eg, proton) imaging, spinal canal and contents, lumbar; without contrast material

9. **73725** Magnetic resonance angiography, lower extremity, with or without contrast material(s)

Chapter 6 – Pathology and Laboratory

1. False. When reporting the Panel codes, ALL of the components listed under the code descriptor MUST be performed, with no substitutions.

2. True. The components in the organ or disease-oriented panel codes are not intended to limit the performance of other tests. If tests are performed in addition to those specifically listed for a particular panel, those tests should be reported separately in addition to the panel code.

3. True. Code **88332** is reported only when a **single** specimen requires **multiple** frozen section tissue blocks. CPT code **88332** is an add-on code and cannot be reported for a specimen that has not already been examined initially, as indicated by code **88331**. If more than one specimen is submitted for consultation, the services for each specimen would be separately coded, as appropriate.

4. False. When reporting a non-automated urinalysis dip stick test performed without microscopy, code **81002** is the appropriate code. In order to select the appropriate code, one must know whether the testing was automated or not and whether the testing was performed with or without microscopy. Code **81000** would not be appropriate to report since the code descriptor states the urinalysis by dip stick is non-automated and with microscopy.

Appendix B

5. True. The unit of service for Surgical Pathology codes **88300** through **88309** is the specimen. The codes are defined by unit.

6. a

7. b

8. specimen

9. unlisted

10. unbundled

11. Surgical Pathology

Chapter 7 – Medicine

1. True. Many services and procedures provided by nonphysician health care providers are also located in the Medicine section.

2. False. There are two basic types of subsections: those that are procedure oriented and those that refer to particular medical specialties.

3. False. Codes in a specialty subsection, such as gastroenterology, are not limited to use by gastroenterologists.

4. False. Code **90389** is reported for the tetanus immune globulin (Tig), human, for intramuscular use. Code **90471** is reported for the immunization administration. Codes **90281-90399** identify the immune globulin product only and must be reported in addition to the administration codes **96365-96368**, **96372**, **96374**, and **96375**, as appropriate.

5. False. Code **96360**, *Intravenous infusion, hydration; initial, 31 minutes to 1 hour* and code **96361**, *Intravenous infusion, hydration; each additional hour (List separately in addition to code for primary procedure)* are intended to report IV infusions of prepackaged fluid and/or electrolytes but are not used to report infusion of drugs or other substances. Code **96360** is an initial service. Code **96361** is reported for hydration each additional hour.

6. False. Chemotherapy administration codes **96401-96549** apply to parenteral administration of nonradionuclide antineoplastic drugs and also to antineoplastic agents provided for treatment of noncancer diagnoses (eg, cyclophosphamide for autoimmune conditions) or to substances such as monoclonal antibody agents and other biologic response modifiers.

7. False. The guidelines for reporting acupuncture state that reporting is based on 15-minute increments of personal (face-to-face) contact with the patient, not the duration of acupuncture needle(s) placement.

8. False. When providing moderate sedation, the administration of the agent(s) is included and not separately reportable.

9. **96365** Intravenous infusion, for therapy, prophylaxis, or diagnosis (specify substance or drug); initial, up to 1 hour

+96368 concurrent infusion (List separately in addition to code for primary procedure)

+96375 Therapeutic, prophylactic, or diagnostic injection (specify substance or drug); each additional sequential intravenous push of a new substance/drug (List separately in addition to code for primary procedure)

Rationale for Code Selection: Code **96365** is reported for the initial service of the antibiotic infusion (not hydration and not chemotherapy). Code **+96368** is reported for the concurrent infusion of simultaneous antibiotic. If an injection or infusion is of a subsequent or concurrent nature, even if it is the first such service within that group or services, then a subsequent or concurrent code from the appropriate section should be reported (eg, the first IV push given subsequent to an initial one-hour infusion is reported using a subsequent IV push code). Code **+96375** is reported for the sequential IV push drug. An IV or intra-arterial push is defined as an injection in which the health care professional who administers the substance or drug is continuously present to administer the injection and observe the patient, or an infusion of 15 minutes or less.

10. **92014** Ophthalmological services: medical examination and evaluation, with initiation or continuation of diagnostic and treatment program; comprehensive, established patient, 1 or more visits

Rationale for Code Selection: Code **92014** is reported for comprehensive ophthalmological services and describes a general evaluation of the complete visual system. A new patient is one who has received no professional services from the physician or another physician of the same specialty who belongs to the same group practice within the past three years. Because the patient is an established patient, code **92014** is appropriate for this service.

11. Code **99172**, *Visual function screening, automated or semi-automated bilateral quantitative determination of visual acuity, ocular alignment, color vision by pseudoisochromatic plates, and field of vision (may include all or some screening of the determination[s] for contrast sensitivity, vision under glare)*, is located in the Medicine section, under the subsection Other Services and Procedures in the CPT codebook. Remember, just because the first digit in the code is a "9" does not necessarily mean that the code is an E/M code. The Medicine section codes all start with the digit "9."

Chapter 8 – Category II Codes

1. Category II codes are intended to help collect data by encoding specific services and/or test results that have an evidence base for contributing to positive health outcomes and quality patient care.

2. True for all questions.

3. False. Category II codes consist of five characters with the letter **"F"** as the last character (eg, 1234F) to distinguish it from Category I and Category III CPT codes.

Appendix B

4. Category II codes are located immediately following the final Category I subsection (Medicine) in the CPT codebook.

Chapter 9 – Category III Codes

1. A set of temporary codes for emerging technology

2. Five, with the fifth alpha character "T"

3. Early January or July of a given CPT cycle

4. Five

5. False

6. False

7. False

8. d

9. d

10. b

Chapter 10 – Modifiers

1. False. HCPCS Level II modifiers are updated by the Centers for Medicare & Medicaid Services (CMS).

2. True. In the CPT Surgical Package Definition, local infiltration, metacarpal/metatarsal/digital block, or topical anesthesia is included.

3. False. Certain codes in the CPT nomenclature represent services performed under anesthesia (eg, **57410**, *Pelvic examination under anesthesia [other than local]*); for these codes, modifier **23** would not be appended.

4. True. Modifier **25** is used to indicate that a significant, separately identifiable E/M service is performed by the same physician on the day of a procedure. As stated in the definition, the E/M service must be "above and beyond" the other service or "beyond" the usual preoperative and postoperative care associated with the procedure. For this circumstance, modifier **57** is used.

5. Code **20600 50**

6. Modifier **24**

7. Modifier **51**

8. Modifier **91**

9. Modifier **62**

Chapter 11 – Appendixes

1. h
2. m
3. a
4. k
5. g
6. d
7. b
8. j
9. f
10. i
11. l
12. e

The HCPCS Coding System

The Healthcare Common Procedure Coding System (HCPCS) comprises both CPT Level I codes and national Level II alphanumeric codes. This system was developed in 1983 by HCFA (now CMS) to standardize the coding systems used to process Medicare claims on a national basis. The HCPCS coding system is structured in two levels. Each of the two HCPCS levels is its own unique coding system.

Level I: CPT Code Set

Level I is the AMA's CPT code set, which is described in this book and makes up the majority of the HCPCS coding system. Most of the procedures and services performed by physicians and other health care professionals, even with respect to Medicare patients, are reported with CPT codes.

Level II: National Codes

In addition to using the Level I (CPT) codes for procedures, the (Level II) HCPCS national codes are used to report supplies. These Level II codes are assigned, updated, and maintained by CMS. The AMA does not develop or maintain HCPCS Level II codes.

These codes describe services and supplies *not* found in the CPT code set. Some examples of the procedures and services described by Level II national codes include durable medical equipment, ambulance services, medical and surgical supplies, drugs, orthotics and prosthetics, dental procedures, and vision services. Highlights of the Level II national codes are as follows:

- Five-character alphanumeric codes are used; the first character is a letter (**A** through **V**, except **I** and **S**) followed by four numeric digits.
- Alpha (eg, **LT**) and alphanumeric (eg, **E1**) modifiers are used.

- The codes are updated annually by CMS.
- The codes are required for reporting most medical services and supplies provided to Medicare and Medicaid patients.

Example of a HCPCS Level II code:

G0103 Prostate cancer screening, prostate specific antigen test (PSA)

How to Search for HCPCS Level II Codes

Knowing how to efficiently and quickly search for a code or codes is important and saves time. The HCPCS Level II codes are not in the CPT codebook, but here are the following locations within the HCPCS Level II coding book that can be used to efficiently and quickly search for HCPCS Level II codes. It is also helpful to review the summary of the different steps provided to locate the specific code(s).

Index

The index **in a HCPCS coding book** enables the user to locate any code without looking through individual ranges of codes. In order to find the appropriate code, one should look up the medical or surgical supply, service, orthotic prostethic, or generic or brand name drug in question.

Table of Drugs

The Table of Drugs **in a HCPCS coding book** lists the brand and generic names of drugs with amount, route of administration, and code numbers. This table, although extensive, is not comprehensive.

Steps to Locate HCPCS Codes

The following steps should be taken to locate a HCPCS code:

- Identify the services or procedures that the patient received.
- Look up the appropriate term in the index.
- Assign a tentative code.
- Locate the code or codes in the appropriate section. When multiple codes are listed in the index, be sure to read the narrative of all codes listed to find the appropriate code based on the service performed.
- Check for symbols, notes, and references.
- Review the appendixes for the reference definitions and other guidelines for coverage issues that apply.
- Determine whether any modifiers should be used.
- Assign the code.

I and S Codes

The **I** codes are reserved for use by the Health Insurance Association of America to fulfill their member companies' unique coding needs. The **S** codes are created and maintained by the Blue Cross and Blue Shield Association for their needs.

National Correct Coding Initiative (NCCI)

On January 1, 1996, the Centers for Medicare & Medicaid Services (CMS) implemented its National Correct Coding Initiative (NCCI) of code edits in an attempt to eliminate unbundling or other inappropriate reporting of CPT® codes. This initiative detects inappropriate coding on claims and thus denies payment for them. The NCCI edits indentify procedures and services that typically should not be reported at the same time when provided by the same provider for the same patient on the same date of service.

CMS developed and maintains the Healthcare Common Procedure Coding System (HCPCS), from which it developed HCPCS CPT (procedure-to-procedure) code edits and correct coding policies that are used nationally by all Medicare Administrative Contractors. These coding edits and policies are known as the NCCI. These correct coding edits are incorporated into claims processing systems used by Medicare Administrative Contractors and other third-party payers to determine payments to physicians.

Translating NCCI Edits

The NCCI contains two tables with code pairs of HCPCS and CPT codes that in general should not be reported together. The codes listed in the Column 1/Column 2 Edits table cannot be reported to Medicare on the same date of service. If a provider reports the two codes of an edit pair, the Column 2 code would be denied, and the Column 1 code would be eligible for payment. The codes listed in the Mutually Exclusive Edits table include procedures that cannot be logically performed together by the same physician on the same patient, during the same encounter, or at the same anatomic site.

Each code listed in the Column 1/Column 2 Edits or Mutually Exclusive Edits table has a *correct coding modifier (CCM) indicator* appended to further explain. For example, CCM indicator 0 indicates that there are no circumstances in which a CPT modifier would be appropriate. The services represented by the code combination will not be paid separately under any circumstances. CCM indicator 1 indicates that a modifier is allowed in order to differentiate between the services provided. Assuming the modifier is used correctly and appropriately, this specificity provides the basis upon which separate payment for the services reported may be considered justifiable. CCM indicator 9 means that the code pair is no longer active; the code combination is billable separately and no modifier is needed.

CPT Modifiers may be appended to CPT codes in order to bypass the NCCI edit if the code pair has a CCM indicator of a "1". A listing of modifiers that may be appended to the code pair under appropriate clinical circumstances can be found in the NCCI guidelines located on the CMS Web site.

It is important for physicians and coders to be aware of the most common code pairs in the NCCI that may affect their practice and claim payments. With this information, physicians should be sure to accurately provide documentation to support the necessity for the procedures reported and the reasons for the separate services.

The NCCI edits are released on a quarterly basis, updates are available on the CMS Web site at www.cms.gov/NationalCorrectCodInitEd/.

Other Resources

Evaluation and Management Documentation Guidelines

The determination of which E/M Services code to assign is made by the physician and should be documented in the patient record. There are two sets of E/M guidelines that are utilized, one is the 1995 E/M Guidelines and the other is the 1997 E/M Guidelines. The 1995 and 1997 E/M Guidelines were created by the Center for Medicare & Medicaid Services (CMS) and may be obtained from the CMS Web site. You may visit CMS Web site at www.cms.gov for further information and updates. While each physician's office requires specific reference materials, the following is a suggested list of coding resources.

Resource Materials for the Physician Office

It is crucial for every physician's office to have comprehensive medical reference material to code diagnoses and procedures appropriately. Many of the questions answered at the American Medical Association (AMA) can be researched in common reference books that are easy to use and provide additional information on choosing correct code(s). All references listed here are distributed or published by the AMA. To obtain these publications, please see the ordering information listed in the following pages. The following publications provide further educational guidance on appropriate coding and may be obtained through the ordering information provided.

(Please note: The AMA does not endorse any specific nonAMA reference book. The books listed are examples of commonly used reference materials and guidebooks.)

Ordering Information

Call toll-free: (800) 621-8335
AMA members call: (800) 262-3211

Mail orders:
Order Department
American Medical Association
P.O. Box 930876
Atlanta, GA 31193-0876

Fax orders: (312) 464-5600
Secure online orders: www.amabookstore.com

Current Procedural Terminology (CPT) Professional Edition

Stay in compliance with code changes each year with AMA's official coding resource for procedural codes, rules, and guidelines.

CPT Changes: An Insider's View

Serves as the definitive text on additions, revisions, and deletions to the CPT code set. To assist CPT users in applying new and revised CPT codes, this book includes clinical examples (vignettes) that describe typical patients who might undergo the procedure, including detailed descriptions.

CPT Reference of Clinical Examples

This is the only reference organized by CPT codebook section and provides more than 1000 detailed case studies of codes pulled from the proprietary CPT database and Medicare claims data.

CPT Assistant Newsletter

A direct link to AMA coding experts, this essential monthly resource will help you stay on top of the latest critical coding changes and trends, answer day-to-day coding questions, train coding staff through case studies and clinical examples, validate coding to auditors, and assist in appeals folowing insurance denials. Have your specific coding questions answered! Subscribers are encouraged to submit questions that will be answered through a yearly bonus issue.

CPT Network

An Internet-based inquiry system that allows one to search an online knowledge base of CPT code information filled with frequently asked questions and clinical examples (vignettes). This service is provided to AMA members as a benefit of membership and is also available as a subscription fee-based service for nonmembers and subscribers. The different packages available can be viewed at www.cptnetwork.com.

Coding with Modifiers

The most definitive book on modifiers, filled with the largest number of modifier changes since 2000. This best-selling edition contains CMS, third-party payer, and AMA-modifier guidelines to assist in coding accurately. Helpful clinical examples guide readers in determining the correct modifier to use, along with coding tips to clear up confusion surrounding modifier usage.

HCPCS Level II Professional Edition

Efficient and effective coding is made possible with the AMA's new *HCPCS 2011 Professional Edition* codebook. Organized to help you code more quickly and accurately, this reference includes the most current HCPCS codes and regulations and provides all the coding reference essentials needed for medical billing and maximum reimbursement.

ICD-9-CM, Volumes 1 and 2

Lists diagnosis codes and descriptions. The ICD-9-CM diagnoses must be reported on the insurance claim form for Medicare and most other third-party payers.

Medicare RBRVS: The Physicians' Guide

The twentieth edition of this concise, authoritative text provides all of the up-to-date information on new 2011 payment rules and how they may affect your practice. This reference will quickly prove its value by providing the insights and tools you need to understand the RBRVS system and helping to ensure that your office is calculating payment schedules accurately.

Medical Dictionaries

These references provide definitions of procedures and diagnoses. *Stedman's Medical Dictionary, Stedman's CPT Dictionary,* and *Dorland's Illustrated Medical Dictionary* are three frequently used medical dictionaries. If a description is not found in the CPT codebook index, often there may be another word to describe the procedure that can be located in the dictionary.

Netter's Atlas of Human Anatomy for CPT® Coding, Second Edition

Designed to provide a better understanding of anatomic structures described within CPT® codes, this unique resource includes true-to-life Frank Netter illustrations associated with official CPT codes and their complete procedural descriptions. Each chapter delves into a particular anatomical region from head to toe by providing a brief introduction that explains the region and provides notes on anatomical and medical terminology.

Tables, Flow Charts, and Illustrations

This appendix consists of helpful tables, flow charts, and illustrations to assist users of CPT codebook in selecting the appropriate CPT code(s).

Figure AF-1 assists CPT users to select the appropriate Evaluation and Management (E/M) level of service based on the key components performed.

FIGURE AF-1 *Evaluation and Management Tables*

Office or Other Outpatient Services

Patient: New
Required Components: 3/3

Required Key Components	Code	99201	99202	99203	99204	99205
	History and Exam (#1 and #2)					
	Problem Focused	x				
	Expanded Problem Focused		x			
	Detailed			x		
	Comprehensive				x	x
	Medical Decision Making (#3)					
	Straightforward	x	x			
	Low			x		
	Moderate				x	
	High					x

Contributory Factors	**Presenting Problem (Severity) (#1)**					
	Self-Limited or Minor	x				
	Low to Moderate		x			
	Moderate			x		
	Moderate to High				x	x
	Counseling and Coordination of Care (#2 and #3) See E/M Guidelines					
	Typical Face-to-Face Time (#4)					
	Minutes	10	20	30	45	60

Office or Other Outpatient Services

Patient: Established
Required Components: 2/3

Required Key Components	Code	99211	99212	99213	99214	99215
	History and Exam (#1 and #2)					
	Problem Focused	N/A	x			
	Expanded Problem Focused			x		
	Detailed				x	
	Comprehensive					x
	Medical Decision Making (#3)					
	Straightforward	N/A	x			
	Low			x		
	Moderate				x	
	High					x

Contributory Factors	**Presenting Problem (Severity) (#1)**					
	Minimal	x				
	Self-Limited or Minor		x			
	Low to Moderate			x		
	Moderate to High				x	x
	Counseling and Coordination of Care (#2 and #3) See E/M Guidelines					
	Typical Face-to-Face Time (#4)					
	Minutes	5	10	15	25	40

(Continued)

FIGURE AF-1 *(Continued)*

Initial Observation Care

Patient: New or Established
Required Components: 3/3

Code	99218	99219	99220
History and Exam (#1 and #2)			
Detailed or Comprehensive	x		
Comprehensive		x	x
Medical Decision Making (#3)			
Straightforward or Low	x		
Moderate		x	
High			x
Presenting Problem (Severity) (#1)			
Low	x		
Moderate		x	
High			x
Counseling and Coordination of Care (#2 and #3) See E/M Guidelines			
Typical Face-to-Face Time (#4) - N/A			

Required Key Components / Contributory Factors

Initial Hospital Care

Patient: New or Established
Required Components: 3/3

Code	99221	99222	99223
History and Exam (#1 and #2)			
Detailed or Comprehensive	x		
Comprehensive		x	x
Medical Decision Making (#3)			
Straightforward or Low	x		
Moderate		x	
High			x
Presenting Problem (Severity) (#1)			
Low	x		
Moderate		x	
High			x
Counseling and Coordination of Care (#2 and #3) See E/M Guidelines			
Typical Face-to-Face Time (#4)			
Minutes	30	50	70

Required Key Components / Contributory Factors

Subsequent Observation Care

Patient: New or Established
Required Components: 2/3

Code	99224	99225	99226
Interval History and Exam (#1 and #2)			
Problem Focused	x		
Expanded Problem Focused		x	
Detailed			x
Medical Decision Making (#3)			
Straightforward or Low	x		
Moderate		x	
High			x
Presenting Problem (Severity) (#1)			
Stable/Recovering/Improving	x		
Responding Inadequately/ Minor Complication		x	
Unstable/Significant Complication/ New Problem			x
Counseling and Coordination of Care (#2 and #3) See E/M Guidelines			
Typical Face-to-Face Time (#4)			
Minutes	15	25	35

Required Key Components / Contributory Factors

Subsequent Hospital Care

Patient: New or Established
Required Components: 2/3

Code	99231	99232	99233
Interval History and Exam (#1 and #2)			
Problem Focused	x		
Expanded Problem Focused		x	
Detailed			x
Medical Decision Making (#3)			
Straightforward or Low	x		
Moderate		x	
High			x
Presenting Problem (Severity) (#1)			
Stable/Recovering/Improving	x		
Responding Inadequately/ Minor Complication		x	
Unstable/Significant Complication/ New Problem			x
Counseling and Coordination of Care (#2 and #3) See E/M Guidelines			
Typical Face-to-Face Time (#4)			
Minutes	15	25	35

Required Key Components / Contributory Factors

(Continued)

FIGURE AF-1 *(Continued)*

Office or Other Outpatient Consultations					
Patient: New or Established					
Required Components: 3/3					
Code	99241	99242	99243	99244	99245

Required Key Components

History and Exam (#1 and #2)	99241	99242	99243	99244	99245
Problem Focused	x				
Expanded Problem Focused		x			
Detailed			x		
Comprehensive				x	x
Medical Decision Making (#3)					
Straightforward	x	x			
Low			x		
Moderate				x	
High					x

Contributory Factors

Presenting Problem (Severity) (#1)	99241	99242	99243	99244	99245
Self-Limited or Minor	x				
Low		x			
Moderate			x		
Moderate to High				x	x
Counseling and Coordination of Care (#2 and #3) See E/M Guidelines					
Typical Face-to-Face Time (#4)					
Minutes	15	30	40	60	80

Observation or Inpatient Care Services (Including Admission and Discharge Services)			
Patient: New or Established			
Required Components: 3/3			
Code	99234	99235	99236

Required Key Components

History and Exam (#1 and #2)	99234	99235	99236
Detailed or Comprehensive	x		
Comprehensive		x	x
Medical Decision Making (#3)			
Straightforward or Low	x		
Moderate		x	
High			x

Contributory Factors

Presenting Problem (Severity) (#1)	99234	99235	99236
Low	x		
Moderate		x	
High			x
Counseling and Coordination of Care (#2 and #3) See E/M Guidelines			
Typical Face-to-Face Time (#4) - N/A			

Critical Care Time Reporting	
Total Duration of Critical Care	**CPT Codes**
Less than 30 minutes	Appropriate E/M codes
30-74 minutes (1/2 hour – 1 hour 14 minutes)	99291 X 1
75-104 minutes (1 hour 15 minutes – 1 hour 44 minutes)	99291 X 1 and 99292 X 1
105-134 minutes (1 hour 45 minutes – 2 hours 14 minutes)	99291 X 1 and 99292 X 2
135-164 minutes (2 hours 15 minutes – 2 hours 44 minutes)	99291 X 1 and 99292 X 3
165-194 minutes (2 hours 45 minutes – 3 hours 14 minutes)	99291 X 1 and 99292 X 4
195 minutes or more (3 hours 15 minutes or more)	99291 and 99292 as appropriate

Appendix F

(Continued)

FIGURE AF-1 *(Continued)*

Inpatient Consultations

Patient: New or Established					
Required Components: 3/3					
Code	99251	99252	99253	99254	99255

Required Key Components

History and Exam (#1 and #2)

	99251	99252	99253	99254	99255
Problem Focused	x				
Expanded Problem Focused		x			
Detailed			x		
Comprehensive				x	x

Medical Decision Making (#3)

	99251	99252	99253	99254	99255
Straightforward	x	x			
Low			x		
Moderate				x	
High					x

Contributory Factors

Presenting Problem (Severity) (#1)

	99251	99252	99253	99254	99255
Self-Limited or Minor	x				
Low		x			
Moderate			x		
Moderate to High				x	x

Counseling and Coordination of Care (#2 and #3) See E/M Guidelines

Typical Face-to-Face Time (#4)

	99251	99252	99253	99254	99255
Minutes	20	40	55	80	110

Subsequent Nursing Facility Care

Patient: New or Established				
Required Components: 2/3				
Code	99307	99308	99309	99310

Required Key Components

Interval History and Exam (#1 and #2)

	99307	99308	99309	99310
Problem Focused	x			
Expanded Problem Focused		x		
Detailed			x	
Comprehensive				x

Medical Decision Making (#3)

	99307	99308	99309	99310
Straightforward	x			
Low		x		
Moderate			x	
High				x

Contributory Factors

Presenting Problem (Severity) (#1)

	99307	99308	99309	99310
Stable/Recovering/Improving	x			
Responding Inadequately to Therapy/Minor Complication			x	
Significant Complication/ Significant New Problem			x	
Unstable/Significant New Problem Requiring Immediate Physician Attention				x

Counseling and Coordination of Care (#2 and #3)
Counseling and/or coordination of care with other providers or agencies are provided consistent with the nature of the problem(s) and the patient's and/or family's needs.

Typical Face-to-Face Time (#4)

	99307	99308	99309	99310
Minutes	10	15	25	35

Emergency Department Services

Patient: New or Established					
Required Components: 3/3					
Code	99281	99282	99283	99284	99285

Required Key Components

History and Exam (#1 and #2)

	99281	99282	99283	99284	99285
Problem Focused	x				
Expanded Problem Focused		x	x		
Detailed				x	
Comprehensive					x

Medical Decision Making (#3)

	99281	99282	99283	99284	99285
Straightforward	x				
Low		x			
Moderate			x	x	
High					x

Contributory Factors

Presenting Problem (Severity) (#1)

	99281	99282	99283	99284	99285
Self-Limited or Minor	x				
Low to Moderate		x			
Moderate			x		
High				x	
High Severity/ Immediate Significant Threat to Life or Physiological Function					x

Counseling and Coordination of Care (#2 and #3)
Counseling and/or coordination of care with other providers or agencies are provided consistent with the nature of the problem(s) and the patient's and/or family's needs.

Typical Face-to-Face Time (#4) - N/A

Initial Nursing Facility Care

Patient: New or Established			
Required Components: 3/3			
Code	99304	99305	99306

Required Key Components

History and Exam (#1 and #2)

	99304	99305	99306
Detailed or Comprehensive	x		
Comprehensive		x	x

Medical Decision Making (#3)

	99304	99305	99306
Straightforward or Low	x		
Moderate		x	
High			x

Contributory Factors

Presenting Problem (Severity) (#1)

	99304	99305	99306
Low	x		
Moderate		x	
High			x

Counseling and Coordination of Care (#2 and #3)
Counseling and/or coordination of care with other providers or agencies are provided consistent with the nature of the problem(s) and the patient's and/or family's needs.

Typical Face-to-Face Time (#4)

	99304	99305	99306
Minutes	25	35	45

(Continued)

Appendix F

FIGURE AF-1 *(Continued)*

Domiciliary, Rest Home (eg, Boarding Home), or Custodial Care Services

Patient: New
Required Components: 3/3

Code	99324	99325	99326	99327	99328
History and Exam (#1 and #2)					
Problem Focused	X				
Expanded Problem Focused		X			
Detailed			X		
Comprehensive				X	X
Medical Decision Making (#3)					
Straightforward	X				
Low		X			
Moderate			X	X	
High					X
Presenting Problem (Severity) (#1)					
Low	X				
Moderate		X			
Moderate to High			X		
High				X	
Unstable/Significant New Problem Requiring Immediate Physician Attention					X
Counseling and Coordination of Care (#2 and #3) See E/M Guidelines					
Typical Face-to-Face Time (#4)					
Minutes	20	30	45	60	75

Required Key Components / Contributory Factors

Domiciliary, Rest Home (eg, Boarding Home), or Custodial Care Services

Patient: Established
Required Components: 2/3

Code	99334	99335	99336	99337
Interval History and Exam (#1 and #2)				
Problem Focused	X			
Expanded Problem Focused		X		
Detailed			X	
Comprehensive				X
Medical Decision Making (#3)				
Straightforward	X			
Low		X		
Moderate			X	
Moderate to High				X
Presenting Problem (Severity) (#1)				
Self-Limited or Minor	X			
Low to Moderate		X		
Moderate to High			X	
Moderate to High/Unstable/Significant New Problem				X
Counseling and Coordination of Care (#2 and #3) See E/M Guidelines				
Typical Face-to-Face Time (#4)				
Minutes	15	25	40	60

Required Key Components / Contributory Factors

Home Services

Patient: New
Required Components: 3/3

Code	99341	99342	99343	99344	99345
History and Exam (#1 and #2)					
Problem Focused	X				
Expanded Problem Focused		X			
Detailed			X		
Comprehensive				X	X
Medical Decision Making (#3)					
Straightforward	X				
Low		X			
Moderate			X	X	
High					X
Presenting Problem (Severity) (#1)					
Low	X				
Moderate		X			
Moderate to High			X		
High				X	
Unstable/Significant New Problem					X
Counseling and Coordination of Care (#2 and #3) See E/M Guidelines					
Typical Face-to-Face Time (#4)					
Minutes	20	30	45	60	75

Required Key Components / Contributory Factors

Home Services

Patient: Established
Required Components: 2/3

Code	99347	99348	99349	99350
Interval History and Exam (#1 and #2)				
Problem Focused	X			
Expanded Problem Focused		X		
Detailed			X	
Comprehensive				X
Medical Decision Making (#3)				
Straightforward	X			
Low		X		
Moderate			X	
Moderate to High				X
Presenting Problem (Severity) (#1)				
Self-Limited or Minor	X			
Low to Moderate		X		
Moderate to High			X	
Moderate to High/Unstable/Significant New Problem				X
Counseling and Coordination of Care (#2 and #3) See E/M Guidelines				
Typical Face-to-Face Time (#4)				
Minutes	15	25	40	60

Required Key Components / Contributory Factors

Appendix F

Appendix F

Figure AF-2 illustrates the requirements for reporting CPT codes **99354-99357** depending on the type of E/M services provided.

Figure AF-3 is helpful in determining whether to report the E/M service provided as a new or an established patient encounter.

FIGURE AF-2 *Reporting CPT Codes 99354-99357*

To Report Code	For	One of These E/M Services Must Be Provided:
99354	Prolonged physician service in the office or other outpatient setting; first hour	99201-99205 99212-99215 99241-99245 99324-99337 99341-99350 90809 90815
99355	Prolonged physician service in the office or other outpatient setting; each additional 30 minutes	99354 plus one of the E/M codes required for use with 99354
99356	Prolonged physician service in the inpatient setting; first hour	99221-99223 99231-99233 99251-99255 99304-99306 99307-99310
99357	Prolonged physician service in the inpatient setting; each additional 30 minutes	99356 plus one of the E/M codes required for use with 99356

FIGURE AF-3 *Decision Tree for New vs Established Patients*

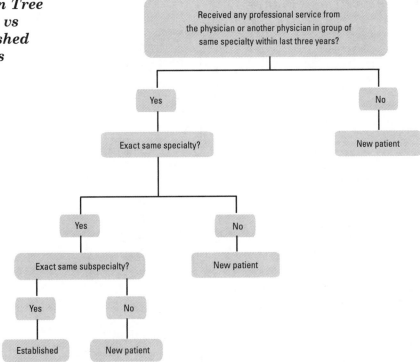

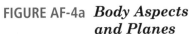
Appendix F

Figures AF-4a–c are useful illustrations that are helpful in the selection of appropriate CPT codes.

FIGURE AF-4a *Body Aspects and Planes*

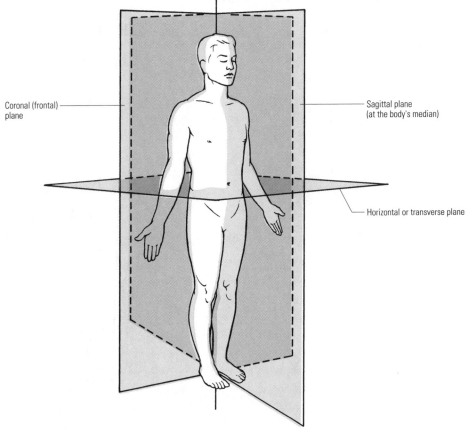

FIGURE AF-4b *Body Aspects and Planes*

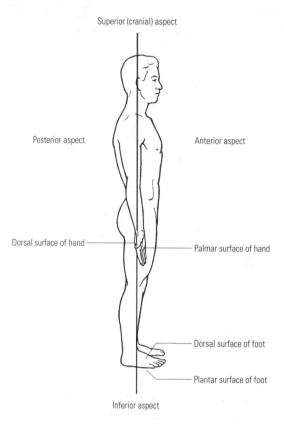

FIGURE AF-4c *Body Aspects and Planes*

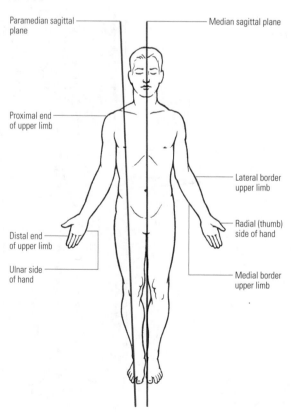

Development of the CPT Code Set

The American Medical Association (AMA) first developed and published the CPT code set in 1966. (See Figure AG-1.) The first edition helped encourage the use of standard terms and descriptors to document procedures in the medical record, helped communicate accurate information on procedures and services to agencies concerned with insurance claims, provided the basis for a computer-oriented system to evaluate operative procedures, and contributed basic information for actuarial and statistical purposes.

The first edition of *Current Procedural Terminology*, published in 1966, contained primarily surgical procedures, with limited sections on medicine, radiology, and laboratory procedures. When first published, CPT coding used a four-digit system. The second edition, published in 1970, presented an expanded system of terms and codes to designate diagnostic and therapeutic procedures in surgery, medicine, and the specialties. It was at that time that the five-digit codes were introduced, replacing the former four-digit system. Another significant change to the book was the inclusion of procedures related to internal medicine.

FIGURE AG-1 *The First Edition of* Current Procedural Terminology

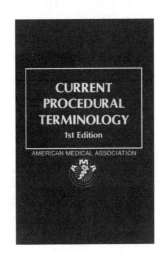

In the mid- to late 1970s, the third and fourth editions of CPT nomenclature were introduced. The fourth edition, published in 1977, represented significant updates in medical technology, and a system of periodic updating was introduced to keep pace with the rapidly changing medical environment.

In 1983, CPT nomenclature was adopted as part of the Healthcare Common Procedure Coding System (HCPCS) developed by the Centers for Medicare and Medicaid Services (CMS) (formerly the Health Care Financing Administration [HCFA]). (Refer to discussions later in this appendix for more detail on HCPCS.) With this adoption, the CMS mandated the use of HCPCS to report services for Part B of the Medicare program. In October 1986, CMS also required state Medicaid agencies to use HCPCS in the Medicaid Management Information System. In July 1987, as part of the Omnibus Budget Reconciliation Act, CMS mandated the use of CPT codes for reporting outpatient hospital surgical procedures.

Today, in addition to use in federal programs (Medicare and Medicaid), the CPT code set is used extensively throughout the United States as the preferred system of coding to describe health care services. In August 2000, the CPT code set was named as a national standard under the Health Insurance Portability and Accountability Act of 1996 (HIPAA).

Maintenance of the CPT Code Set

The AMA's CPT Editorial Panel is responsible for maintaining the CPT code set. This panel is authorized to revise, delete, update, and modify CPT codes. The panel is made up of 17 members. Eleven are nominated by the AMA. Designated seats on the CPT Editorial Panel consist of the following:

- One member is a representative of the Performance Measures development organizations.
- Two members are nonphysicians, representing the Health Care Professionals Advisory Committee (HCPAC).
- One is nominated by the Blue Cross and Blue Shield Association.
- One is nominated by the health insurance plans.
- One is nominated by CMS.
- One is nominated by the American Hospital Association.

The AMA's Board of Trustees appoints the panel members. Of the 11 AMA seats on the panel, 7 are regular seats, having a maximum tenure of two four-year terms, or a total of eight years for any one individual. One of these seats is designated for a physician who can represent the performance measures development organizations. The four remaining seats, called *rotating seats*, each have one four-year term. These rotating seats allow for diverse specialty input.

Five members of the Editorial Panel serve as the panel's Executive Committee. The Executive Committee includes the chair, the vice chair, and three panel members-at-large, as elected by the entire panel. One of the three members-at-large of the executive committee must be a third-party payer representative.

The AMA provides staff support for the CPT Editorial Panel and appoints a staff secretary who records the minutes of the meetings and keeps records.

The CPT Advisory Committee

In addition to the CPT Editorial Panel, there is a larger body of CPT advisers that supports the CPT Editorial Panel in its work. The CPT Advisory Committee members are primarily physicians nominated by the national medical specialty societies represented in the AMA House of Delegates. Currently, the Advisory Committee is limited to national medical specialty societies seated in the AMA House of Delegates and to the AMA HCPAC organizations representing limited-license practitioners and other allied health professionals. Additionally, a group of individuals, the Performance Measures Advisory Group (PMAG), who represent various organizations concerned with performance measures, also provide expertise.

The Advisory Committee's primary objectives are as follows:

- To serve as a resource to the CPT Editorial Panel by giving advice on procedure coding and appropriate nomenclature as relevant to the member's specialty or practice.
- To provide documentation to AMA staff and the CPT Editorial Panel regarding the appropriateness of various medical and surgical procedures under consideration as CPT codes.
- To suggest revisions to the CPT nomenclature. (The Advisory Committee meets annually to discuss items of shared concern and keep informed on current issues in coding and nomenclature.)
- To assist in the review and further development of relevant coding issues and in the preparation of technical education material and articles pertaining to CPT coding.
- To promote and educate its membership on the use and benefits of CPT coding.

AMA Health Care Professionals Advisory Committee

The current CPT code set contains many codes that are used by both physicians (ie, doctors of medicine [MDs] and doctors of osteopathy [DOs]) and nonphysicians. In some instances, use of CPT codes by non-physicians is required by legislation and regulation. In other instances, third-party payers have retained limiting policies governing how non-physicians report their services by means of CPT codes. In 1992, the AMA Board of Trustees concluded that the HCPAC should be established for the CPT Editorial Panel and the Relative Value Scale Update Committee (RUC) to open up the processes for code set maintenance to all the groups legally required to use CPT codes to report their services.

Responding to this recommendation, organizations representing physician assistants, nurses, occupational and physical therapists, optometrists, podiatrists, psychologists, social workers, audiologists, speech pathologists, chiropractors, dietitians, and, most recently, respiratory therapists, naturopaths, and genetic counselors were invited to nominate representatives to the HCPAC.

The HCPAC allows for participation of organizations representing limited-license practitioners and allied health professionals in the CPT and RUC processes. The co-chair and one member of the HCPAC are also voting members of the CPT Editorial Panel.

Requests for CPT Code Set Changes

Anyone can request a change to CPT coding. The effectiveness of the CPT code set depends on constant updating to reflect changes in medical practice. Suggestions of physicians, medical specialty societies, state medical associations, and those who deal regularly with health care information are the only way to ensure that the CPT code set reflects current practice.

The AMA welcomes correspondence, inquiries, and suggestions concerning old and new procedures. Specific procedures exist for addressing suggestions to revise CPT coding, add or delete codes, or modify existing nomenclature. Coding change request forms are available on the CPT page of the AMA Web site and are required to initiate a review of a proposed coding change by the CPT Advisory Committee. These forms play a vital role in maintaining and increasing the efficiency of the CPT process. One can visit the CPT Web site at www .ama-assn.org for information regarding submitting suggestions for changes to the CPT code set.

The CPT Code Set Change Process

Before submitting suggestions for changes to the CPT code set, the requester should consider the following questions:
- Is the suggestion a fragmentation of an existing procedure or service?
- Can the suggested procedure or service be reported by using one or more existing codes?
- Is the suggested procedure or service performed by many physicians or practitioners across the United States, or is it highly regionalized?
- Does the suggested procedure or service represent a distinct physician service?
- Is the suggested procedure or service merely a means to report extraordinary circumstances related to the performance of a procedure or service already having a specific CPT code?
- Why are the existing CPT codes inadequate?

As indicated in the CPT Process flow chart (see Figure AG-2), the review of code change applications is a multistep process. Being a multistep process naturally means that deadlines are very important. The deadlines for coding change requests and the Advisory Committee's

FIGURE AG-2 *CPT Code Set Change Process*

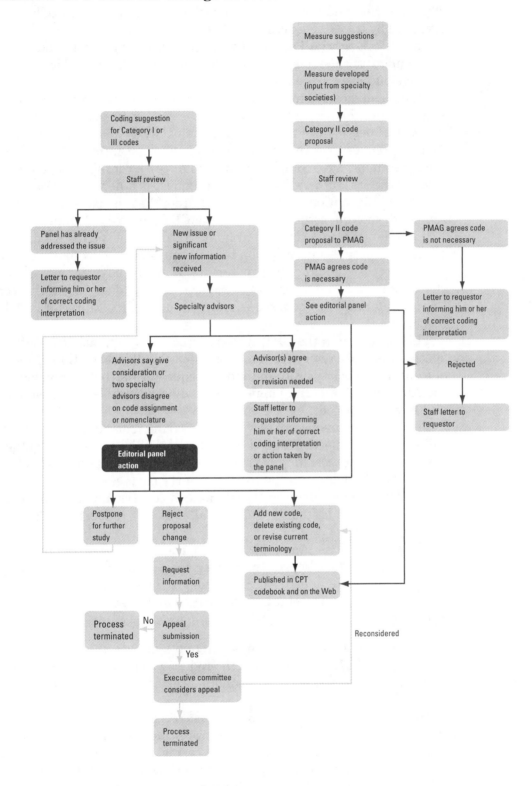

comments are based on a schedule that allows at least three months of preparation and processing time before the issue is ready to be reviewed by the CPT Editorial Panel.

The CPT Editorial Panel meets three times each year to address the complexities associated with new and emerging technologies and to manage outdated procedures.

When a suggestion to revise CPT nomenclature is received, AMA staff reviews the proposal to evaluate the coding suggestion. If the AMA staff determines that the panel has already addressed the question, the requester is informed of the panel's prior interpretation. The requester must have completed and submitted a coding change request form. If the staff determines that the request is a new issue or significant new information is received on an item that the panel previously reviewed, the request is referred to the CPT Advisory Committee.

If the advisers determine that no new code or revision is needed, the AMA staff provides information to the requester on how to use existing codes to report the procedure or service. If all the advisers agree that a change should be made or if two or more advisers disagree or give conflicting information, the issue is referred to the CPT Editorial Panel for resolution.

This first step in the CPT proposal process, which includes staff and specialty adviser review, is complete when (1) all information requested of a specialty society or an individual requester has been provided to the AMA staff, and (2) all appropriate advisers have been contacted and have responded.

The next step involves AMA staff preparing materials for the CPT Editorial Panel meeting agenda. The topics for the agenda are gathered from several sources. Medical specialty or other professional societies, individual physicians, hospitals, third-party payers, and other interested parties may submit materials for consideration by the Editorial Panel. Each agenda item includes a ballot for the request to be acted upon by the panel.

The panel actions can result in one of the following three outcomes:
• Add a new code or revise an existing code, in which case the change would appear in a forthcoming edition of the CPT codebook,
• Postpone an item to obtain further information, or
• Reject an item.

Once the panel has taken an action and approved the minutes of the meeting, the AMA staff informs the requester of the outcome. If the requester wishes to appeal the panel's decision, there is an appeal process to follow.

To appeal a decision, AMA staff must receive a written request for reconsideration. The request must contain the reason the requester believes that the panel's actions are incorrect and should respond to the panel's stated rationale. Once this information is received, the issue is referred to the CPT Executive Committee for a decision to reconsider. A proposal whose appeal is rejected by the Executive Committee and/ or panel cannot be reconsidered for one year from the date of that meeting. (See Figure AG-3.)

FIGURE AG-3 *Appeals Process*

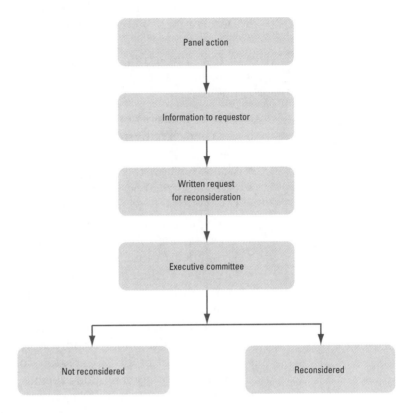

Categories of CPT Codes

To adapt the CPT code set to allow maximum participation of users and key stakeholders, the AMA began a project that used the workgroup process to assess the ability of the CPT code set to address issues of clinical practice, data management, government, organized medicine, and coding. This project, called CPT-5, examined issues such as coding for nonphysician professionals, coding to facilitate the collection of data for quality health services and public health research, the elimination of ambiguity and enhanced specificity, the development of uniform coding rules, and changes to the editorial process to allow greater participation and efficient development of new descriptions of service. New ways to maintain the CPT code set were also examined, including enhanced databases and other new technologies.

The final recommendations of the CPT-5 workgroup were that CPT processes should: (1) enhance the existing functionality of the CPT nomenclature; (2) correct problem areas; and (3) expand the codes and descriptors to accommodate emerging demands in the provision of health care. The recommendations of the CPT-5 workgroup have been introduced into the code set in an incremental fashion since the conclusion of the workgroup. The changes resulting from these recommendations preserve the core elements that define CPT nomenclature as the language to communicate clinical information for administrative and financial purposes. These core elements include the following:

- Descriptions of clinically recognized and generally accepted health care services,
- A five-character core with concept extenders (modifiers), and
- Professional responsibility for a mechanism for periodic review and updating.

On the basis of the activities of the workgroup, CPT code set attributes that have been developed or continue to evolve include the following:

- Codes for new technology
- Standardized codes for performance measures
- Codes to capture preventive medicine or screening services
- Codes to capture education or counseling services
- Development of nonphysician health professional evaluation services
- Expanded Editorial Panel process
- Decrease of the time frame involved in obtaining a CPT code through Web and Internet communications
- Expansion of the CPT Advisory Committee
- Improvement of CPT code set instructions and guidelines to be more comprehensive, user-friendly, and specific
- Development of a CPT glossary to standardize definitions and differentiate use of synonymous terms
- Maintenance of the CPT code set through a database that incorporates data modeling tools and vocabulary structures to formalize the hierarchical relationships within the CPT code set
- Computer management of intellectual content data and transition into various print publication processes
- Development of CPT educational material and training for postgraduate medical education, health care professional societies, and others who use CPT terminology

As a part of the drive to extend the functionality of CPT nomenclature, in which CPT nomenclature would meet the needs of data reporting in the areas of enrollment, encounter, outcomes, and quality data, and to enhance data collection with CPT codes without significantly altering the current structure and payment focus of CPT nomenclature, the workgroups involved in the CPT-5 project recommended that CPT codes be tiered to accommodate inclusion of codes to report performance measures and codes for emerging technology, services, and procedures.

With the implementation of the workgroup recommendations, CPT codes have been introduced to facilitate collection of data for performance measures (Category II codes) and to report emerging technology, services, and procedures (Category III codes). These codes appear after the Medicine section and before Appendix A of the CPT codebook. All five-character codes other than these are considered to be CPT Category I codes.

Glossary

abortion. The premature expulsion from the uterus of the products of conception, the embryo, or a nonviable fetus.

allograft (homograft). Tissue transplanted from one individual to another of the same species.

allograft. A donor bone obtained from a bone bank.

analyte. The actual drug or chemical substance one is testing for (eg, glucose, sodium theophylline)

anesthesia. The induction or administration of a drug to obtain partial or complete loss of sensation.

anesthesia modifiers. Modifiers used to indicate the patient's condition at the time anesthesia is administered.

aneurysm. Circumscribed dilation of an artery or a cardiac chamber, usually resulting from an acquired or congenital weakness of the wall of the artery or chamber.

angioplasty. Surgical reconstitution or recanalization of a blood vessel.

anoscopy. The examination of the anal canal and lower rectum.

antepartum care. Care during the first trimester.

aphakia. The absence of the crystalline lens of the eye.

approach procedure(s). Described according to anatomical area involved, ie, anterior cranial fossa, middle cranial fossa, posterior cranial fossa, and brain stem or upper spinal cord.

array. The collection of electrodes or contacts that are on one catheter.

arthrodesis. Surgical fusion or fixation of a joint.

assay. The determination of the amount of a particular part of a mixture, or the determination of the biological or pharmacological potency of a drug.

attended surveillance. The immediate availability of a remote technician to respond to rhythm or device alert transmissions from a patient, either from an implanted or wearable monitoring or therapy device, as they are generated and transmitted to the remote surveillance location or center.

autograft. Tissue transplanted from one part of the body to another in the same patient, or cancellous bone or bone cortex surgically removed from another area of the patient's own body.

bariatrics. The branch of medicine concerned with the management (prevention or control) of obesity and allied diseases.

benign. In reference to a neoplasm, being nonmalignant in character.

Bethesda system. A system for reporting cervical-vaginal cytologic diagnoses in a certain format.

block. Radiation-shielding device placed into the radiation beam that allows for a change in the shape or projected configuration of the port.

bypass. A shunt or auxiliary flow.

catheter. A tubular instrument to allow passage of fluid.

catheterization. The use or introduction of a catheter.

central nervous system. The brain and spinal cord.

claim edits. A set of business rules that the health insurer establishes to ensure that specific fields are completed and CPT codes are paid in accordance with the health insurer's business design.

clean claim. A paper claim that meets all the health insurer's standard submission requirements and that the health insurer has accepted for processing. When an electronic claim is submitted and is covered by the Health Insurance Portability and Accountability Act of 1996 (HIPAA), then this clean claim meets all the HIPAA submission requirements and is in compliance with that Act. A clean claim is a complete and error-free claim submitted to the health insurer on the health insurer's claim form.

clearinghouse. An entity that submits electronic claims on behalf of providers while maintaining the health insurer requirements for claim submission specified by each payer.

closed treatment. A fracture or dislocation site that is not surgically opened.

CMS-1500. The universal claim form that physicians and other health care professionals use to submit claims to Medicare. It is the claim form most health insurers accept.

colonoscopy. The examination of the entire colon, from the rectum to the cecum, and may include the examination of the terminal ileum.

complex repair. A repair that requires more than layered closure, namely, scar revision, debridement (eg, traumatic lacerations or avulsions), extensive undermining, stents, or retention sutures. Necessary preparation includes creation of a limited defect for repairs or the debridement of complicated lacerations or avulsions. Complex repair does not include excision of benign or malignant lesions, excisional preparation of a wound bed, or debridement of an open fracture or open dislocation.

computed tomographic angiography (CTA). A noninvasive technique for imaging vessels.

computed tomography (CT) imaging. Combines the use of a computer and a rotating X-ray device to obtain image data from different angles around the body. Computer processing of the image data is then performed to show a cross-section of body tissue, bone, and organs.

concurrent. Two or more things occurring at the same time, as when multiple infusions are provided simultaneously through the same IV line.

concurrent care. Provision of similar services (eg, hospital visits) to the same patient by more than one physician on the same day.

contact. The portion of a stimulator array that allows the flow of electrical current between the electrodes and the adjacent patient tissue.

contract amount. The amount agreed upon by the provider and insurer.

contractual adjustments. Amounts not covered by the insurer that the patient is not responsible to pay.

cryosurgery. An operation using freezing temperature (achieved by liquid nitrogen or carbon dioxide) as an independent agent or in an instrument to destroy tissue.

cryotherapy. The use of cold in the treatment of disease.

curettement (curettage). Scraping, usually of the interior of a cavity or tract, for the removal of new growth or other abnormal tissue, or to obtain material for tissue diagnosis.

debridement. The removal of loose, devitalized, necrotic, and/or contaminated tissue, foreign bodies, and other debris on the wound, using mechanical or sharp techniques.

defect. An imperfection, malformation, dysfunction, or absence; an attribute of quality, in contrast with deficiency, which is an attribute of quantity.

defibrillation. The delivery of an electrical impulse to the heart.

definitive procedure(s). Describes the repair, biopsy, resection, or excision of various lesions of the skull base and, when appropriate, primary closure of the dura, mucous membranes, and skin.

dermal. Grafts composed of the dermis, the second layer of skin immediately below the epidermis.

destruction. The ablation of benign, premalignant, or malignant tissues by any method, with or without curettement, including local anesthesia and not usually requiring closure.

Glossary

device, dual-lead. A pacemaker or implantable cardioverter-defibrillator (ICD) with pacing and sensing function in only two chambers of the heart.

device, multiple-lead. A pacemaker or implantable cardioverter-defibrillator (ICD) with pacing and sensing function in three or more chambers of the heart.

device, single-lead. A pacemaker or implantable cardioverter-defibrillator (ICD) with pacing and sensing function in only one chamber of the heart.

electrode. The conductor that allows transmission of electrical impulses (created by the generator and carried by the lead) to be translated into energy in the tissue of the patient.

electrosurgery. The division of tissues by high-frequency current applied locally with a metal instrument or needle.

endoscopy. A method of exploration and treatment for conditions and diseases that allows viewing of the site without requiring an open surgical incision.

endoscopic retrograde cholangiopancreatography. The examination of the hepatobiliary system and gallbladder.

endothelial. Replacement of only the innermost layer of the cornea containing the corneal endothelium.

enteroscopy (or small intestinal endoscopy). The examination of the small intestine beyond the second portion of the duodenum.

epidermal. Grafts composed of the epidermis, the outermost layer of the two layers that make up the skin.

epigastric hernia. A hernia through the linea alba above the navel.

esophagogastroduodenoscopy (EGD). An examination in which the pyloric channel is traversed.

esophagoscopy. A limited study of the esophagus. When the endoscope passes the diaphragm into the stomach, the procedure is an *esophagogastroscopy*.

established patient. A patient who has received professional services from the physician or another physician of the same specialty who belongs to the same group practice within the past three years.

excision. Full-thickness (through the dermis) removal of a lesion including margins.

explanation of benefits (EOB). A explanation of the health insurer's (third-party payers) benefits, detailing the processing of codes on claims submitted. Including the allowed and covered charges, the amount the patient may owe (from their deductible, coinsurance, or copayment amount), any contractual adjustments (amounts not covered by the insurer that the patient is not responsible to pay), and if applicable, the reason for denial.

fascial or subfascial soft tissue tumors. These involve the resection of tumors confined to the tissue within or below the deep fascia, but not involving the muscle or bone. Included are digital (ie, fingers and toes) subfascial tumors that involve the tendons, tendon sheaths, or joints of the digit.

femoral hernia. A hernia through the femoral ring.

fluoroscopy. An imaging technique commonly used by physicians to obtain real-time images of the internal structures of a patient through the use of a fluoroscope.

fraction. Term for treatment sessions for radiation therapy management.

full-thickness skin grafts. Grafts composed of the full layer of both the epidermis and dermis.

general anesthesia. A drug-induced loss of consciousness during which patients are not arousable, even by painful stimulation. Assistance in maintaining a patent airway is usually required. General anesthesia requires the undivided attention of a separate provider who is well trained and appropriately licensed in the monitoring and rescue functions inherently required for the safe provision of general anesthesia.

gravida. A pregnant woman. Called gravida I or primigravida during the first pregnancy.

Health Insurance Portability and Accountability Act (HIPAA). A law that, among other things, requires all third-party payers to use and accept CPT codes and modifiers for procedure coding and ICD-9-CM codes for diagnosis coding.

hysteroscopy. A visual instrumental inspection of the uterine cavity.

immunotherapy. The parenteral administration of allergenic extracts as antigens at periodic intervals, usually on an increasing dosage scale, to a dose that is selected as maintenance therapy.

implantable cardiovascular monitor (ICM). An implantable cardiovascular device used to assist the physician in the management of non–rhythm-related cardiac conditions such as heart failure. The device collects longitudinal physiologic cardiovascular data elements from one or more internal sensors (such as right ventricular pressure, left atrial pressure, or an index of lung water) and/or external sensors (such as blood pressure or body weight) for patient assessment and management. The data are stored and transmitted to the physician by either local telemetry or remotely to an Internet-based file server or surveillance technician.

implantable cardioverter-defibrillator (ICD). An implantable device that provides high-energy and low-energy stimulation to one or more chambers of the heart to terminate rapid heart rhythms called *tachycardia* or *fibrillation*. ICDs also have pacemaker functions to treat slow heart rhythms, called *bradycardia*.

implantable loop recorder (ILR). An implantable device that continuously records the electrocardiographic (ECG) rhythm triggered automatically by rapid and slow heart rates or by the patient during a symptomatic episode. The ILR function may be the only function of the device or it may be part of a pacemaker or implantable cardioverter-defibrillator (ICD) device. The data are stored and transmitted to the physician by either local telemetry or remotely to an Internet-based file server or surveillance technician. Extraction of data and compilation or report for physician interpretation is usually performed in the office setting.

in vitro fertilization. Procedures in which egg cells are fertilized outside the woman's body.

incarcerated. The abnormal entrapment of a part (ie, a hernia that is nonreducible).

incisional or ventral hernia. Ventral or incisional hernias occur in the area of a prior abdominal incision. They develop as the result of a thinning, separation, or tear in the muscle or tendon closure from prior surgery.

indirect. An inguinal hernia that leaves the abdomen, protrudes through the inguinal ring, and passes down obliquely through the inguinal canal, lateral to the inferior epigastric artery.

inguinal hernia. A hernia that occurs in the groin (the area between the abdomen and thigh). It is called *inguinal* because the intestines push through a weak spot in the inguinal canal. Obesity, pregnancy, heavy lifting, or straining to pass stool can cause the intestine to push against the inguinal canal.

initial. The key or primary reason for the encounter.

initial hernia. A hernia that has not required previous repair(s).

intermediate repair. The repair of wounds that require layered closure of one or more of the deeper layers of subcutaneous tissue and superficial (nonmuscle) fascia in addition to the skin (epidermal and dermal) closure. Single-layer closure of heavily contaminated wounds that have required extensive cleaning or removal of particulate matter also constitutes intermediate repair.

International Classification of Disease, 9th Edition, Clinical Modification (ICD-9-CM). The universal diagnosis coding system for health care claims coordinated by the National Centers for Vital and Health Statistics, ICD-9-CM codes assist physicians in transforming verbal descriptions of diseases, injuries, conditions, and certain procedures into numerical destinations (diagnostic coding). They are 3-5 characters in length and number over 14,000.

International Classification of Disease, 10th Edition Clinical Modification (ICD-10-CM). ICD-10-CM is the diagnosis code set that will be replacing ICD-9-CM Volumes 1 and 2. ICD-10-CM will be used to report diagnoses in all clinical settings. They are 3-7 characters in length and total 68,000.

interrogation device evaluation. An evaluation of an implantable device, such as a cardiac pacemaker, implantable cardioverter-defibrillator (ICD), implantable cardiovascular monitor (ICM), or implantable loop recorder (ILR). Using an office, hospital, or emergency department (ED) instrument or via a remote interrogation system, stored and measured information about the lead(s) when present, sensor(s) when present, battery and the implanted device function, as well as data collected about the patient's heart rhythm and heart rate are retrieved.

interspace. The nonbony compartment between two adjacent vertebral bodies that contains the intervertebral disk and includes the nucleus pulposus, annulus fibrosus, and two cartilaginous endplates.

key components. History, examination, and medical decision making.

kyphoplasty. A new, minimally invasive surgical technique for treating fractures of the spine that occur because of osteoporosis, usually in postmenopausal women.

lamellar. Transplant method that removes the anterior layers of the diseased cornea and replaces them with a piece of donor cornea cut to the same size and shape.

lesions. A pathological change in the tissues, eg, wound, cyst, abscess, or boil.

ligament. A band or sheet of fibrous tissue connecting two or more bones, cartilages, or other structures or serving as support for fasciae or muscles.

local anesthesia. The use of local anesthetics to numb sensory nerves that are in proximity to their terminations. This will result in only a small area being numbed, such as a circumscribed area of the integumentary or part of a foot or hand. Motor nerve blockage occurs significantly less frequently with local anesthesia.

lumbar hernia. A protrusion between the last rib and the iliac crest where the transverse muscle is covered by the latissimus dorsi. Lumbar hernias rarely result in strangulation, and hence the prognosis is good.

lung allotransplantation. Cadaver donor pneumonectomy.

magnetic resonance angiography (MRA). A noninvasive diagnostic study used to evaluate disorders of the arterial and venous structures.

malignant. In reference to a neoplasm, having the property of locally invasive and destructive growth and metastasis.

manipulation. The attempted reduction or restoration of a fracture or joint dislocation to its normal anatomic alignment by applying forces. Please note that this definition applies to codes in the Musculoskeletal System section.

mobile cardiovascular telemetry (MCT). The continuous recording of the electrocardiographic (ECG) rhythm from external electrodes placed on the patient's body. Segments of the ECG data are automatically (without patient intervention) transmitted to a remote surveillance location by cellular or land-line telephone signal.

modality. Any physical agent applied to produce therapeutic changes to biologic tissue, including but not limited to thermal, acoustic, light, mechanical, or electric energy.

moderate (conscious) sedation. A drug-induced depression of consciousness during which patients respond purposefully to oral commands, either alone or accompanied by light tactile stimulation.

Mohs micrographic surgery. A technique for the removal of skin cancer in a critical location (ie, periorbital, perioral, periauricular, perinasal, hands and feet, genitalia), recurrent tumors (ie, tumors that have recurred after prior treatment), ill-defined skin cancer (eg, tumor has ill-defined margins), and large (ie, greater than 2 cm) or aggressive tumors with histologic examination of 100% of the surgical margins (all of the peripheral and deep margins are examined).

monitored anesthesia care (MAC). MAC is a specific anesthesia service for a diagnostic or therapeutic procedure that involves giving sedatives through an intravenous catheter (IV) into the patient's blood stream and may be indicated when there may be the need to convert to general or regional anesthesia.

morselized bone graft. A graft that consists of small pieces of bone obtained either from a bone bank or from the patient's own body.

new patient. A patient who has not received any professional services from the physician or another physician of the same specialty who belongs to the same group practice within the past three years.

non-Bethesda system. The manual screening of conventional Pap smears.

nonreducible hernia. A hernia that cannot be reduced by manual manipulation. In these types of hernias, the hernial contents are fixed in the hernial sac.

nonsegmental instrumentation. Fixation at each end of the construct, possibly spanning several vertebral segments without attachment to the intervening segments.

omphalocele/gastroschisis. Presence of congenital outpouching of the umbilicus containing internal organs in the fetus or newborn infant.

open treatment. A fracture or dislocation site that is surgically opened to allow for visualization and internal fixation.

pacemaker. An implantable device that provides low-energy localized stimulation to one or more chambers of the heart to initiate contraction in that chamber.

para. A woman who has produced viable young regardless of whether the child was living at birth. Used with Roman numerals to designate the number of pregnancies that have resulted in the birth of viable offspring, as para 0 (none), para I (one), para II (two), para III (three), para IV (four), etc. Since the number indicates how many pregnancies, a multiple birth counts as just one in the calculation.

penetrating. Full-thickness replacement of the cornea following removal of the diseased corneal tissue.

percutaneous skeletal fixation. Utilizes a type of treatment that holds the position of a fracture by the use of external pins inserted across the skin into bone.

percutaneous vertebroplasty. A procedure in which a sterile biomaterial such as methyl methacrylate is injected from one side or both sides into the damaged vertebral body to act as a bone cement to reinforce the fractured or collapsed vertebra.

peripheral nervous system. The voluntary and autonomic systems.

physical status modifiers. Modifiers that describe the presurgery status of a patient and thereby distinguish among various levels of complexity of the anesthesia service provided.

plate/paddle. Four or more contacts or electrodes providing electrical stimulation in the epidural space; this design allows a large and complex stimulation design to be used to try to "cover" the patient's pain distribution.

port. The area encompassed by a single radiation beam.

postpartum care. Care, including hospital and office visits, following a vaginal or cesarean delivery.

proctosigmoidoscopy. The examination of the rectum and sigmoid colon.

professional (physician) component. Includes physician work and associated overhead and professional liability insurance costs involved in the diagnostic or therapeutic radiological service.

professional services. Face-to-face services rendered by a physician and reported by a specific CPT code.

primigravida. A woman pregnant for the first time; also written gravida I.

qualifying circumstances. Important qualifying circumstances that significantly affect the character of the anesthesia service provided.

qualitative assays. Tests that detect whether a particular analyte, constituent, or condition is present or absent. They are reported with the drug testing codes.

quantitative assays. Tests that give results expressing the specific numerical amount of an analyte in a specimen. They are reported with the therapeutic drug assay or chemistry codes.

radical resection of bone tumors. The resection of the tumor with wide margins of normal tissue. Radical resection of bone tumors is usually performed for malignant tumors or very aggressive tumors.

radical resection of soft tissue tumors. The resection of a tumor, usually malignant, with wide margins of normal tissue.

radiologic examination. Conventional X rays.

recipient lung allotransplantation. Transplantation of a single or double lung allograft and care of the recipient.

reconstruction/repair. Reported separately if extensive dural grafting, cranioplasty, local or regional myocutaneous pedicle flaps, or extensive skin grafts are required.

recurrent hernia. A hernia that has required previous repair(s).

reducible hernia. A hernia that can be corrected by manual manipulation; there is free mobility of the hernia contents through the hernial orifice.

regional anesthesia. The use of local anesthetics to temporarily block large groups of sensory nerves or the spinal cord so that the pain signal cannot reach the brain. Regional anesthesia also often results in blockage of motor neurons. This technique is separate and distinct from the use of local anesthesia to numb distal parts of the extremities by numbing nerves that are in proximity to their terminations. Thus, for the purposes of CPT definitions, regional anesthesia does not include use of local anesthesia below the elbow or ankle.

remittance advice (RA). A report, generally electronic, that outlines reimbursement data for single- or multiple-patient claims. Generally includes the patient name, insurer member identification number, group number, dates of service, charges with fees, the covered amount (or allowed charges), the noncovered amount due to contractual agreements (patient is not responsible for) or not covered for policy exclusion or other reasons, as well as the portion that patient is responsible for (eg, deductible, coinsurance, copayment), and the amount the insurer will pay.

secondary implant procedures. Implants that are placed in the orbit at a time **after** the initial surgery to enucleate or eviscerate the eye.

segment. The basic constituent part into which the spine may be divided. It represents a single complete vertebral bone with its associated articular processes and laminae.

segmental instrumentation. Fixation at each end of the construct and at least one additional interposed bony attachment.

shaving. The sharp removal by transverse incision or horizontal slicing to remove epidermal and dermal lesions without a full-thickness dermal excision.

sheaths. Any enveloping structure, such as the membranous covering of a muscle, nerve, or blood vessel; any sheathlike structure.

sigmoidoscopy. The examination of the entire rectum and sigmoid colon, and it may include examination of a portion of the descending colon.

simple repair. Repair of wounds that are superficial, eg, involving primarily epidermis or dermis, or subcutaneous tissues without significant involvement of deeper structures, and requires simple one-layer closure. This includes local anesthesia and chemical or electrocauterization of wounds not closed.

skin replacement. A tissue or graft that permanently replaces lost skin with healthy skin.

skin substitute. A biomaterial, engineered tissue, or combination of materials and cells or tissues that can be substituted for skin autograft or allograft in a clinical procedure.

skin tags, removal of. The removal by scissoring or any sharp method, ligature strangulation, electrosurgical destruction, or combination of treatment modalities including chemical destruction and electrocauterization.

specimen. Tissue(s) that is submitted for individual and separate attention, requiring individual examination and pathologic diagnosis.

spigelian hernia. A rare lateral ventral hernia.

split-thickness skin grafts. Grafts composed of the full layer of epidermis and part of the dermis.

stereotactic radiation therapy. General term for stereotactic-based radiation treatment. This treatment usually consists of one to five high-dose radiation treatments delivered by either a linear accelerator or a cobalt 60 unit.

strangulated. The most serious complication related to the hernia. Congestion or strangulation at the hernial ring impairs the blood supply to the herniated part. Once the vessels are obstructed, a simple incarceration becomes a strangulation.

structural bone graft. A whole piece of cancellous and/or bone cortex obtained from a bone bank or removed from the patient's own body.

subcutaneous soft tissue tumors. The simple or marginal resection of tumors confined to subcutaneous fatty tissue below the skin, but above the deep fascia.

subsequent. Infusion or injection of a second or subsequent drug after the initial drug.

super bill. A form a physician practice or other facility uses to record services rendered by a physician or health care professional during the patient encounter. This form generally lists the most common diagnostic codes (ICD-9) and service and procedural codes performed in the practice or facility.

technical component. Includes the cost of equipment, supplies, technician salaries, etc. The global charge refers to both the professional and technical components when billed together.

temporary wound closure. Not the final resurfacing material but provides closure of the wound surface until the skin surface can be permanently replaced.

third-party payers. Insurance carriers, both private and public (ie, Medicare and Medicaid), that provide medical coverage to their members.

thromboendarterectomy. A procedure that involves opening an artery, removing an occluding thrombus along with the intima and atheromatous material.

tissue block. A portion of tissue from a specimen that is frozen or encased in a support medium such as paraffin or plastic, from which sections are prepared.

tissue cultured autograft. Cultured first in the laboratory from skin cells harvested from the patient and then, once grown into sheets of graft material, are shipped in sterile containers by the laboratory to arrive in the operating room where they are applied to the recipient site(s).

tissue section. A thin slice of tissue from a block prepared for microscopic examination.

transfer of care. Process whereby a physician who is providing management for some or all of a patient's problems relinquishes this responsibility to another physician who explicitly agrees to accept this responsibility and who, from the initial encounter, is not providing consultative services.

transurethral microwave thermotherapy. The process of delivering sufficient microwave heating to destroy prostatic tissue without causing unnecessary damage to surrounding structures.

transurethral resection of the prostate (TURP). A procedure that uses electrical current to heat a wire loop on a resectoscope that slices through urethral or prostatic tissue like a knife.

trigger point. A specific point or area where stimulation by touch, pain, or pressure induces a painful response.

ultrasound. Noninvasive imaging technique that uses high-frequency sound waves and their echoes.

umbilical hernia. A protrusion of the intestine and omentum through a hernia in the abdominal wall near the navel, usually self-correcting after birth.

ureteral stents. Thin catheters threaded into the ureter for diversion of the urine either internally into the bladder or externally into a collection system.

vertebral components. The vertebral body, spinous process, laminae, facets, and intervertebral disc.

xenograft (heterograft). Tissue transplanted from one species to an unlike species (eg, baboon to human).

Index

B

Index

N

Index

U

V

W

X

Index

Code Index

Index

Category II Performance Measurement (F) Codes

Category III New/Emerging Technology (T) Codes

Modifiers

Index